MANUAL OF CLINICAL PROBLEMS IN OPHTHALMOLOGY
WITH ANNOTATED KEY REFERENCES

MANUAL OF CLINICAL PROBLEMS IN OPHTHALMOLOGY
WITH ANNOTATED KEY REFERENCES

JOHN W. GITTINGER, JR., M.D.
Professor of Surgery (Ophthalmology) and Neurology and Chairman, Division of Ophthalmology, University of Massachusetts Medical School, Worcester; Chief of Ophthalmology, University of Massachusetts Medical Center, Worcester

GEORGE K. ASDOURIAN, M.D.
Associate Professor of Surgery (Ophthalmology), University of Massachusetts Medical School, Worcester; Director, Vitreous-Retinal Service, University of Massachusetts Medical Center, Worcester

LITTLE, BROWN AND COMPANY   BOSTON/TORONTO

To Anne and Elizabeth Gittinger and Angelique and Raffi Asdourian, in affectionate recognition of our children's sacrifice of their fathers' time and attention to this work

CONTENTS

With thousands of journals, the medical literature has reached such size that it is difficult for individual physicians to keep up with new developments in their discipline and still have time to see patients. I have been aware of the lack of a compact source for selected current references in ophthalmology and was pleased when Ms. Susan Pioli, the able editor of the Little, Brown Spiral® series, approached me about putting together a manual of clinical problems in ophthalmology to stand beside the *Manual of Ocular Diagnosis and Therapy* edited by Dr. Deborah Pavan-Langston.

In order to keep a uniform style, I decided to write as much as possible myself, but I asked my colleague at the University of Massachusetts Medical School, Dr. George K. Asdourian, to write the parts on vitreo-retinal disease and on uveitis. In addition, Dr. Melvin G. Alper of Washington Hospital Center and George Washington University reviewed the part on orbital disease, and Dr. Michael A. Kass of Washington University Medical Center and Washington University School of Medicine reviewed the parts on the anterior chamber and glaucoma and on the lens. Their input was invaluable, but any errors in fact or emphasis are my responsibility.

Of course one could not, as one of my colleagues suggested ironically, hope to rewrite Duke Elder. Instead, we identified a number of topics of clinical interest on which new information is available and then prepared short essays emphasizing the pathogenesis, diagnosis, and treatment of those entities. These discussions are accompanied by a limited number of annotated references from the English language literature, with emphasis on recent publications rather than "classic" papers.

This is a source book, not a textbook, and its goal is to unravel only a few of the threads from the fabric of current ophthalmic literature. The *Manual of Clinical Problems in Ophthalmology* is intended to serve as a guide and review, not as a definitive reference. We have done our best to reflect the current views expressed in the literature on therapy, but new information becomes available every day, and practical decisions on patient management in areas where the ophthalmologist has limited personal experience are usually best made after discussion or formal consultation with a knowledgeable subspecialist.

J.W.G.

I. LIDS AND ADNEXAE

John W. Gittinger, Jr.

1. NEONATAL CONJUNCTIVITIS

Ophthalmia neonatorum is the term traditionally applied to neonatal conjunctivitis of any etiology. Historically, gonococcal ophthalmia neonatorum was an important cause of blindness. Infection with *Neisseria gonorrheae* acquired during passage through the birth canal presents as a hyperacute conjunctivitis, developing characteristically two to four days after birth. Because of the potentially devastating nature of gonococcal infection—the bacterium is able to penetrate even intact epithelium, resulting in corneal ulceration and even perforation—newborns in the United States receive prophylaxis with silver nitrate 1% solution (Credé prophylaxis) or an antibiotic. Prophylaxis reduces but does not eliminate the incidence of gonococcal ophthalmia neonatorum, which should be suspected in any conjunctivitis of the newborn period.

When silver nitrate is administered, the solution itself is the commonest cause of ophthalmia neonatorum. This chemical conjunctivitis, with swelling of the lids and a serous discharge, occurs frequently during the first day or two of life and does not require treatment. Wax ampules with single doses should be used for administration of silver nitrate because of the risk of inadvertent concentration of bulk solutions, with resulting skin and ocular burns.

Some developed countries have discontinued routine prophylaxis because of a declining incidence of gonococcal infection in their childbearing women. Canadian authorities recommend that 1% silver nitrate, 1% tetracycline, or 0.5% erythromycin be administered as soon as possible after birth, along with intramuscular or intravenous penicillin if the mother has a known infection.

Silver nitrate is not an effective prophylactic against the most common infectious agent producing neonatal conjunctivitis: *Chlamydia trachomatis*. Chlamydial ophthalmia neonatorum is often called *inclusion blenorrhea* because of the basophilic cytoplasmic inclusions seen on Giemsa staining of conjunctival scrapings (Halberstadter-Prowazek inclusion bodies). Clinically, chlamydial infection presents as a mucopurulent conjunctivitis, usually mild but sometimes severe. Because of the possibility of a chronic course with corneal pannus formation and an associated systemic infection with otitis, rhinitis, and even pneumonitis, treatment with topical erythromycin, tetracycline, or sulfonamides and systemic erythromycin is warranted. The parents should also be treated systemically, avoiding oral tetracycline in nursing mothers because it is secreted in milk and will produce a yellowish discoloration in developing teeth. Similarly, systemic tetracycline should not be prescribed for infants and children, although topical tetracycline is tolerated well.

Herpesvirus hominis is an uncommon but potentially devastating cause of neonatal infection; when it is untreated, the mortality exceeds 50%. To avoid this, women with known genital herpes are often delivered by cesarean section. Neonates with suspected herpetic infections should be isolated to prevent nosocomial spread. In addition to the conjunctivitis, which may be associated with skin vesicles, keratitis (either typical dendritic or diffuse), uveitis, chorioretinitis, and optic neuritis may occur.

Bacteria other than *N. gonorrheae* are another major cause of neonatal conjunctivitis. A variety of species have been isolated; *Staphylococcus aureus, Streptococcus* sp., *Haemophilus* sp., coliform bacilli, and *Pseudomonas aeruginosa* are prominent among them. Pseudomonas infection is encountered in premature infants and may evolve into systemic sepsis. Gram stain of conjunctival discharge will usually allow selection of an appropriate antibiotic.

Bacterial cultures with antibiotic sensitivities should be obtained for all neonates with purulent eye discharges. If *Neisseria* is suspected, administer parenteral antibiotics. The appearance of penicillin-resistant gonococci means that the choice of initial antibiotic should be determined by the sensitivities of strains prevalent in the patient's geographical area. At this writing, amoxicillin or ceftriaxone is recommended in Massachusetts.

Authorities debate the necessity of topical antibiotics for gonococcal infection. An appropriate systemic medication and saline irrigation of the culs-de-sac to wash out the purulent discharge are probably sufficient. Gram-positive organisms and *Hemophilus* usually respond to topical erythromycin ointment, and gram-negative organisms respond to gentamicin ointment. If herpesvirus infection is suspected, begin topical antivirals and consult a pediatrician as to the advisability of systemic vidarabine.

1. American Academy of Pediatrics, Committee on Drugs, Committee on Fetus and Newborn, Committee on Infectious Disease. Prophylaxis and treatment of neonatal gonococcal infections. *Pediatrics* 65:1047–1048, 1980.
   These specific recommendations were agreed upon by 28 pediatricians, who conclude that "topical antibiotics are superfluous" in gonococcal ophthalmia neonatorum.
2. Cohen, K.L., McCarthy, L.R. *Haemophilus influenzae* ophthalmia neonatorum. *Arch. Ophthalmol.* 98:1214–1215, 1980.
   A case report occasions a discussion of epidemiology.
3. Friendly, D.S. Ophthalmia neonatorum. *Pediatr. Clin. North Am.* 30:1033–1042, 1983.
   Friendly provides a well-referenced clinical review.
4. Gammon, J.A., Nahmias, A.J. *Herpes simplex* ocular infections in the newborn. In R.W. Darrell (ed.), *Viral Diseases of the Eye.* Philadelphia: Lea & Febiger, 1985. Pp. 46–58.
   A thorough discussion of the diagnosis and therapy of Herpesvirus hominis *infections, emphasizing the role of the ophthalmologist in the management of affected infants.*
5. Hobson, D., Rees, E., Viswalingam, N.D. Chlamydial infections in neonates and older children. *Br. Med. Bull.* 39:128–132, 1983.
   An overview of diagnosis and treatment of chlamydial infections, including conjunctivitis.
6. Laga, M., Naamara, W., Brunham, R.C., et al. Single-dose therapy of gonococcal ophthalmia neonatorum with ceftriaxone. *N.E.J.M.* 315:1382–1385, 1986.
   *In this clinical trial undertaken in Nairobi, Kenya, where no prophylaxis is used, a single intramuscular injection of 125 mg of ceftriaxone was an effective treatment for gonococcal ophthalmia neonatorum. An accompanying editorial by Dillon (*N.E.J.M. *315:1414–1415, 1986) offers a perspective on the problem in underdeveloped countries.*
7. Oriel, J.D. Ophthalmia neonatorum: relative efficacy of current prophylactic practices and treatment. *J. Antimicrob. Chemother.* 14:209–220, 1984.
   Oriel reviews the controversies over antibiotic choice in prophylaxis and management of neonatal conjunctivitis. Kanamycin, gentamicin, erythromycin, cefazolin, and cefotaxime have all been used in the treatment of penicillin-resistant gonococcal ophthalmia neonatorum.
8. Pierce, J.M., Ward, M.E., Seal, D.V. Ophthalmia neonatorum in the 1980's: incidence, aetiology and treatment. *Br. J. Ophthalmol.* 66:728–731, 1982.
   Twelve percent of 450 consecutive births in Southampton developed neonatal conjunctivitis. None were gonococcal, and most were treated with chloramphenicol by general practitioners. (For another English perspective on ophthalmia neonatorum, see the editorial "Ophthalmia neonatorum today" in The Lancet, *December 15, 1984, pp. 1375–1376.)*
9. Rapoza, P.A., Quinn, T.C., Kiessling, L.A., et al. Epidemiology of neonatal conjunctivitis. *Ophthalmology* 93:456–461, 1986.
   Chlamydial conjunctivitis, often difficult to distinguish clinically from bacterial causes, is very common in the low-income black population served by the Johns Hopkins Hospital.
10. Raucher, H.S., Newton, M.J. New issues in the prevention and treatment of ophthalmia neonatorum. *Ann. Ophthalmol.* 15:1004–1009, 1983.
    Raucher and Newton suggest intramuscular penicillin plus topical tetracycline as prophylaxis, but report a case of penicillin-resistant gonococcal infection in an infant who received such an injection and a case of sequential gonococcal then chlamydial infection when silver nitrate was used.

11. Sandstrom, K.I., Bell, T.A., Chandler, J.W., et al. Microbial causes of neonatal conjunctivitis. *J. Pediatrics* 105:706–711, 1984.
    No gonococcal infection was found among 61 cases of neonatal conjunctivitis in Seattle. Chlamydia, S. aureus, S. pneumoniae, and Haemophilus sp. were most often identified.
12. Traboulsi, E.I., Shammas, I.V., Ratl, H.E., et al. *Pseudomonas aeruginosa* ophthalmia neonatorum. *Am. J. Ophthalmol.* 98:801–802, 1984.
    Four premature infants in a neonatal intensive care unit developed Pseudomonas *conjunctivitis within a two-week period and responded to topical and systemic therapy.*

2. HERPES ZOSTER OPHTHALMICUS

Herpes zoster ophthalmicus is a rash in the distribution of the first (ophthalmic) division of the trigeminal nerve, caused by the varicella-zoster virus and often associated with pain and malaise. The varicella-zoster virus lies dormant in the trigeminal ganglion after the initial infection—chicken pox—and then reactivates. This can happen at any age, although it most often occurs in older adults. The ophthalmic division of the trigeminal nerve is the second most common site of zoster after the thoracic dermatomes in aggregate. The first division of the fifth nerve is the single dermatome most likely to develop zoster.

Diagnosis
Facial pain often precedes by a few days the appearance of a rash, which is initially macular and then rapidly progresses to vesicular. Several days into the attack, crusting develops. The crusted, swollen skin resembles a bacterial cellulitis, and superinfection is a possibility. Lymphoma, immunosuppression, acquired immunodeficiency syndrome, and trauma serve as triggers, but most cases have no obvious precipitant.

Ocular involvement is especially likely when vesicles appear on the tip of the nose (Hutchinson's sign), skin that is innervated by the same branch of V-1 that supplies the globe, the nasociliary nerve. In the acute phase the eye findings are a keratoconjunctivitis, a uveitis, or both. The keratitis may be dendritiform, but the zoster dendrite is small, thin, and raised, and often peripheral, an appearance distinct from that of simplex dendritic keratitis. A more chronic epithelial keratitis manifests as linear or branching gray plaques, mucus plaque keratitis.

Multiple fine, granular infiltrates in the superficial stroma constitute superficial stromal punctate keratitis or nummular keratitis, present in about one-third of cases. This may evolve into a disciform keratitis over a period of weeks, and rarely, inflammation of the deep stroma resembles that encountered in congenital syphilis, an interstitial keratitis. Chronic zoster keratitis is probably the leading cause of lipid keratopathy.

The pleomorphic nature of herpes zoster keratitis results from the combination of factors involved in its pathogenesis: the virus itself, the host response, and the superimposition of the effects of viral injury-induced denervation on the cornea. The exact contribution of each of these factors is difficult to assess, especially in late-developing sequelae such as marginal corneal ulcers.

Many patients with ophthalmic zoster develop iritis, which varies widely in severity and duration. Characteristic of herpes zoster iritis is segmental infarction of the iris, producing areas of iris atrophy, which are best seen by retroillumination. The presence of such iris changes helps in the differential diagnosis from herpes simplex disciform keratitis.

Ophthalmic zoster is usually self-limited, but in some patients, particularly those with underlying systemic disease, serious acute and chronic complications ensue. Inflammation may result in necrosis of ciliary body and choroid with overlying retina. An acute secondary glaucoma is occasionally encountered, and both scleritis and anterior segment necrosis are reported.

Neuro-ophthalmologic complications include optic neuritis and ocular motor palsies, both probably on an ischemic basis as the result of vaculitis. The prognosis for recovery of motor function is good; of vision, poor. A transient facial palsy may develop after ophthalmic zoster. (This should be distinguished from facial nerve palsy in combination with herpetic eruption in the external auditory meatus, known as the *Ramsay Hunt syndrome* or *Herpes zoster oticus*.) The most common neurologic sequela of ophthalmic zoster is postherpetic neuralgia, which may be very severe and disabling [12]. Rarely, encephalitis, myelitis, and polyradiculitis are encountered. Postherpetic cerebral vasculitis may be responsible for a syndrome of delayed contralateral hemiplegia [7].

Treatment

Management of an attack of *Herpes zoster ophthalmicus* initially consists of analgesia and topical treatment of the skin. Cool compresses are applied, and steroid and antibiotic ointments may reduce scarring and superinfection. If the patient is on immunosuppressants, the dosage is decreased if possible.

There is now some evidence that an immunosuppressed patient should be given systemic antivirals as soon as possible [1]. At present, intravenous acyclovir has been released for use in the United States; however, other drugs and methods of delivery are under investigation. A short course of systemic steroids in immunocompetent patients may lessen the severity of the disease and decrease the incidence of complications [2].

Uveitis is managed with topical steroids and cycloplegia. Keratoconjunctivitis is treated with topical steroids when indicated. Evidence that topical antivirals are effective in zoster keratitis is not convincing. Antivirals are sometimes prescribed with the justification that there might be concurrent simplex infection, but this is poorly documented. Topical steroids should be tapered slowly because keratitis often recrudesces when the dosage is rapidly decreased. The distinction between zoster and simplex keratitis is critical, as topical steroids are contraindicated in epithelial herpes simplex.

The development of corneal anesthesia adds an additional factor to consider in management. Steroids are relatively contraindicated in neurotrophic keratitis, which is initially treated with artificial tears or bland ointments and may require tarsorrhaphy. Bacterial superinfection is a complication of neurotrophic keratitis [13].

1. Cobo, L.M., Foulks, G.N., Liesegang, T., et al. Oral acyclovir in the treatment of acute herpes zoster ophthalmicus. *Ophthalmology* 93:763–770, 1986.
   A double-masked study of oral acyclovir in non-immunosuppressed patients indicates that this drug is well tolerated and reduces the incidence and severity of the ocular complications. (See also Am. J. Ophthalmol. *102:531–532, 1986.)*
2. Dickinson, J.A. Should we treat herpes zoster with corticosteroid agents? *Med J. Aust.* 144:375, 378–380, 1986.
   A position paper that concludes that systemic steroids should be used.
3. Easty, D.L. Ocular disease in varicella zoster infections. In *Virus Disease of the Eye.* Chicago: Year Book, 1985. Pp. 228–256.
   A clinical review with excellent illustrations, some in color.
4. Edgerton, A.E. Herpes zoster ophthalmicus: Report of cases and review of literature. *Arch. Ophthalmol.* 34:40–62, 114–153, 1945.
   An enormous review that is still the gold standard of clinical description.
5. Giles, K.E. Herpes zoster and cimetidine. *Med. J. Aust.* 142:283, 1985.
   Giles comments on the problems with anecdotal reports of improvement after cimetidine administration.
6. Hedges, T.R., III, and Albert, D.M. The progression of the ocular abnormalities of herpes zoster: Histopathologic observation of nine cases. *Ophthalmology* 89:165–177, 1982.
   Material from an ocular pathology laboratory that gives an insight into the pathophysiology of zoster.
7. Hilt, D.C., Bucholz, D., Krumholz, A., et al. Herpes zoster ophthalmicus and delayed

contralateral hemiparesis caused by cerebral angiitis: Diagnosis and management approaches. *Ann. Neurol.* 14:543–553, 1983.
These authors describe a devastating neurologic syndrome that is being recognized more often.

8. Liesegang, T.J. Herpes zoster ophthalmicus. *International Ophthalmology Clinics* 25(1):77–96, 1985.
Liesegang provides a good discussion of therapeutic options.

9. Marsh, R.J. Ophthalmic herpes zoster. In Darrell, R.W. *Viral Diseases of the Eye.* Lea & Febiger, Philadelphia, 1985. Pp. 78–89.
Marsh offers another perspective.

10. Mondino, B.J. Corneal manifestations of herpes zoster. In Darrell, R.W. *Viral Diseases of the Eye.* Lea & Febiger, Philadelphia, 1985. Pp. 90–96.
A succinct and nicely illustrated description of the various corneal manifestations.

11. Sandor, E.V., Millman, A., Croxon, T.S., et al. Herpes zoster ophthalmicus in patients at risk for the acquired immune deficiency syndrome (AIDS). *Am. J. Ophthalmol.* 101:153–155, 1986.
A consecutive case series indicating that Herpes zoster ophthalmicus with ocular complications may be a marker for AIDS in high-risk populations.

12. Watson, P.N., Evans, R.J. Postherpetic neuralgia: A review. *Arch. Neurol.* 43:836–840, 1986.
This debilitating complication has an increased incidence in older patients and may be very difficult to manage. Watson and Evans review prophylaxis, pathogenesis, and treatment.

13. Webb, R.M., Duke, M.A. Bacterial infection of a neurotrophic cornea in an immunocompromised subject. *Cornea* 4:14–18, 1985–6.
A case report that describes successful management of an infectious ulcer.

14. Womack, L.W., and Liesegang, T.J. Complications of herpes zoster ophthalmicus. *Arch. Ophthalmol.* 101:42–45, 1983.
A series of 86 patients from the Mayo Clinic illustrates the spectrum of clinical problems encountered.

15. Yeo, J.H., Pepose, J.S., Stewart, J.A., et al. Acute retinal necrosis syndrome following herpes zoster dermatitis. *Ophthalmology* 93:1418–1422, 1986.
The acute retinal necrosis syndrome is a newly recognized complication of Herpes zoster ophthalmicus.

3. BLEPHAROSPASM

Blepharospasm is an involuntary contraction of the orbicularis oculi muscle that narrows the palpebral fissure or closes the eyes. Blepharospasm is a normal response to ocular irritation or inflammation, when it is often accompanied by photophobia, and also develops in otherwise healthy persons as a response to bright light or manipulation of the eyes. An exaggerated form of this reflex blepharospasm may follow certain hemiplegic strokes and is encountered as a familial trait.

Pathogenesis

Most people with blepharospasm who seek medical advice have an involuntary dyskinesia. This may be a feature of idiopathic and especially postencephalitic Parkinson's disease and occasionally of other basal ganglia disorders, including kernicterus and Wilson's disease. There have been reports of a few cases of appearance of blepharospasm after upper brain stem strokes, usually at an interval after the event, or development of blepharospasm in a patient with known multiple sclerosis [7, 8]. Blepharospasm is a dose-related side effect of levodopa and is one component of the tardive dyskinesia that may be a consequence of treatment with antipsychotic drugs.

In the majority of patients, there is no definable etiology. Because the symptoms vary and are made worse by stress, a psychiatric cause is often considered. Reinforcing this impression in some patients is the history that sleep, talking, humming, or pulling on the lids produces temporary improvement. While hysterical blepharospasm may develop in young persons with emotional problems, relatively few cases are purely psychogenic.

Isolated blepharospasm is called *essential blepharospasm* or *benign essential blepharospasm*. When blepharospasm is accompanied by dystonic spasms of other facial, lingual, and cervical muscles, this is termed *idiopathic orofacial dystonia* or *Meige syndrome* [16]. Other types of dystonia may be associated: oculogyric crises, torticollis or retrocollis, or spasms of other muscle groups.

Diagnosis

Blepharospasm should be distinguished from apraxia of lid opening, in which the problem is an inability to initiate eye opening. Most likely an involuntary inhibition of the levator palpebrae, apraxia of lid opening is encountered in Parkinson's disease and related extrapyramidal disorders such as progressive supranuclear palsy and Shy-Drager syndrome [9]. In blepharospasm, contraction of the orbicularis brings the eyebrows below the orbital rim (Charcot's sign), while in apraxia of lid opening the brows are characteristically elevated. Apraxia of lid opening and blepharospasm, however, may coexist in the same patient.

Hemifacial spasm refers to unilateral contraction of the facial muscles that develops spontaneously or after facial palsy. In its early stages, blepharospasm may be unilateral, but eventually virtually all cases become bilateral. Treatment of hemifacial spasm and blepharospasm is similar.

Treatment

Blepharospasm is potentially blinding; if the eyelids won't open, the eyes can't see. Management of patients with blepharospasm is difficult. Various drugs have been used with only limited success. A few patients experience marked improvement after administration of trihexyphenidyl (Artane), lorazepam (Ativan), clonazepam (Clonopin), diazepam (Valium), deanol (Deaner), baclofen (Lioresal), or levodopa-carbidopa (Sinemet) [4, 5]. No drug is consistently effective. This has led to the use of alternative therapies such as biofeedback, acupuncture, hypnosis, and psychotherapy, again with only occasional success.

Until recently the procedure of choice in severe blepharospasm unresponsive to conservative treatment was surgical weakening of the orbicularis, either by direct removal of the muscle or by selective ablation of the seventh nerve [18]. Such iatrogenic facial palsy has the same potential risks as other causes of facial paralysis: corneal exposure, ectropion, dermatochalasis, and brow droop. In addition, especially after selective ablation, the blepharospasm often recurs because of incomplete removal or regeneration of the nerve.

Relief of blepharospasm may be accomplished temporarily by facial nerve block with local anesthetics or alcohol injection. Recently, one type of neurotoxin produced by the bacterium *Clostridium botulinum* has replaced alcohol as the long-acting agent of choice. Botulinum A toxin is injected in dilute solution into the orbicularis oculi and other facial muscles through a small-gauge needle. Four or more sites are usually chosen. Even though botulinum is a potentially lethal neurotoxin, no systemic side effects have been reported, presumably because of the low dosages used and rapid local binding by muscle. Transient ptosis is commonly reported, and care must be taken to treat exposure keratitis. The risk of significant exposure increases if the patient has had prior neurectomy or orbicularis stripping.

The duration of the paralysis produced by injection of botulinum toxin varies, both individually and with the dosage used. On average, reinjections are required every two to three months. This does not necessarily reflect the true duration of action of the toxin, as the subjective complaints of the patient are the most common criteria used to time the injections. Early reinjections may be less effective than initial injections, and some investigators increase the reinjection dosage when necessary.

Despite the enthusiastic endorsement of this treatment in all published reports, with estimates of success as high as 98%, botulinum toxin was not available in the United

States for a time, even as an investigational drug, as the result of liability problems associated with its manufacture (see *Time*, October 27, 1986, p. 71). These have apparently been resolved.

1. Dutton, J.J., Buckley, E.G. Botulinum toxin in the management of blepharospasm. *Arch. Neurol.* 43:380–382, 1986.
   A continuation of the series reported by Tsoy, Buckley, and Dutton (see below).
2. Gillum, W.N., Anderson, R.L. Blepharospasm: An anatomical approach. *Arch. Ophthalmol.* 99:1056–1062, 1981.
   These surgeons report excellent short-term relief of blepharospasm from their surgical procedure.
3. Hurwitz, J.J., Kazdan, M., Codere, F., et al. The orbicularis stripping operation for intractable blepharospasm: Surgical results in eighteen patients. *Can. J. Ophthalmol.* 21:167–169, 1986.
   Four surgeons pool their experience and report good results, but estimate that each operation took four hours. They recommend surgery only when botulinum toxin injection fails.
4. Jankovic, J., Havins, W.E., Wilkins, R.B. Blinking and blepharospasm: Mechanism, diagnosis, and management. *J.A.M.A.* 249:3160–3164, 1982.
   A clinical overview of blinking and blepharospasm just prior to the introduction of botulinum toxin, with 88 references.
5. Jankovic, J., Ford, J. Blepharospasm and orofacial-cervical dystonia: Clinical and pharmacological findings in 100 patients. *Ann. Neurol.* 13:402–411, 1983.
   Sixty-nine percent of patients in this series had some improvement from medical treatment, but in only 22 percent was the effect clinically satisfactory.
6. Jankovic, J., Orman, J. Blepharospasm: Demographic and clinical survey of 250 patients. *Ann. Ophthalmol.* 16:371–376, 1984.
   This paper tabulates the results of a questionnaire mailed to patients with blepharospasm.
7. Jankovic, J., Patel, S.C. Blepharospasm associated with brainstem lesions. *Neurology* 33:1237–1240, 1983.
   Six patients, four with brain stem strokes and two with multiple sclerosis, had blepharospasm.
8. Keane, J.R., Young, J.A. Blepharospasm with bilateral basal ganglia infarction. *Arch. Neurol.* 42:1206–1208, 1985.
   Blepharospasm, dystonia, and rigidity were features of a hypoxic encephalopathy in a 31-year-old man following self-administration of rat poison.
9. Lepore, F.E., Duvoisin, R.C. "Apraxia" of eyelid opening: An involuntary levator inhibition. *Neurology* 35:423–427, 1985.
   Apraxia of lid opening is seen with parkinsonism and related disorders, sometimes in association with blepharospasm.
10. Mauriello, J.A. Jr. Blepharospasm, Meige syndrome, and hemifacial spasm: Treatment with botulinum toxin. *Neurology* 35:1499–1500, 1985.
    Another series with a total of 50 patients reports good results.
11. McCord, C.D. Jr., Coles, W.H., Shore, J.W., et al. Treatment of essential blepharospasm. I. Comparison of facial nerve avulsion and eyebrow-eyelid muscle stripping procedure. *Arch. Ophthalmol.* 102:266–268, 1984.
    The number of reoperations was lower in these surgeons' hands when they performed muscle stripping rather than seventh nerve ablation.
12. McCord, C.D., Jr., Shore, J., Putnam, J.R. Treatment of essential blepharospasm. II. A modification of exposure for the muscle stripping technique. *Arch. Ophthalmol.* 102:269–273, 1984.
    In this companion paper, the surgical technique used is described.
13. Perman, K.I., Baylis, H.I., Rosenbaum, A.L., et al. The use of botulinum toxin in the medical management of benign essential blepharospasm. *Ophthalmology* 93:1–3, 1986.

Twenty-seven of 28 patients with blepharospasm experienced relief with botulinum toxin injections.

14. Scott, A.B., Kennedy, R.A., Stubbs, H.A. Botulinum A toxin injection as a treatment for blepharospasm. *Arch. Ophthalmol.* 103:347–350, 1985.
    This series of 39 patients was treated by the originator of botulinum therapy.
15. Shorr, N., Seiff, S.R., Kopelman, J. The use of botulinum toxin in blepharospasm. *Am. J. Ophthalmol.* 99:542–546, 1985.
    Relief of symptoms occurred about three days after injection and lasted 6 to 12 weeks.
16. Tolosa, E.S. Clinical features of Meige's disease (idiopathic orofacial dystonia): A report of 17 cases. *Arch. Neurol.* 38:147–151, 1981.
    Tolosa feels that Meige's disease may be a distinct dystonic disorder rather than a forme fruste of idiopathic torsion dystonia.
17. Tsoy, E.A., Buckley, E.G., Dutton, J.J. Treatment of blepharospasm with botulinum toxin. *Am. J. Ophthalmol.* 99:176–179, 1985.
    The mean interval between reinjections in this series of 43 patients with essential blepharospasm or hemifacial spasm was 65 days.
18. Waller, R.R., Kennedy, R.H., Henderson, J.W., et al. Management of blepharospasm. *Tr. Am. Ophthalmol. Soc.* 88:367–386, 1985.
    These authors' review of the Mayo Clinic experience from 1950 to 1984 suggests that myectomy is preferable to neurectomy as a surgical procedure.

4. CONJUNCTIVAL KAPOSI'S SARCOMA

Multiple idiopathic hemorrhagic sarcoma, also known as *Kaposi's sarcoma,* is a tumor of vascular origin, perhaps derived from endothelial cells. In the form most often encountered in the United States until recently, elderly patients, usually men of Jewish or Italian ancestry, presented with blue-red nodules on the skin, especially that of the lower extremities, associated with lymphedema. The disease ran an indolent course.

Occasionally involvement of the eyelids or conjunctiva was reported. In several cases of conjunctival Kaposi's sarcoma, there was a history of prolonged use of topical ocular medications. The appearance was that of a black or red vascular mass, sometimes associated with subconjunctival hemorrhage. As the tumor was superficial, complete excision was usually possible. Even partially excised tumors sometimes regressed after surgery. Radiotherapy and chemotherapy were also used in selected cases.

An endemic focus was also recognized in natives of equatorial Africa. This disease was often more aggressive than that encountered in elderly Americans and could be divided into four groups: a nodular type (the indolent form); a florid type (an exophytic, ulcerating tumor); an infiltrative type (involving underlying bone); and generalized disease. Generalized African Kaposi's sarcoma characteristically developed in children and young adults, with predominantly visceral rather than dermatologic involvement and eventual death, usually within three years. In some areas of the Congo and Uganda, Kaposi's sarcoma accounted for up to 10 percent of reported tumor deaths. An immune deficiency was suspected in the pathogenesis of the more severe forms of Kaposi's sarcoma in Africa, a hypothesis supported by the four- to fivefold increase in the incidence of the disease among renal transplant patients in the United States and its occurrence in other patients on immunosuppression.

In the early 1980s an aggressive form of Kaposi's sarcoma was recognized in increasing numbers of young homosexual men in the United States. It soon became apparent that Kaposi's sarcoma was an index for the acquired immune deficiency syndrome (AIDS). The other risk groups for AIDS—intravenous drug users, Haitians, and users of blood products such as hemophiliacs—also were more likely than the general population to have Kaposi's sarcoma.

In AIDS patients Kaposi's sarcoma appears after multiple infections with opportunistic organisms, including *Pneumocystis carinii, Candida,* and cytomegalovirus. The geographic distribution of Kaposi's sarcoma in Africa parallels that of African Burkitt's lymphoma, which has a known association with the Epstein-Barr virus. Also, Kaposi's sarcoma patients without AIDS have an increased incidence of a second cancer, either a carcinoma or a lymphoreticular malignancy. These epidemiologic observations support the possibility that Kaposi's sarcoma is caused by an oncogenic virus, and the leading candidate for this role is cytomegalovirus.

Because of the AIDS epidemic, an individual ophthalmologist is now much more likely to encounter cases of Kaposi's sarcoma. Unfortunately, there is at present no effective treatment for the severe generalized form found in association with AIDS. A patient who presents with Kaposi's sarcoma must be examined carefully for other ocular signs of AIDS—cotton-wool spots, cytomegalovirus retinitis, retinal periphlebitis, and neuroophthalmologic abnormalities as the result of central nervous system involvement by lymphoma, opportunistic infections, or even the sarcoma itself. Such patients should then be referred for further medical management.

1. Bedrick, J.J., Savino, P.J., Schatz, N.J. Conjunctival Kaposi's sarcoma in a patient with myasthenia gravis. *Arch. Ophthalmol.* 99:1607–1609, 1981.
   Conjunctival Kaposi's sarcoma developed in a myasthenic patient on immunosuppressive therapy; excellent color illustrations.
2. Gorin, F.A., Bale, J.F., Jr., Halks-Miller, M., et al. Kaposi's sarcoma metastatic to the CNS. *Arch. Neurol.* 42:162–165, 1985.
   Clinicopathologic verification of brain metastases, with a discussion of the potential for neurologic involvement by Kaposi's sarcoma.
3. Holland, G.N., Gottlieb, M.S., Yee, R.D., et al. Ocular disorders associated with a new severe acquired cellular immunodeficiency syndrome. *Am. J. Ophthalmol.* 93:393–402, 1982.
   One of the first reports of the ophthalmologic findings with AIDS, including a case of conjunctival Kaposi's sarcoma.
4. Howard, G.M., Jakobiec, F.A., DeVoe, A.G. Kaposi's sarcoma of the conjunctiva. *Am. J. Ophthalmol.* 79:420–423, 1975.
   Report of a case with diffuse conjunctival involvement treated with radiotherapy.
5. Jaimovich, L., Calb, I., Kaminsky, A. Kaposi's sarcoma of the conjunctiva. *J. Am. Acad. Dermatol.* 14:589–592, 1986.
   Three cases from the dermatologic literature.
6. Lieberman, P.H., Llovera, I.N. Kaposi's sarcoma of the bulbar conjunctiva. *Arch. Ophthalmol.* 88:44–45, 1972.
   Conjunctival Kaposi's sarcoma developed after prolonged treatment of Herpes simplex keratitis and uveitis.
7. Modlin, R.L., Crissey, J.T., Rea, T.H. Kaposi's sarcoma. *Int. J. Dermatol.* 22:443–448, 1983.
   A succinct review of the nonophthalmologic aspects of Kaposi's sarcoma.
8. Nicholson, D.H., Lane, L. Epibulbar Kaposi sarcoma. *Arch. Ophthalmol.* 96:95–96, 1978.
   An elderly woman being treated for open-angle glaucoma developed a rapidly growing, isolated conjunctival Kaposi's sarcoma that was treated by excision.
9. Nicolitz, E. Kaposi's sarcoma of the conjuntiva. *Ann. Ophthalmol.* 13:205–207, 1981.
   A conjunctival tumor in an elderly American man being treated for open-angle glaucoma was successfully treated by surgical excision.
10. Palestine, A.G., Rodrigues, M.M., Macher, A.M., et al. Ophthalmic involvement in acquired immunodeficiency syndrome. *Ophthalmology* 91:1092–1099, 1984.
    A large series with 20 autopsies suggests that Kaposi's sarcoma and neuroophthalmic findings occur late in the disease process.
11. Weiter, J.J., Jakobiec, F.A., Iwamoto, T. The clinical and morphologic characteristics of Kaposi's sarcoma of the conjunctiva. *Am. J. Ophthalmol.* 89:546–552, 1980.
    A case report with a review of the status of Kaposi's sarcoma just prior to the discovery of AIDS.

5. CONJUNCTIVAL MELANOSIS AND MELANOMA

To understand the significance of conjunctival pigmentation, a considerable terminology must be deciphered. One group of investigators has acknowledged a "Tower of Babel" effect in the naming of melanocytic disorders [8]. To begin with, conjunctival pigmentation alone is a normal racial variant in blacks and orientals. Also, the various forms of acquired melanosis must be distinguished from ocular melanocytosis or melanosis oculi, congenital conjunctival pigmentation that is not associated with conjunctival melanoma but may increase the risk of choroidal and orbital melanoma [7]. When the skin of the lid is involved, the condition is known as *oculodermal melanocytosis* or the *nevus of Ota.* Both the upper and lower lids often have a blue or slate gray color (kissing nevi). The iris of the involved eye may be hyperpigmented. Oculodermal melanocytosis is more common in orientals than in blacks or whites.

Primary acquired melanosis, also called *precancerous melanosis* or *benign acquired melanosis,* refers to pigmentation arising in the conjunctiva of white adults and often is a precursor to conjunctival melanoma. Conjunctival pigmentation as the result of conjunctival inflammation (as in trachoma), from chemicals or toxins (argyrosis, radiation, arsenic, thorazine, or adrenochrome deposits), or in pregnancy and Addison's disease is not premalignant. When the pigment deposited is melanin, this is termed *secondary acquired melanosis.*

Pathogenesis
Conjunctival malignant melanomas are potentially fatal tumors whose management is no less difficult or controversial than that of the more common choroidal melanomas. Conjunctival melanomas can arise de novo, or from preexisting nevi, or in primary acquired melanosis. The inference that a melanoma is derived from a nevus is often made from histologic criteria alone, in the absence of a known preexisting pigmented lesion. The percentage of conjunctival melanomas attributable to each of the three possible sources is thus uncertain. It is estimated that about one-half arise de novo, one-fourth from nevi, and one-fourth from acquired melanosis.

Despite the association of conjunctival melanomas with nevi, conjunctival nevi that appear during childhood are generally considered benign lesions. Only if the nevus grows or changes is biopsy warranted. This is in contrast to primary acquired melanosis, for which orbital exenteration was once advocated as a prophylactic measure.

Diagnosis
Although difficult to recognize in blacks or orientals, primary acquired melanosis is considered a potentially premalignant lesion in whites. Primary acquired melanosis usually appears as a diffuse, unilateral, brown, conjunctival pigmentation in adults between the ages of 40 and 50 years. In contrast with congenital ocular melanocytosis, the lesion moves with the conjunctiva and tends to change its appearance over time. Only a minority of patients with primary acquired melanosis develop conjunctival malignant melanomas. Identification of a subpopulation likely to undergo malignant change is possible histologically, and an initial biopsy may be warranted. Biopsies that reveal cellular atypia predict development of a malignant melanoma within an average of 2.5 years. Thickening or vascularization of the involved conjunctiva is an indication for rebiopsy.

Treatment
Treatment of primary conjunctival melanosis with atypia is difficult and controversial. Surgical removal of the entire involved conjunctiva results in severe alterations in ocular function. Most ophthalmologists consider orbital exenteration—removal of the globe, conjunctiva, and orbital contents—too mutilating to be justifiable as prophylaxis. Even advocates of prophylactic cryotherapy and radiotherapy admit that these approaches are far from ideal [11, 13].

A conjunctival melanoma arising in the absence of acquired melanosis is usually treated by local excision. Because of discouragingly high recurrence rates, some European surgeons use exfoliative cytology for diagnosis to minimize manipulation and irrigate the tumor bed with a cytotoxic solution immediately after excision to prevent tumor seeding [1].

Conjunctival melanomas metastasize through local lymphatics to regional nodes, and they also metastasize hematogenously. Unlike choroidal melanomas, conjunctival melanomas show no special predilection to metastasize to the liver. The morbidity of patients with conjunctival melanomas ranges from 14 to 42 percent in reported series. Tumors on the globe itself that are thin and well localized have a relatively favorable prognosis.

When extensive excision fails to produce tumor-free margins, adjunctive radiotherapy or cryotherapy may be used. One protocol delivers 6000 to 10,000 rad of beta irradiation over a five-week period, reserving exenteration for invasive, bulky tumors or large recurrences after radiation therapy. The users of cryotherapy suggest that this treatment eliminates the need for exenterations. If exenteration is undertaken, consideration should be given to radical excision of regional lymph nodes, the most likely sites for metastasis. There is no clear evidence that even such vigorous therapy improves prognosis when metastatic disease is already present.

1. de Wolff-Rouendaal, D. Management of conjunctival tumors. In Oosterhuis, J.A. (ed.), *Ophthalmic Tumours*. Dordrecht: W. Junk Publishers, 1985.
   A clinician presents his approach.
2. de Wolff-Rouendaal, D., Oosterhuis, J.A. Conjunctival melanomas in The Netherlands: a follow-up study. *Documenta Ophthalmol.* 56:49–54, 1983.
   In this series of 45 patients the recurrence rate was 80 percent.
3. Dutton, J.J., Anderson, R.L., Schelper, R.I., et al. Orbital malignant melanoma and oculodermal melanocytosis: Report of two cases and review of the literature. *Ophthalmology* 91:497–507, 1984.
   Based on their cases and those previously reported, the authors calculate an incidence of malignant degeneration of 4.6 percent in oculodermal melanocytosis. Their cases represent the fifth and perhaps the sixth instances of orbital, as opposed to choroidal, malignant melanoma.
4. Folberg, R., McLean, I.W., Zimmerman, L.E. Conjunctival melanosis and melanoma. *Ophthalmology* 91:673–678, 1984.
   Drawing on their large experience, these authors attempt to answer a series of questions about conjunctival melanosis and melanoma.
5. Folberg, R., McLean, I.W., Zimmerman, L.E. Primary acquired melanosis of the conjunctiva. *Hum. Pathol.* 16:129–135, 1985.
   Analysis of 41 cases from the A.F.I.P. suggests that primary acquired melanosis with cytologic atypia should be totally extirpated because of the risk of melanoma.
6. Folberg, R., McLean, I.W., Zimmerman, L.E. Malignant melanoma of the conjunctiva. *Hum. Pathol.* 16:136–143, 1985.
   In this series of 131 cases, the presence or absence of nevi had no effect on prognosis. When primary acquired melanosis was associated (75 percent of cases), pagetoid invasion was a sensitive indication of metastatic potential.
7. Gonder, J.R., Nichol, J., Augsberger, J.J., et al. Ocular and oculodermal melanocytosis. *Can. J. Ophthalmol.* 20:176–178, 1985.
   Ten of 33 cases of ocular or oculodermal melanocytosis had uveal melanomas.
8. Gonder, J.R., Wagoner, M.D., Albert, D.M. Idiopathic acquired melanosis. *Ophthalmology* 87:835–840, 1980.
   A nicely illustrated case report emphasizes the difficulties in nomenclature and management.
9. Guillen, F.J., Albert, D.M., Mihm, M.C. Jr. Pigmented melanocytic lesions of the conjunctiva—a new approach to their classification. *Pathology* 17:275–280, 1985.
   Another attempt to sort out the pathology and nomenclature.
10. Jakobiec, F.A. Conjunctival melanoma; Unfinished business. *Arch. Ophthalmol.* 98:1378–1384, 1980.
    Jakobiec offers an editorial expatiation.

11. Jakobiec, F.A., Brownstein, S., Albert, W., et al. The role of cryotherapy in the management of conjunctival melanoma. *Ophthalmology* 89:502–515, 1982.
    This paper provides an extensive analysis of one therapeutic modality.
12. Jeffrey, I.J.M., Lucas, D.R., McEwan, C., et al. Malignant melanomas of the conjunctiva. *Histopathology* 10:363–378, 1986.
    In this series of 37 patients, prognosis was related to subsite and size. Origin in the fornix or caruncle conferred a poor prognosis.
13. Lederman, M., Wybar, K., Busby, E. Malignant epibulbar melanoma: Natural history and treatment by radiotherapy. *Br. J. Ophthalmol.* 68:605–617, 1984.
    A posthumous paper reviews the lifetime experience of the principal proponent of radiotherapy.
14. Liesegang, T.J., Campell, J. Mayo Clinic experience with conjunctival melanomas. *Arch. Ophthalmol.* 98:1385–1389, 1980.
    In this series of 42 cases, tumor deaths did not occur in melanomas that arose from nevi.
15. Morris, D.A., Jackobiec, F.A., Henkind, P., et al. Recurrent conjunctival melanoma with neuroidal spindle cell features. *Ophthalmology* 94:56–60, 1987.
    A recurrent melanoma arising in an eye with primary acquired melanosis had unusual pathologic features.
16. Oosterhuis, J.A., de Wolff-Rouendaal, D. Local metastasis in conjunctival melanoma. *Documenta Ophthalmol.* 56:55–59, 1983.
    A case report occasions an outline of the authors' approach.
17. Stefani, F.H. A prognostic index for patients with malignant melanoma of the conjunctiva. *Graefe's Arch. Clin. Exp. Ophthalmol.* 224:580–582, 1986.
    Mitoses and thickness predicted metastatic potential.

II. ORBIT

John W. Gittinger, Jr.

5. ORBITAL CELLULITIS

Bacterial infections involving the orbit may be divided into five types: preseptal or periorbital cellulitis, inflammatory edema or true orbital cellulitis, orbital abscess, subperiosteal abscess, and cavernous sinus thrombosis. Any orbital infection is a threat to both vision and life.

Pathogenesis

Orbital infections most often arise from bacterial sinusitis, but other facial infections including dental abscesses, nasal furuncles, and facial cellulitis may serve as precursors. Dental surgery and infections occasionally lead to orbital cellulitis, usually by inciting a sinusitis [2, 4, 20]. An insect bite or laceration of the skin of the lid can also cause local suppuration. The possibility of an occult intraorbital foreign body or orbital fracture must also be considered. Orbital or strabismus surgery is seldom complicated by infection [11].

Diagnosis

Preseptal or Periorbital Cellulitis

Preseptal or periorbital cellulitis presents as inflammatory swelling of the upper lid. This most common form of orbital infection can occur at any age but characteristically occurs in children. Either the eye is white and quiet, or conjunctival injection and chemosis may be present. Some authorities consider periorbital cellulitis with chemosis to be an intermediate stage between periorbital cellulitis and true orbital cellulitis, and they report less consistent response to antibiotics when chemosis is present [3].

In children under the age of 4 years, preseptal cellulitis with a purplish blue discoloration of the lid suggests *Haemophilus influenzae* infection. Children with this disease are acutely ill, with fever and leukocytosis. Blood cultures are often positive. Recognition of this possibility is important because of its implications in the selection of antibiotic treatment. Ampicillin was considered the drug of choice for haemophilus infections until resistant strains appeared. Chloramphenicol or cefamandole are also effective against haemophilus. Physicians treating young children with orbital cellulitis should consult an authority on infectious disease for the current antibiotic of choice.

Orbital Cellulitis

In a true *orbital cellulitis* the characteristic finding is a nonneurogenic ophthalmoplegia. Chemosis and proptosis are often present, but the conjunctiva and sclera may be near normal in appearance. Differential diagnosis must be made from infections of the lacrimal gland (dacryoadenitis) or the lacrimal sac (dacryocystitis). In children, rhabdomyosarcomas and, rarely, retinoblastomas or neuroblastomas may mimic orbital inflammations. Severe idiopathic orbital inflammation (see Chap. 8) must also be considered in the differential diagnosis.

Subperiosteal and Orbital Abscess

Subperiosteal abscess and the rarer orbital abscess are complications of orbital cellulitis. A subperiosteal abscess is an accumulation of pus between the orbital bone and its periosteum, usually adjacent to an infected sinus [12–15]. A true orbital abscess lies in the soft tissues of the orbit. The presence of a subperiosteal abscess should be suspected when a patient with orbital cellulitis fails to improve when treated with parenteral antibiotics or has visual loss or displacement of the globe. If the abscess is located anteriorly in the orbit, a fluctuant mass may be palpable. Subperiosteal abscesses may develop during antibiotic treatment, resulting in subacute and atypical presentations [15].

Cavernous Sinus Thrombosis

Cavernous sinus thrombosis is encountered both as a complication of orbital cellulitis and as the initial manifestation of spread of local infection through the valveless veins tributary to the cavernous sinus. Cavernous sinus thrombosis should be suspected when there is evidence of neurologic dysfunction: pupillary dilation, numbness in the distribution of the first two divisions of the facial nerve, or, most significantly, bilateral ophthalmoplegia. The cavernous sinuses lie on either side of the sella turcica and are usually interconnected, with the consequence that infection in one sinus quickly spreads to the other. A contralateral sixth nerve palsy is often the first sign of bilaterality since the sixth nerve passes through the sinus itself, whereas the third, fourth, and fifth nerves have relatively protected locations in its wall. The meninges are frequently involved in cavernous sinus thrombosis, and a lumbar puncture should be considered Magnetic resonance imaging and computed tomography may help demonstrate septic thrombosis [16, 18, 23].

Septic cavernous sinus thrombosis must be distinguished from fungal infections (see Chap. 2) and pituitary apoplexy, the latter resulting from hemorrhagic enlargement of a preexisting pituitary tumor. Even when recognized early and treated appropriately with antibiotics, corticosteroids (because inflammation of the adjacent pituitary produces hypopituitarism), and perhaps anticoagulants, cavernous sinus thrombosis is associated with serious complications such as visual loss, permanent ophthalmoplegia septic thrombosis of the internal carotid in its intracavernous portion [22], or even death.

Treatment

Most patients with orbital infections should be hospitalized to receive parenteral antibiotics. Staphylococci (coagulase positive and negative), streptococci, and haemophilus are the most common bacteria cultured. A wide range of other species is encountered, however, and broad-spectrum antibiotic coverage is warranted until specific sensitivities are available. Conjunctival cultures are rarely helpful, but cultures of the nasopharynx, sinuses, blood, and (if relevant) cerebrospinal fluid should be taken.

Preseptal or true orbital cellulitis usually responds to antibiotics alone. If there is not prompt improvement, then computed tomography or magnetic resonance imaging of the orbits and sinuses and perhaps orbital ultrasonography should be performed. Localization of associated sinusitis and recognition of subperiosteal abscess formation can be achieved by such studies. Lack of response to antibiotics is an indication for surgical drainage of infected sinuses.

Inflammatory edema is sometimes difficult to distinguish from abscess by computed tomography, but if there is a localizable process that is not steadily improving in patients on antibiotics, surgical exploration of the orbit should be undertaken with the expectation of draining an abscess. The presence of a presumed subperiosteal abscess on computed tomography is not, however, an absolute indication for surgery, since resolution may occur with medical treatment alone [12]. When there is significant visual loss or a marked increase in intraorbital, and thus intraocular, pressure, urgent surgical intervention is mandated.

General

1. Bergin, D.J., Wright, J.E. Orbital cellulitis. *Br. J. Ophthalmol.* 70:174–178, 1986.
   The clinical lessons from this series of 49 patients include the subacute onset of symptoms, the value of evaluation of the sinuses, and the unreliability of cultures in identifying the causative organism.
2. Bullock, J.D., Fleischmen, J.A. Orbital cellulitis following dental extraction. *Trans. Am. Ophthalmol. Soc.* 82:111–133, 1984.
   Four cases of orbital cellulitis follow extractions of maxillary molars. In most cases of odontogenic orbital infection, a sinusitis intermediates.
3. Eustis, H.S., Armstrong, D.C., Buncic, J.R., et al. Staging of orbital cellulitis in children: Computerized tomography characteristics and treatment guidelines. *J. Pediatr. Ophthalmol. Strab.* 23:246–251, 1986.
   Several patients thought to represent a transitional stage between inflammatory cellulitis and subperiosteal abscess and two patients with presumed subperiosteal abscesses on computed tomography responded to medical treatment alone, although they required a longer course of antibiotics than those whose abscesses were surgically drained. One patient was explored without finding an abscess.

4. Flood, T.P., Brande, L.S., Jampol, L.M., et al. Computed tomography in the management of orbital infections associated with dental disease. *Br. J. Ophthalmol.* 66:269–274, 1982.
   Two cases of orbital infections followed dental procedures.
5. Jackson, K., Baker, S.R. Clinical implications of orbital cellulitis. *Laryngoscope* 96:568–574, 1986.
   In this series of 137 patients, 98 had periorbital cellulitis and 39 had orbital cellulitis. Almost half of the patients with orbital cellulitis had abscesses drained.
6. Schramm, V.L., Jr., Curtin, H.D., Kennerdell, J.S. Evaluation of orbital cellulitis and results of treatment. *Laryngoscope* 92:732–738, 1982.
   A review of 303 cases.
7. Simon, M.W., Broughton, R.A. Orbital cellulitis; A presentation of two cases with unusual features. *Clin. Pediatr.* 24:226–228, 1985.
   Cases reported from the pediatrician's perspective.
8. Slavin, M.L., Glaser, J.S. Acute severe irreversible visual loss with sphenoethmoiditis—'posterior' orbital cellulitis. *Arch. Ophthalmol.* 105:345–348, 1987.
   In these three cases, sinusitis caused severe, permanent visual loss with minimal signs of orbital inflammation.
9. Spires, J.R., Smith, R.J.H. Bacterial infections of the orbital and periorbital soft-tissues in children. *Laryngoscope* 96:763–767, 1986.
   As in other series, periorbital infection is much more common than true orbital cellulitis and usually responds promptly to antibiotics.
10. Weiss, A., Friendly, D., Eglin, K., et al. Bacterial periorbital cellulitis in childhood. *Ophthalmology* 90:195–203, 1983.
    Details diagnosis and management of 158 children, most with preseptal cellulitis. An appended discussion by D. Jones clarifies and expands on the topic.
11. Wilson, M.E., Paul, T.O. Orbital cellulitis following strabismus surgery. *Ophthalmic. Surg.* 18:92–94, 1987.
    The seventh reported case of orbital cellulitis after strabismus surgery.

Orbital and Subperiosteal Abscess

12. Goodwin, W.J., Jr., Weinshall, M., Chandler, J.R. The role of high resolution computerized tomography and standardized ultrasound in the evaluation of orbital cellulitis. *Laryngoscope* 92:728–731, 1982.
    Three patients with the presumptive diagnosis of subperiosteal abscess by computed tomography responded to antibiotic therapy alone.
13. Harris, G.J. Subperiosteal abscess of the orbit. *Arch. Ophthalmol.* 101:751–757, 1983.
14. Hornblass, A., Herschorn, B.J., Stern, K., et al. Orbital abscess. *Surv. Ophthalmol.* 29:169–178, 1984.
    Both of these case series cover diagnosis and therapeusis. (See also Tannenbaum, M., Tenzel, M.D.J., Byrne, S.F., et al. Medical management of orbital abscess. Surv. Ophthalmol. 30:211–212, 1985.)
15. Krohel, G.B., Krauss, H.R., Winnick, J. Orbital abscess; Presentation, diagnosis, therapy, and sequelae. *Ophthalmology* 89:492–498, 1982.
    Various atypical presentations are emphasized.

Cavernous Sinus Thrombosis

16. Ahmadi, J., Keane, J.R., Segall, H.D., et al. CT observations pertinent to septic cavernous sinus thrombosis. *A.J.N.R.* 6:755–758, 1985.
    Multiple irregular filling defects in the enhanced cavernous sinus and enlargement of the superior ophthalmic vein were demonstrated on axial computed tomography.
17. Clifford-Jones, R.E., Ellis, C.J.K., Stevens, J.M., et al. Cavernous sinus thrombosis. *J. Neurol. Neurosurg. Psychiatry.* 45:1092–1097, 1982.
    Four cases produced by sinusitis presented with severe headache, obtundation, and orbital swelling. The patients were treated with antibiotics and corticosteroids.
18. Curnes, J.T., Creasy, J.L., Whaley, R.L., et al. Air in the cavernous sinus: A new sign of septic cavernous sinus thrombosis. *A.J.N.R.* 8:176–177, 1987.

A brief report of a rapidly fatal case caused by bacterial sinusitis with intracavernous air demonstrated on computed tomography.

19. Fiandaca, M.S., Spector, R.H., Hartmann, T.M., et al. Unilateral septic cavernous sinus thrombosis; A case report with digital orbital venographic documentation. *J. Clin. Neuro-ophthalmol.* 6:35–38, 1986.
Computed tomography and digital subtraction venography were used to differentiate unilateral cavernous sinus thrombosis with associated sphenoid osteomyelitis from orbital cellulitis.

20. Harbour, R.C., Trobe, J.D., Ballinger, W.E. Septic cavernous sinus thrombosis associated with gingivitis and parapharyngeal abscess. *Arch. Ophthalmol.* 102:94–97, 1984.
An undiagnosed odontogenic infection led to cavernous sinus thrombosis and death in this 29-year-old man.

21. Karlin, R.J., Robinson, W.A. Septic cavernous sinus thrombosis. *Ann. Emerg. Med.* 13:449–455, 1984.
An extensively referenced clinical review.

22. Mathew, N.T., Abraham, J., Taori, G.M., et al. Internal carotid artery occlusion in cavernous sinus thrombosis. *Arch. Neurol.* 24:11–16, 1971.
Four cases of cavernous sinus thrombosis with an important but seldom discussed major complication.

23. Savino, P.J., Grossman, R.I., Schatz, N.J., et al. High-field magnetic resonance imaging in the diagnosis of cavernous sinus thrombosis. *Arch. Neurol.* 43:1081–1082, 1986.
Magnetic resonance imaging is sensitive to thrombus formation.

24. Yarington, C.T. Cavernous sinus thrombosis revisited. *Proc. R. Soc. Med.* 70:456–459, 1977.
Yarington distills his considerable experience.

7. FUNGAL ORBITAL INFECTION

Fungi usually invade the orbit by extension from the adjacent sinuses. The two genera most often encountered clinically are *Rhizopus* and *Aspergillus*. *Rhizopus* is of the class Phycomycetes, order Mucorales, and its infections are usually reported as mucormycoses or phycomycoses. Clinically similar infections by related fungi (*Mucor* and *Absidia*) are also grouped under these headings, which for practical purposes are used interchangeably. *Aspergillus* infection is known as *aspergillosis;* the fungal mass is an aspergilloma.

Aspergillosis

Pathogenesis
Most aspergillosis is bronchopulmonary disease: asthma, bronchitis, and invasive pulmonary aspergillosis. Paranasal sinus aspergillosis is rare, except in the Sudan where an endemic focus exists; however, it still represents the most common fungal sinusitis. Species of *Aspergillus* are ubiquitous; spores are found in especially high concentrations in composted hay. Marijuana contaminated with aspergillus may be a clinically significant source of sensitization and colonization. Aspergillus sinus infections develop most often in hot and humid climates and should be suspected when a chronic maxillary sinusitis fails to respond to antibiotics.

Orbital aspergillosis is a disease of otherwise healthy adults, although a fulminant form resembling phycomycosis has been observed in immunologically incompetent patients [3]. A chronic sinusitis is often but not invariably associated. The characteristic presentation is slowly progressive unilateral exophthalmos. Pain, ophthalmoplegia, and visual loss signal invasion of the orbital apex [2]. Cases of orbital apex syndrome without proptosis have been reported [5], and intracranial involvement may develop by extension from the orbit or sinuses. Immunocompromised persons or intravenous drug users are at risk for primary intracranial aspergillosis.

Diagnosis
Cultures are unreliable because *Aspergillus* is ubiquitous, and the diagnosis of aspergillosis of the sinuses, orbit, or brain is made by pathologic evaluation of biopsies. These reveal a chronic, fibrosing, granulomatous inflammation containing hyphae. The hyphae have septae, branch dichotomously at a 45-degree angle (forked-stick), and are 3 to 4 μ in diameter. These characteristics are more apparent on special fungal stains (e.g., Gomori methenamine silver) than with routine hematoxylin and eosin preparations. The fructification heads, whose resemblance to the aspergillum, a perforated container used for sprinkling holy water, gave rise to the name of the genus, are not observed. An adequate biopsy specimen may be difficult to obtain, resulting in the finding of only nonspecific acute and chronic inflammatory changes.

Mucormycosis

Pathogenesis
Rhinocerebral mucormycosis, in contrast to the indolent behavior of most aspergillosis infections, is a rapidly fatal infection when left untreated. Even with early diagnosis and aggressive management, the mortality is high. The normally nonpathogenetic fungus is activated in patients with systemic acidosis, which is usually caused by uncontrolled diabetes. Also at risk are persons with renal disease and infants with diarrhea and vomiting, in whom acidosis develops without diabetes. Cases have also been reported in patients with leukemias and lymphoma, especially those receiving chemotherapy, even in the absence of acidosis, presumably because there is suppression of the normal immune mechanisms. A few well-documented instances have no identifiable risk factors [13, 18].

Diagnosis
The characteristic clinical presentation of patients with mucormycosis is lethargy, headache, and visual loss, followed by facial pain and swelling, exophthalmos, and ophthalmoplegia. Because early recognition probably improves prognosis, an apparent orbital cellulitis or acute sinus infection in a susceptible individual should be approached with a high degree of clinical suspicion. The diagnosis should be considered in any diabetic in ketoacidosis who remains lethargic once the metabolic imbalance has been corrected. The fungus has a propensity to invade arteries, producing thrombosis and tissue infarction. Otolaryngologic examination may reveal necrosis of the turbinates or ulcerations of the nasal mucosa and hard palate, and the facial tissues rapidly become involved as the infection progresses.

Computed tomography helps to define the extent of the infection, but biopsy is necessary for definitive diagnosis. The biopsy specimen should be processed for fungal culture and histopathology, with a potassium hydroxide preparation performed on the fresh tissue to look for hyphae. *Rhizopus* hyphae are larger than *Aspergillus* (up to 25 μ) and are thick-walled and nonseptate, branching at right angles. If frozen sections are taken, care must be taken to distinguish the *Rhizopus* hyphae from blood vessels.

Treatment
The treatment of both aspergillosis and mucormycosis is a combination of surgery and antifungal agents. Removal of the fungal mass and the walls of the sinus should cure an aspergilloma of the maxillary sinus. If the infected tissue cannot be completely excised, the patient should be treated with local and systemic amphotericin B. In the more aggressive fulminant aspergillosis and in mucormycosis, the underlying metabolic abnormality should be corrected and any concurrent bacterial infection treated. Debridement of infected and necrotic tissue is desirable; in some, but certainly not all, cases, this means orbital exenteration.

Surgery should establish drainage of the sinuses and involved orbit, thus allowing daily local irrigations of amphotericin B solution, in addition to intravenous amphotericin B treatment. Use of amphotericin B in combination with 5-flucytosine may allow a lower dose of amphotericin which may be beneficial when there is concurrent renal failure [15]. Other antifungal agents such as ketoconazole have also seen limited use. The therapeutic role of hyperbaric oxygenation is not clearly established [14].

Aspergillosis

1. Green, W.R., Font, R.L., Zimmerman, L.E. Aspergillosis of the orbit: Report of ten cases and a review of the literature. *Arch. Ophthalmol.* 82:302–313, 1969.
   The orbital aspergillosis story.
2. Hedges, T.R., Leung, L.E. Parasellar and orbital apex syndrome caused by aspergillosis. *Neurology* 26:117–120, 1976.
   A good discussion of an unusual presentation.
3. McGill, T.J., Simpson, G., Healy, G.B. Fulminant aspergillosis of the nose and paranasal sinuses: A new clinical entity. *Laryngoscope* 90:748–754, 1980.
   Aspergillosis masquerades as phycomycosis.
4. Robb, P.J. Aspergillosis of the paranasal sinuses (a case report and historical perspective). *J. Laryngol. Otol.* 100:1071–1077, 1986.
   Robb provides access to the otolaryngological literature on aspergillosis of the paranasal sinuses.
5. Weinstein, J.M., Sattler, F.A., Towfighi, J., et al. Optic neuropathy and paratrigeminal syndrome due to *Aspergillus fumigatus*. *Arch. Neurol.* 39:582–585, 1982.
   Aspergillosis presents in unusual ways, too.
6. Whitehurst, F.O., Liston, T.E. Orbital aspergillosis: Report of a case in a child. *J. Pediatr. Ophthalmol. Strab.* 18:50–54, 1981.
   A fungal infection, felt to be aspergillosis, developed in a healthy 9-year-old and eventually led to exenteration. The initial diagnoses were abscess, eosinophilic granuloma, malignancy, and then inflammatory pseudotumor.

Mucormycosis

7. Abedi, E., Sismanis, A., Choi, K., et al. Twenty-five years' experience treating cerebro-rhino-orbital mucormycosis. *Laryngoscope* 94:1060–1062, 1984.
   An approach to management from the otolaryngologic literature.
8. Ferry, A.P., Abedi, S. Diagnosis and management of rhino-orbitocerebral mucormycosis (phycomycosis): A report of 16 personally observed cases. *Ophthalmology* 90:1096–1104, 1983.
   The ophthalmologic perspective from the same institution as Abedi et al. (above).
9. Finn, D.G., Farmer, J.C. Jr. Chronic mucormycosis. *Laryngoscope* 92:761–763, 1982.
   Two patients had osteomyelitis and bony sequestration 8 months and 2 years after apparently successful treatment. Despite the pathologic diagnosis, the initial presentation of neither case is typical.
10. Kohn, R., Hepler, R. Management of limited rhino-orbital mucormycosis without exenteration. *Ophthalmology* 92:1440–1444, 1985.
    A series of eight cases where relatively conservative management was successful.
11. Lehrer, R.I., Howard, D.H., Sypherd, P.S., et al. Mucormycosis. *Ann. Intern. Med.* 93:93–108, 1980.
    Mycology is thoroughly discussed in this summary based on an interdepartmental symposium at U.C.L.A.
12. Maniglia, A.J., Mintz, D.H., Novak, S. Cephalic phycomycosis: A report of eight cases. *Laryngoscope* 92:755–760, 1982.
    A tabulation of eight cases associated with diabetes and leukemia, with discussion of management.
13. O'Keefe, M., Haining, W.M., Young, J.D.H., et al. Orbital mucormycosis with survival. *Br. J. Ophthalmol.* 70:634–636, 1986.
    Mucormycosis in an otherwise healthy 61-year-old man was successfully treated with orbital exenteration-ethmoidectomy, amphotericin B, and ketoconazole.
14. Price, J.C., Stevens, D.L. Hyperbaric oxygen in the treatment of rhinocerebral mucormycosis. *Laryngoscope* 90:737–747, 1980.

A single case report allows some tentative conclusions: hyperbaric oxygen may be useful, especially in patients who refuse surgery.

15. Rangel-Guerra, R., Martinez, H.R., Saenz, C. Mucormycosis: Report of 11 cases. *Arch. Neurol.* 42:578–581, 1985.
    This series of 11 cases confirms previous experience.

16. Schwartz, J.N., Donnelly, E.H., Klintworth, G.K. Ocular and orbital phycomycosis. *Surv. Ophthalmol.* 22:3–28, 1977.
    An extensive review of cases reported up until 1976.

17. Schwartze, G.M., Kilgo, G.R., Ford, C.S. Internal ophthalmoplegia resulting from acute orbital phycomycosis. *J. Clin. Neuro-ophthalmol.* 4:105–108, 1984.
    Mucormycosis presents as internal ophthalmoplegia during treatment for ketoacidosis.

18. Zak, S.M., Katz, B. Successfully treated spheno-orbital mucormycosis in an otherwise healthy adult. *Ann. Ophthalmol.* 17:344–348, 1985.
    Biopsy of a mass found during evaluation of an optic neuropathy revealed nonseptate branching hyphae. This was treated with amphotericin B, and no other problems developed.

8. INFLAMMATORY PSEUDOTUMOR OF THE ORBIT

The term *pseudotumor* is used in several contexts in medicine. Of ophthalmic interest are *pseudotumor cerebri* (see Ch. 51) and *inflammatory pseudotumor of the orbit,* two unrelated processes. Orbital pseudotumor is "an idiopathic, localized, inflammatory disease characterized by a lymphocytic infiltration, a polymorphonuclear response, and a fibrovascular tissue reaction that has a variable but self-limited course" [2]. Some authorities prefer to avoid the term pseudotumor and classify the same process as *diffuse* or *localized nonspecific orbital inflammation* to exclude reactive or atypical lymphoid hyperplasia [10]. Others group all nonneoplastic processes together as *pseudolymphomas* [11].

Diagnosis
The classic clinical presentation of orbital pseudotumor is with signs of orbital inflammation: pain, proptosis, conjunctival injection and chemosis, and periorbital swelling. Differentiation must be made from infections, especially those arising in the adjacent sinuses and affecting the orbit secondarily (see Chaps. 1 and 2), and from specific inflammations. This second category includes vasculitides, orbital amyloid, sclerosing angioma, nodular fasciitis, histiocytosis, and Graves' orbitopathy.

Distinguishing pseudotumor of the orbit from ophthalmic Graves' disease, in which thyroid studies are entirely normal, may be difficult. Usually, but not always, pain is not prominent in Graves' orbitopathy. Also, pseudotumor tends to be unilateral, whereas Graves' orbitopathy is usually bilateral, although occasionally quite asymmetrical (see Chap. 10).

Differentiation of pseudotumor from true tumor may be impossible on clinical grounds. True orbital tumors tend to be slow growing and generally without inflammatory signs, but some pseudotumors present as noninflammatory mass lesions. Particularly in children, inflammation is seen with true tumors: rhabdomyosarcoma (see Chap. 4), a common orbital tumor of childhood, may initially mimic a cellulitis, and a ruptured dermoid cyst characteristically causes orbital inflammation.

The clinical picture encountered will depend on which orbital structures are primarily affected. One syndrome is that of *orbital myositis* [2, 5, 21]. This is largely a disorder of young adults, who have pain, ophthalmoplegia, and enlargement of an ocular muscle or muscles on computed tomography. Orbital pseudotumor also presents as a *dacryoadenitis,* with inflammation localized to the superolateral orbit, downward displacement of the globe, and minimal proptosis. The optic nerve, posterior sclera (see Chap. 18), and orbital fat may also be loci of inflammation. Associated intraocular inflammation—uveitis or papillitis—is also observed.

The same pathologic process that characterizes inflammatory pseudotumor of the orbit has been identified in the walls of the cavernous sinus. This syndrome of painful ophthalmoplegia has come to be known as the *Tolosa-Hunt syndrome*. Care must be taken to distinguish a true Tolosa-Hunt syndrome from other processes involving multiple ocular motor nerves and the first and second division of the trigeminal nerve, especially tumors and aneurysms.

Treatment

All patients with signs of pseudotumor of the orbit should undergo high-resolution computed tomography or magnetic resonance imaging. These studies help to localize and define the orbital process and permit evaluation of the contiguous bones and sinuses. If both the clinical findings and the imaging are consistent with inflammatory pseudotumor of the orbit, then a trial of steroid treatment is probably warranted before biopsy, except perhaps in children. In many instances, a moderately high dosage of prednisone (40–60 mg/day) produces dramatic improvement in signs and symptoms, a response that supports the diagnosis of pseudotumor. Malignant lymphoma and other diseases also sometimes temporarily improve with steroid administration.

An attempt should then be made to taper the steroids. If there are no atypical features, biopsy should probably be avoided. Orbital biopsies are never a trivial undertaking, and instances are reported in which the biopsy appeared to exacerbate the orbital inflammation acutely, leading to visual loss and ophthalmoplegia. A partial response or an accessible anterior mass argues for biopsy [15]. If biopsy reveals lymphocytes, the tissue should be processed for cell surface markers, if available [12]. Monoclonal lesions suggest malignant lymphoma; polyclonal lesions are characteristic of benign processes.

Lymphomas localized to the orbit and biopsy-proven pseudotumor that cannot be controlled with steroids are candidates for local radiotherapy [11, 20]. Most but not all improve with administration of low-dose (1000–2000 rad), high-voltage radiotherapy. The correlation between steroid responsiveness and radiation responsiveness is not perfect. Some pseudotumors not controlled with steroids or radiation respond to chemotherapy with drugs such as chlorambucil or cyclophosphamide [4]. A few biopsy-proven inflammatory pseudotumors evolve into lymphomas or vasculitides, and the patients must be followed.

1. Atlas, S.W., Grossman, R.I., Savino, P.J., et al. Surface-coil MR of orbital pseudotumor. *A.J.N.R.* 8:141–146, 1987.
   Although technically more demanding than computed tomography, magnetic resonance imaging allows differentiation between inflammatory pseudotumor and metastases or hemorrhage.
2. Bullen, C.L., Younge, B.R. Chronic orbital myositis. *Arch. Ophthalmol.* 100:1749–1751, 1982.
   A larger series of patients with clinical features similar to those of the patients of Slavin and Glaser (ref. 21).
3. Chavis, R.M., Garner, A., Wright, J.E. Inflammatory orbital pseudotumor: A clinicopathologic study. *Arch. Ophthalmol.* 96:1817–1822, 1978.
   A large clinical series (where biopsies were undertaken) from the era before computed tomography.
4. Clay, C., Bilaniuk, L.T., Vignaud, J. Orbital pseudotumors: Preliminary report on a new type of therapy. *Neuro-ophthalmology* 1:101–107, 1980.
   Description of the use of chlorambucil in pseudotumor not controlled by steroids.
5. Dresner, S.C., Rothfus, W.E., Slamovits, T.L., et al. Computed tomography of orbital myositis. *A.J.N.R.* 5:351–354, 1984.
   In 11 cases, bilaterality and multiple muscle involvement was recognized more often than in previous reports.
6. Dua, H.S., Smith, F.W., Singh, A.K., et al. Diagnosis of orbital myositis by nuclear magnetic resonance imaging. *Br. J. Ophthalmol.* 71:54–57, 1987.

Magnetic resonance imaging was used to define the lesion and to follow its response to corticosteroids.

7. Frohman, L.P., Kupersmith, M.J., Lang, J., et al. Intracranial extension and bone destruction in orbital pseudotumor. *Arch. Ophthalmol.* 104:380–384, 1986.
   Three cases where a process pathologically defined as pseudotumor behaved aggressively.

8. Fujii, H., Fujisada, H., Kondo, T., et al. Orbital pseudotumor: Histopathological classification and treatment. *Ophthalmologica* 190:230–242, 1985.
   On the basis of 43 cases studied histopathologically, these authors divide pseudotumor into lymphoid, granulomatous, and sclerosing types, with transitions between types. Lymphoid pseudotumors responded well to radiotherapy; the granulomatous type responded to systemic corticosteroids; and the sclerosing type responded to neither.

9. Garner, A. Pathology of 'pseudotumors' of the orbit: A review. *J. Clin. Pathol.* 26:639–648, 1973.
   An excellent overview of the differential diagnosis.

10. Garner, A., Rahi, A.H.S., Wright, J.E. Lymphoproliferative disorders of the orbit: An immunological approach to diagnosis and pathogenesis. *Br. J. Ophthalmol.* 67:561–569, 1983.
    This prospective study attempts to correlate clinical features with histologic and immunologic evidence to separate inflammation from neoplasia.

11. Gordon, P.S., Juillard, G.J.F., Selch, M.T., et al. Orbital lymphomas and pseudolymphomas: Treatment with radiation therapy. *Radiology* 159:797–799, 1986.
    Sixteen patients with lymphomas and pseudolymphomas responded well to radiotherapy.

12. Harmon, D.C., Aisenber, A.C., Harris, N.L., et al. Lymphocyte surface markers in orbital lymphoid neoplasms. *J. Clin. Oncol.* 2:856–860, 1984.
    In 23 consecutive patients with lymphoid orbital tumors, monoclonal surface immunoglobulin was found in 15 and helped distinguish between benign lymphoid infiltrates and malignant lymphomas.

13. Jakobiec, F.A., Jones, I.S. Orbital inflammations. In T.D. Duane and E.A. Jaeger (eds.), *Clinical Ophthalmology* (Vol. 2). Philadelphia: Harper & Row, 1985. Chap. 35, pp. 1–75.
    A well-written and extensive clinicopathologic review taking a perspective from early in the computed tomography era.

14. Kennerdell, J.S., Dresner, S.C. The nonspecific orbital inflammatory syndromes. *Surv. Ophthalmol.* 29:93–103, 1984.
    The authors discard the term "pseudotumor," preferring classification according to the structure primarily involved and whether the process is acute or chronic.

15. Leone, C.R. Jr., Lloyd, W.C. III. Treatment protocol for orbital inflammatory disease. *Ophthalmology* 92:1325–1331, 1985.
    An outline of a specific approach to management, supporting early biopsy in steroid-unresponsive cases.

16. Mauriello, J.A. Jr., Flanagan, J.C. Management of orbital inflammatory disease. A protocol. *Surv. Ophthalmol.* 29:104–116, 1984.
    Another approach to the management of patients with pseudotumor and related disorders.

17. Noble, S.C., Chandler, W.F., Lloyd, R.V. Intracranial extension of orbital pseudotumor: A case report. *Neurosurgery* 18:798–801, 1986.
    From the neurosurgical literature, a report of an orbital pseudotumor invading the anterior cranial fossa.

18. Orcutt, J.C., Garner, A., Henk, J.M., et al. Treatment of idiopathic inflammatory orbital pseudotumors by radiotherapy. *Br. J. Ophthalmol.* 67:570–574, 1983.
    Seventy-five percent of patients responded to radiotherapy. Polymorphonuclear leukocytes and eosinophils on biopsy were predictive of a poor response.

19. Rootman, J., Nugent, R. The classification and management of acute orbital pseudotumors. *Ophthalmology* 89:1040–1048, 1982.
    An attempt to group pseudotumor by clinical manifestations.

20. Sergott, R.C., Glaser, J.S., Charyulu, K. Radiotherapy for idiopathic inflammatory

orbital pseudotumor: Indications and results. *Arch. Ophthalmol.* 99:853–856, 1981.
The title says it all.
21. Slavin, M.S., Glaser, J.S. Idiopathic orbital myositis: Report of six cases. *Arch. Ophthalmol.* 100:1261–1265, 1982.
Delineates a subgroup of idiopathic inflammatory orbital pseudotumor now frequently recognized by computed tomography.

9. RHABDOMYOSARCOMA

Rhabdomyosarcomas are malignant tumors that arise from undifferentiated mesenchymal cells, which have morphologic similarities to developing skeletal muscle. In approximate order of frequency, rhabdomyosarcomas arise in the head and neck, orbit, genitourinary tract, extremities, trunk, retroperitoneum, perineum and anus, and elsewhere. Those primary to the head and neck may cause cranial neuropathies [2, 11], but it is the orbital tumors that are of major ophthalmic interest. Orbital rhabdomyosarcomas are the commonest primary orbital malignancy of childhood. Some are congenital; 75 percent develop before the patient has reached the age of 10 years. The average age at discovery is 8 years.

Pathogenesis
Orbital rhabdomyosarcoma is not a tumor of the extraocular muscles, but arises in undifferentiated cells elsewhere in the orbit [8]. No hereditary predisposition has been recognized.

Diagnosis
The most common presentation is exophthalmos, which may progress rapidly. Orbital rhabdomyosarcomas sometimes mimic orbital cellulitis or hemorrhage and should be considered in the differential diagnosis of these entities. Hemangiomas, lymphangiomas, optic nerve gliomas, and dermoid cysts are benign orbital tumors of childhood that also present with exophthalmos. Neuroblastomas, whose primary tumors arise in the sympathetic chains or the adrenal glands, characteristically metastasize to the orbits, producing bilateral hemorrhagic exophthalmos. Granulocytic sarcoma, a variant of granulocytic (myeloid) leukemia in which the malignant cells behave as an invasive and destructive mass, involves the orbits in children of exactly the same age range as those who are susceptible to rhabdomyosarcoma. Hematologic evidence of leukemia may not develop until months later. Rarely, in younger children, orbital signs are the initial presentation of retinoblastomas.

Rhabdomyosarcomas commonly present as a ptosis or lid mass, often in the upper, inner quadrant of the orbit. Because they are both malignant and treatable, a high degree of clinical suspicion is warranted. Nicholson and Green [10] put it well, "Any time a lid lump, conjunctival elevation, or evidence of a space-occupying disease process is seen in a child under the age of 16 years, the clinician should ask, 'Could this be rhabdomyosarcoma?' A chalazion that does not have quite the expected consistency at the time of curettage, acute orbital cellulitis that does not begin to improve rapidly after the institution of systemic antibiotic therapy, and suspected orbital hemorrhage after a fall from a bicycle are examples of observations leading to the suspicion and detection of orbital rhabdomyosarcoma."

Initial evaluation of a child suspected to have orbital rhabdomyosarcoma should include complete ophthalmologic examination, blood count and chemistries, and computed tomography or magnetic resonance imaging of the orbit. The computed tomography may demonstrate bony destruction. Physicians experienced in the management of rhabdomyosarcomas emphasize the rapidity with which the tumor mass enlarges in some children, lending an urgency to obtaining a biopsy and commencing therapy. At some centers, if biopsy must be delayed over a weekend in a child with rapidly progressive proptosis, a low dose of radiotherapy is delivered in the interim to retard tumor growth.

The diagnosis of rhabdomyosarcoma is made by histopathology. The four major histologic types are pleomorphic, embryonal, alveolar, and botryoid. Most orbital rhabdomyosarcomas are of the embryonal type; alveolar and differentiated tumors also occur. Characteristic cross striations may not be present on routine histologic preparations, and electron microscopy to demonstrate myosin fibers confirms the diagnosis.

Treatment

The traditional treatment for rhabdomyosarcoma was exenteration of the orbit. There is now good evidence that a more conservative regimen of chemotherapy and radiotherapy results in excellent survival, obviating the need for mutilating surgery in most children. Because of disfiguring osseous growth retardation after radiotherapy in very young children and relative resistance to radiation in adolescents, some physicians suggest consideration of exenteration as a primary therapy in these two groups. Of all primary sites, the orbit has the best prognosis, with a three-year relapse-free survival rate of 91 percent in the Intergroup Rhabdomyosarcoma Study in the United States [6, 12] and a five-year survival of 94 percent in the British Children's Solid Tumour Group study [7]. These excellent results are attributed to the early detection of orbital neoplasms and the absence of orbital lymphatics to facilitate metastases.

The current therapeutic regimen for orbital rhabdomyosarcoma consists of megavoltage irradiation delivered to the orbits and adjacent sinuses combined with courses of chemotherapy using combinations of adriamycin, carmustine (BCNU), vincristine, cyclophosphamide, and dactinomycin. High-dose irradiation frequently induces cataracts and may result in a keratitis so severe that enucleation or evisceration is required. As in other situations when radiotherapy must be delivered to the unprotected eye, the lids should be open during treatment to afford the exquisitely radiosensitive corneal epithelium the surface-sparing effect. A secondary malignancy, which is a frequent problem in children treated with radiation for retinoblastomas, has been reported only once—a malignant melanoma of the orbit developing 45 years after treatment [9].

1. Abramson, D.H., Ellsworth, R.M., Tretter, P., et al. The treatment of orbital rhabdomyosarcoma with irradiation and chemotherapy. *Ophthalmology* 86:1330–1335, 1979.
   A brief discussion of the Columbia-Presbyterian Medical Center experience.
2. Breen, L.A., Kline, L.B., Hart, W.M., Jr., et al. Rhabdomyosarcoma causing rapid bilateral visual loss in children. *J. Clin. Neuro-ophthalmol.* 4:185–188, 1984.
   Two cases where rhabdomyosarcomas of the nasopharynx presented with visual loss and ophthalmoplegia, initially mimicking optic neuritis.
3. Cameron, J.D., Wick, M.R. Embryonal rhabdomyosarcoma of the conjunctiva: A clinicopathologic and immunohistochemical study. *Arch. Ophthalmol.* 104:1203–1204, 1986.
   A tumor arose in a 16-year-old girl at an unusual site.
4. Ghafoor, S.Y.A., Dudgeon, J. Orbital rhabdomyosarcoma: Improved survival with combined pulsed chemotherapy and irradiation. *Br. J. Ophthalmol.* 69:557–561, 1985.
   A report of the successful treatment of three children, two with intracranial extension.
5. Haik, B.G., Jereb, B., Smith, M.E., et al. Radiation and chemotherapy of parameningeal rhabdomyosarcoma involving the orbit. *Ophthalmology* 93:1001–1009, 1986.
   In this series of 18 patients with rhabdomyosarcomas arising in and around the orbit, a combination of chemotherapy and comparatively low-dose radiotherapy resulted in good survival and relatively low ocular morbidity.
6. Heyn, R., Ragab, A., Raney, R.B., Jr., et al. Late effects of therapy in orbital rhabdomyosarcoma in children: A report from the Intergroup Rhabdomyosarcoma Study. *Cancer* 57:1738–1743, 1986.
   Of 50 children, 6 had primary exenterations and 4 required secondary enucleations.

Ninety percent developed cataracts in the ipsilateral eye, and 20 percent had corneal changes. One developed acute myeloblastic leukemia.

7. Kingston, J.E., McElwain, T.J., Malpas, J.S. Childhood rhabdomyosarcoma: Experience of the Children's Solid Tumour Group. *Br. J. Cancer* 48:195–207, 1983.
   Excellent survival is reported in orbital rhabdomyosarcoma.

8. Knowles, D.M. III, Jakobiec, F.A., Jones, I.S. Rhabdomyosarcoma. In Duane, T.D., Jaeger, E.A. (eds.), *Clinical Ophthalmology* (2nd ed., Vol. 2). Philadelphia: Harper & Row, 1985. Chap. 43, pp. 1–25.
   In the most comprehensive discussion currently available, Knowles and co-authors emphasize the pathologic differential diagnosis.

9. Leff, S.R., Henkind, P. Rhabdomyosarcoma and late malignant melanoma of the orbit. *Ophthalmology* 90:1258–1260, 1983.
   The first report of secondary malignancy.

10. Nicholson, D.H., Green, W.R. Tumors of the eye, lids, and orbit in children. In Harley, R.D. (ed.), *Pediatric Ophthalmology* (2nd ed.). Philadelphia: Saunders, 1983. Pp. 1223–1271.
    This chapter emphasizes the differential diagnosis.

11. Reynard, M., Brinkley, J.R. Cavernous sinus syndrome caused by rhabdomyosarcoma. *Ann. Ophthalmol.* 15:94–97, 1983.
    Metastatic rhabdomyosarcoma from the masseter produced a multiple cranial neuropathy.

12. Wharam, M., Beltangady, M., Hays, D., et al. Localized orbital rhabdomyosarcoma; An interim report of the Intergroup Rhabdomyosarcoma Study Committee. *Ophthalmology* 94:251–254, 1987.
    Analysis of 127 cases of rhabdomyosarcoma confined to the eyelid and orbit encountered between November 1972 and June 1983 confirms the therapeutic efficacy of partial tumor resection followed by chemotherapy and radiotherapy.

10. GRAVES' ORBITOPATHY

Graves' orbitopathy, also referred to as *dysthyroid orbitopathy* or *endocrine exophthalmos,* is a common disorder with multiple manifestations and a variable clinical course. Generally, the ophthalmic signs of Graves' disease can be divided into two categories: *toxic* (primarily lid retraction), which is a function of the hyperthyroid state; and *congestive.* Congestive signs appear independently of the current endocrine status, developing during hyperthyroid, euthyroid, and even hypothyroid states. Congestive Graves' orbitopathy is closely linked to Graves' thyroid disease, but in a subset of patients with typical orbitopathy there are no abnormalities of thyroid function demonstrable by even the most sophisticated testing. Because of the existence of this *ophthalmic Graves' disease,* the clinical and radiologic manifestations are more important than an endocrinologic evaluation in establishing the diagnosis.

The most common toxic sign is lid retraction (Dalrymple's sign) as the result of sympathetic hyperactivity. Lid retraction is also encountered as part of the physiological response to fear, after instillation of sympathomimetic medications, and in lesions of the dorsal midbrain (Collier's sign). It has also been reported with hepatic cirrhosis, Cushing's disease, chronic steroid therapy, and hyperkalemic periodic paralysis. Unilateral lid retraction is also observed when there is contralateral ptosis and compensatory increased innervation. The majority of persons with hyperthyroidism have only lid retraction, which remits when circulating thyroid hormone levels return to normal. Perhaps 10 percent go on to develop an infiltrative orbitopathy.

Pathogenesis

The exact basis for the infiltrative orbitopathy is still uncertain, and various immunologic abnormalities have been demonstrated. No known immunologic parameter, however, correlates well with the severity of the process. Clinically, there is exophthalmos and orbital congestion; pathologically, there is round cell infiltration of orbital tissues. In some cases the inflammatory signs are severe, with pain, periorbital swelling, and conjunctival injection that is most marked over the insertions of the rectus muscles.

Diagnosis

The orbital tissue most characteristically affected is muscle, especially that in the inferior, medial, and superior recti and the levator palpebrae muscles. The rectus muscle enlargement produces a characteristic appearance on computed tomography—fusiform enlargement sparing the tendinous insertions. There are other causes of enlarged ocular muscles (see Chaps. 8 and 12), but asymmetric bilateral extraocular muscle enlargement is most often encountered with Graves' orbitopathy. Volume analysis of computed tomographic sections also reveals an increase in the orbital fat compartment [6]. Because of these findings, the computed tomogram of the orbit, augmented with coronal sections or sagittal reformation, is the most sensitive diagnostic test for Graves' orbitopathy.

lid retraction and exophthalmos predisposes the eye to exposure keratitis. Scarring of the other muscles leads to ophthalmoplegia and diplopia. Because the limitation of eye movement is the result of muscle inelasticity, the ophthalmoplegia is mechanical. This is demonstrated by positive forced ductions or by elevation of intraocular pressure when an attempt is made to move the eye in the direction of the limitation of gaze.

In a few patients the tightness of the orbit and the enlargement of muscles combine to compress the optic nerve, reducing vision [4, 14]. Dysthyroid optic neuropathy is not caused by stretching of the optic nerve. In fact, the incidence of optic neuropathy is low in patients with large degrees of exophthalmos, which serves as a sort of physiologic decompression.

Treatment

Treatment of severe Graves' orbitopathy is extremely difficult. Fortunately, most patients can be managed conservatively, and the orbitopathy runs a self-limited course over one to three years. Exposure keratitis may be controlled with artificial tears and a tape tarsorrhaphy at night. Surgical tarsorrhaphies are sometimes utilized.

When exposure keratitis, inflammation, or optic neuropathy is severe, a trial of systemic corticosteroids is usually considered the first line of treatment. Most authorities do not believe that ophthalmoplegia alone is a sufficient indication for corticosteroid treatment, and there is no convincing evidence that early steroid treatment prevents progression of the ophthalmoplegia. When steroids fail or are contraindicated, orbital decompression or radiation therapy should be considered. The indications for radiation therapy vary considerably from center to center, as do its reported effectiveness and complications [1, 2]. If this modality is used, care must be taken that the method of delivery of the radiation avoids excessive dosage to the retina and optic nerve. Blindness from radiation retinopathy and optic neuropathy in patients with Graves' orbitopathy is now being encountered [12]. As alternative therapies, plasmapheresis and chemotherapy have their enthusiastic supporters. Both must be considered investigative therapies until better clinical studies are available [7, 17].

Orbital decompression is probably still the most widely used treatment in severe Graves' orbitopathy that cannot be controlled with corticosteroids. Various surgical approaches have their advocates, with some variant of the transantral (Ogura) procedure probably the preferred technique. Orbital decompression reduces exophthalmos thus relieving exposure keratitis and bringing about a cosmetic improvement in the patient, while decreasing pressure on the optic nerve. Decompression does not improve, and may exacerbate, motility problems.

Once Graves' orbitopathy has run its course, motility problems and lid retraction can be corrected surgically. During the several years from the onset of the orbitopathy until such intervention is possible, if none of the major complications appears, reassurance and emotional support are often the most important therapies provided by the physician. The alterations in facial appearance and the annoying diplopia of progressive Graves' orbitopathy are upsetting to even the most psychologically stable person.

1. Brenna, M.W., Leone, C.R. Jr., Janaki, L. Radiation therapy for Graves' disease. *Am. J. Ophthalmol.* 96:195–199, 1983.
   The successful results in this series of 14 patients treated with orbital irradiation could reflect favorable patient selection.
2. Char, D.H. *Thyroid Eye Disease.* Baltimore: Williams & Wilkins, 1985.
   The author of this comprehensive monograph advocates relatively aggressive treatment with short-term steroids and high-voltage radiotherapy.
3. Dresner, S.C., Kennerdell, J.S. Dysthroid orbitopathy. *Neurology* 35:1628–1634, 1985.
   This clinical review provides perspectives on diagnosis and management.
4. Feldon, S.E., Lee, C.P., Muramatsu, S., et al. Quantitative computed tomography of Graves' ophthalmopathy: Extraocular muscle and orbital fat in development of optic neuropathy. *Arch. Ophthalmol.* 103:213–215, 1985.
   These investigators find a correlation between high extraocular muscle volume measured by computed tomography and the development of optic neuropathy.
5. Fells, P. Orbital decompression for severe dysthyroid eye disease. *Br. J. Ophthalmol.* 71:107–111, 1987.
   Fells favors corticosteroids and transantral decompression over radiotherapy or plasmapheresis in the acute situation.
6. Forbes, G., Gorman, C.A., Brennan, M.D., et al. Ophthalmopathy of Graves' disease: Computerized volume measurements of the orbital fat and muscle. *A.J.N.R.* 7:651–656, 1986.
   Although there was considerable variation, ocular muscle volume was significantly higher in Graves' orbitopathy, and there was a tendency toward increase in the orbital fat compartment.
7. Glinoer, D., Etienne-Decerf, M., Schrooyen, M., et al. Beneficial effects of intensive plasma exchange followed by immunosuppressive therapy in severe Graves' orbitopathy. *Acta Endocrinol. (Copenh.)* 111:30–38, 1986.
   Plasmapheresis was followed by improvement in soft tissue involvement in eight of nine patients with severe Graves' orbitopathy.
8. Gorman, C.A. Temporal relationship between onset of Graves' ophthalmopathy and diagnosis of thyrotoxicosis. *Mayo Clin. Proc.* 58:515–519, 1983.
   Twenty-nine of 194 patients undergoing orbital decompressions were never hyperthyroid. In the rest, hyperthyroidism occurred in an almost normal distribution around the development of eye symptoms.
9. Gorman, C.A., Waller, R.R., Dyer, J.A. *The Eye and Orbit in Thyroid Disease.* New York: Raven Press, 1984.
   This monograph's 23 chapters offer an interdisciplinary perspective on thyroid eye disease.
10. Hufnagel, T.J., Hickey, W.F., Cobbs, W.H., et al. Immunohistochemical and ultrastructural studies on the exenterated orbital tissues of a patient with Graves' disease. *Ophthalmology* 91:1411–1419, 1984.
    An unexpected death from unrelated causes during treatment provided the opportunity for a pathologic study.
11. Hurwitz, J.J., Birt, D. An individualized approach to orbital decompression in Graves' orbitopathy. *Arch. Ophthalmol.* 103:660–665, 1985.
    These surgeons favor lateral decompression as having less effect on ocular motility, but use a transantral or external ethmoidectomy approach as a secondary procedure for severe optic neuropathy.
12. Kinyoun, J.L., Kalina, R.E., Brower, S.A., et al. Radiation retinopathy after orbital irradiation for Graves' ophthalmopathy. *Arch. Ophthalmol.* 102:1473–1476, 1984.
    Four patients lost vision after radiation therapy. The authors suggest that this complication may be avoided by attention to the details of delivery of the radiotherapy.
13. Leone, C.R. The management of ophthalmic Graves' disease. *Ophthalmology* 91:770–779, 1984.
    Dr. Leone's discussion emphasizes surgical techniques.
14. Panzo, G.J., Tomsak, R.L. A retrospective review of 26 cases of dysthyroid optic neuropathy. *Am. J. Ophthalmol.* 96:190–194, 1983.

A case series details management of dysthyroid optic neuropathy. In these patients, orbital decompression was most successful.

15. Perrild, H., Feldt-Rasmussen, U., Bech, K., et al. The differential diagnostic problems in unilateral Graves' orbitopathy. *Acta Endocrinol. (Copenh.)* 106:471–476, 1984.

Cases that exemplify the difficulty distinguishing, by endocrinologic criteria alone, other causes of exophthalmos from Graves' ophthalmopathy.

16. Riddick, F.A. Update on thyroid disease. *Ophthalmology* 88:467–470, 1981.

In an issue devoted to Graves' orbitopathy, this is the lead article.

17. Weetman, A.P., McGregor, A.M., Hall, R. Ocular manifestations of Graves' disease: A review. *J. R. Soc. Med.* 77:936–942, 1984.

This review emphasizes immunology. Subsequent letters to the editor (J. R. Soc. Med. 78:416–417, 1985) point up the controversies surrounding plasmapheresis and noncorticosteroid immunotherapy.

11. BLOW-OUT FRACTURE

When trauma to the eye and orbit does not fracture the orbital rim but produces a boney defect in the orbital wall, this is an *internal* or *blow-out fracture*. Blow-out fractures most often involve the orbital floor (the maxillary bone), followed by the medial wall (the ethmoid bone), and, rarely, the roof (the sphenoid bone). An associated iritis, pupillary deformation, eyelid laceration, retinal edema and hemorrhage, or ptosis may accompany the blow-out fracture. Hyphema and choroidal rupture also occur, but, because the fracture dissipates the energy of the blow, the globe seldom ruptures.

Medial wall blow-out fractures are a relatively frequent accompaniment of orbital floor fractures. A small number of cases are reported in which entrapment of orbital tissues in the medial wall of the orbit results in retraction of the globe on abduction, a type of acquired Duane's syndrome [5].

Pathogenesis

There are at least two mechanisms postulated for blow-out fractures. The conventional explanation is that blunt trauma by an object slightly larger than the anterior opening of the orbit, such as a fist or baseball, compresses the orbital contents. According to what has been termed the hydraulic theory [8], the forces generated fracture the thin orbital walls into the adjacent sinuses. An alternative mechanism favored by some clinical and experimental evidence is the buckling force theory. Forces transmitted from direct trauma to the orbital rim result in fracture of the adjacent orbital floor. Both explanations may be correct.

Diagnosis

The typical patient with a blow-out fracture of the orbital floor presents with limited elevation of the eye and anesthesia of the skin over the inferior orbital rim. This area is supplied by the infraorbital nerve, which runs in a canal in the floor of the orbit. Elevation is affected more than depression because the ophthalmoplegia is mechanical: the result of tissue entrapment in the fracture or hemorrhage and edema.

Entrapment is suggested by a positive *forced ductions* test. The eye is anesthetized topically, and fine forceps or a suction cup is used to grasp the globe. The patient is instructed to look in the direction of the limitation of movement, and an attempt is made to move the eye passively. With a mechanical, as opposed to a neurogenic, ophthalmoplegia, a resistance is felt by the examiner. Obviously, forced ductions are difficult to interpret in an uncooperative patient. Measurements of saccadic velocities, if available, are helpful in distinguishing those patients with entrapment that is likely to produce permanent diplopia from those with transient deficits [14].

In the presence of clinical signs of a blow-out fracture, radiologic evaluation confirms the presence and extent of the fracture. Clouding of the maxillary sinus is often evident on plain radiographs. Various types of tomography and even positive contrast orbitography, which were once used to demonstrate blow-out fractures, have largely been replaced by computed tomography, which has the unique advantage of simultaneously visualizing both the bony and soft tissues. Both axial and coronal scans may provide clinically useful information. Recent studies suggest that prediction of outcome is possible on the basis of the radiologic findings [4].

Treatment

The management of orbital blow-out fractures is still the subject of considerable controversy. Treatment is intended to decrease the incidence of persistent diplopia and to avoid the development of enophthalmos. The conventional surgical therapy consists of exploring the floor of the orbit, usually through the skin, sometimes combined with an approach via the maxillary sinus (the Caldwell-Luc procedure). Tissue entrapped in the fracture is freed, and larger defects are covered with a plate that is usually made of an alloplastic such as Teflon, Supramid, or silicone.

The indications for such surgery are debated. Some surgeons believe that any blowout fracture should be repaired because of the possibility of late development of enophthalmos, which may be difficult to remedy surgically [17]. This point of view is difficult to support since documentation of such occurrences in asymptomatic fractures is lacking. Also, the surgery itself has well-recognized and serious complications: blindness secondary to postoperative hemorrhage [10], infection, migration of the orbital implant [11], late dacryocystitis [12], and disturbance of the normal lid and lacrimal functions. Other surgeons reserve surgery for those patients with ocular motility disturbances; however, the ophthalmoplegia often spontaneously resolves within a week or two of injury or may continue to improve for months.

The approach that currently finds the most support is to postpone surgical repair for one to four weeks to see whether the ophthalmoplegia resolves. The presence of enophthalmos or of a large fracture where enophthalmos seems likely is also a surgical criterion [7]. Supporting an even more conservative approach are studies of the natural history of blow-out fractures that indicate that the incidence of permanent diplopia and significant enophthalmos may not be as high as that of operative complications [15]. When significant diplopia persists, strabismus surgery can give good functional results even years after the injury, and enophthalmos is not in most cases a major disability.

1. Beyer, C.K., Fabian, R.L., Smith, B. Naso-orbital fractures, complications, and treatment. *Ophthalmology* 89:456–463, 1982.
   An overview of the ophthalmologic aspects of midfacial fractures.
2. Converse, J.M., Smith, B. On the treatment of blowout fractures of the orbit. *Plast. Reconstr. Surg.* 62:100–104, 1978.
   Two surgeons with a long-term interest in the problem provide an editorial perspective.
3. Deutch, T.A., Feller, D.B. *Paton and Goldberg's Management of Ocular Injuries* (2nd ed.). Philadelphia: Saunders, Chap. 3, pp. 37–59.
   This useful monograph provides an approach to blow-out fractures, with a detailed discussion of surgical techniques.
4. Gilbard, S.M., Mafee, M.F., Lagouros, P.A., et al. Orbital blowout fractures: The prognostic significance of computed tomography. *Ophthalmology* 92:1523–1528, 1985.
   Gilbard and co-workers have developed radiologic criteria from computed tomograms that apparently predict the outcome of blow-out fractures.
5. Gittinger, J.W. Jr., Hughes, J.P., Suran, E.L. Medial orbital wall blow-out fracture producing an acquired retraction syndrome. *J. Clin. Neuro-ophthalmol.* 6:153–156, 1986.

Isolated medial wall blow-out fractures may be more common in young black males because of poorly developed ethmoid struts. Most will probably require surgery.

6. Greenwald, H.S., Jr., Keeney, A.H., Shannon, G.M. A review of 128 patients with orbital fractures. *Am. J. Ophthalmol.* 78:655–664, 1974.
   This large series allows an overview of the complications of an aggressive surgical approach.

7. Hawes, M.J., Dortzbach, R.K. Surgery on orbital floor fractures: Influence of time of repair and fracture size. *Ophthalmology* 90:1066–1070, 1983.
   In this series of 51 fractures, repair within two months gave better results, and not surprisingly, fractures involving more than half of the orbital floor were more likely to produce enophthalmos. A prospective study is promised.

8. Kersten, R.C. Blowout fracture of the orbital floor with entrapment caused by isolated trauma to the orbital rim. *Am. J. Ophthalmol.* 103:214–220, 1987.
   A fall that occurred when a postoperative cataract patient was leaving his ophthalmologist's office provides confirmation that isolated trauma to the orbital rim may produce a classic blow-out fracture.

9. Koornneef, L. Current concepts on the management of orbital blow-out fractures. *Ann. Plast. Surg.* 9:185–200, 1982.
   The development of the concept of blow-out fractures is presented, along with the author's anatomic research, which helps justify conservative management.

10. Lederman, I.R. Loss of vision associated with surgical treatment of zygomatic-orbital floor fracture. *Plast. Reconstr. Surg.* 68:94–99, 1981.
    A case report and tabular review of visual loss after surgery.

11. Mauriello, J.A. Jr., Flanagan, J.C., Peyster, R.G. An unusual late complication of orbital floor fracture repair. *Ophthalmology* 91:102–107, 1984.
    Three cases are reported in which, years after the repair of a blow-out fracture with an alloplastic implant, an orbital mass producing exophthalmos proved to be a fibrous cyst around the implant.

12. Mauriello, J.A. Jr., Fiore, P.M., Kotch, M. Dacryocystitis: Late complication of orbital floor fracture repair with implant. *Ophthalmology* 94:248–250, 1987.
    Mauriello and co-workers describe another late complication and suggest modifications in surgical technique to avoid this and other problems.

13. McCartney, D.L., Char, D.H. Return of vision following orbital decompression after 36 hours of postoperative blindness. *Am. J. Ophthalmol.* 100:602–604, 1985.
    Repair of a blow-out fracture seven days after injury for marginal indications ("some observers believed that ductions were limited") resulted in postoperative blindness. A two-wall orbital decompression 36 hours after the initial surgery restored visual acuity to 20/70 and restored a small island of field.

14. Metz, H.S., Scott, W.E., Madson, E., et al. Saccadic velocity and active force studies in blow-out fractures of the orbit. *Am. J. Ophthalmol.* 78:665–670, 1974.
    A group of patients are reported in whom saccadic velocity and quantitative forced ductions were used to predict outcome.

15. Putterman, A.M., Stevens, T., Urist, M.J. Nonsurgical management of blow-out fractures of the orbital floor. *Am. J. Ophthalmol.* 77:232–239, 1974.
    A retrospective and prospective study supports the proposition that the natural history of blow-out fractures is usually one of improvement.

16. Ruttum, M.S., Harris, G.J. Orbital blowout fracture with ipsilateral fourth nerve palsy. *Am. J. Ophthalmol.* 100:343–344, 1985.
    Even in the presence of an orbital floor fracture, not all hypertropias are caused by entrapment.

17. Sacks, A.C., Friedland, J.A. Orbital floor fractures—Should they be explored early? *Plast. Reconstr. Surg.* 64:190–193, 1979.
    The answer offered here is yes, a point of view almost diametrically opposed to that of Putterman and co-workers (ref. 16). In this series, all blow-out fractures required surgery, and no significant complications were encountered.

18. Wilkins, R.B., Havins, W.E. Current treatment of blow-out fractures. *Ophthalmology* 89:464–466, 1982.
    This position paper is based on a poll of the American Society of Ophthalmic Plastic and Reconstructive Surgery and the opinions of the authors.

12. CAVERNOUS SINUS ARTERIOVENOUS FISTULA

The carotid artery passes through the cavernous sinus, a venous structure. Rupture of the carotid or its branches in the cavernous sinus produces, instead of a subarachnoid hemorrhage, a *carotid-cavernous sinus arteriovenous (AV) fistula.* The signs and symptoms of traumatic carotid-cavernous sinus AV fistulae are well known: pulsatile exophthalmos with orbital swelling and arterialization of veins, a bruit, and ocular ischemia as the result of decreased perfusion pressure. These high-flow, high-pressure shunts are commonly encountered after severe head trauma and may be seen with penetrating orbital trauma or following transsphenoidal or carotid surgery.

Another type of AV communication has been recognized with increasing frequency, the *dural AV fistula* or *shunt* [11, 13]. These arise spontaneously or after only minor trauma, especially in middle-aged to elderly women, and often present as a red eye with dilated episcleral vessels. Because these are low-flow, low-pressure shunts, the presence of exophthalmos, bruit, ophthalmoplegia, and orbital pain is variable, leading to diagnostic confusion with conjunctivitis, inflammatory pseudotumor of the orbit, and Graves' orbitopathy.

Pathogenesis
Some authorities distinguish between direct AV communications (fistulas) and indirect AV communications (shunts). The validity of this distinction depends on the mechanism producing the communication. Dural AV shunts or spontaneous carotid-cavernous fistulas derive their arterial contribution from the meningeal branches of the internal (especially the meningohypophyseal and inferolateral trunks) and external (especially the internal maxillary and middle meningeal arteries) carotids. One theory of pathogenesis postulates that the fistulas are caused by the rupture of thin-walled vessels present as a result of vascular disease. This idea draws its strongest support from the increased incidence of dural AV fistulas in connective tissue disorders associated with vascular fragility, e.g., some variants of the Ehlers-Danlos syndrome, pseudoxanthoma elasticum, and fibromuscular dysplasia [2].

An alternative explanation is that the dural AV shunts are normal vessels that become shunts because of abnormal venous drainage [4]. According to this theory, changes in blood coagulation occurring during menopause predispose women to intracranial venous thrombosis, and the shunt opens as an alternative pathway for venous drainage.

Diagnosis
The diagnosis of dural AV shunts depends on an awareness of the clinical syndrome. The characteristic corkscrew appearance of episcleral veins in a patient with a bruit or sixth nerve palsy is virtually pathognomonic. Intraocular pressure is often elevated, and retinal venous congestion with hemorrhages and disk swelling may be present. Unusual presentations include spontaneous choroidal detachments, central serous choroidopathy, and trigeminal sensory neuropathy [6, 15]. Asymptomatic, posteriorly located fistulae are discovered incidentally on angiograms performed for another purpose.

When a dural AV fistula is suspected, the diagnosis may be supported by computed tomography, orbital ultrasound, or intravenous digital subtraction angiography. Computed tomography and orbital ultrasound demonstrate enlargement of the ocular muscles and superior ophthalmic vein. Extraocular muscle enlargement is also a feature of Graves' orbitopathy, inflammatory pseudotumor of the orbit, metastatic or infiltrative neoplasia, and, less commonly, of acromegaly, trauma, and parasitic infections. A dilated superior ophthalmic vein is also seen with other vascular anomalies and causes of orbital venous congestion, but is characteristic of carotid-cavernous fistulas. Digital subtraction angiography confirms the presence of a fistula, but does not enable the vessels involved to be identified [10]. The definitive diagnostic test for fistulas in the region of the cavernous sinus is selective carotid angiography.

Sudden worsening of the symptoms of dural-cavernous AV fistulas may be an effect of thrombosis of the superior ophthalmic vein, which may be demonstrated as an absence of the normal flow void on T1-weighted, surface-coil magnetic resonance orbital images

[16]. Such thrombosis, however, is often the harbinger of spontaneous improvement, and intervention is not indicated.

Treatment

High-flow carotid-cavernous fistulas represent an imminent threat to vision. Ophthalmoplegia and proptosis predispose the eye to exposure; the eye is ischemic, with the attendant risk of anterior segment infarction, neovascular glaucoma, and proliferative retinopathy. High-flow carotid-cavernous fistulas must be closed by one of various surgical techniques [1].

The indications for intervention in dural AV fistulas are less clear. Although vision may be threatened by glaucoma and ocular hypoxia, many patients do well without treatment, and these low-flow shunts often close spontaneously. Angiography is not necessarily indicated in mild cases, but when vision is threatened, selective carotid angiography has both diagnostic and therapeutic value, as the fistula may close as an effect of the angiogram.

Balloon embolization techniques used for high-flow fistulas have not been as successful with low-flow fistulas, but some centers have obtained good results from carotid embolization with suspensions of polyvinyl alcohol or similar particles, even if the arterial feeders to the fistula can be only partially occluded [3, 17]. Japanese physicians report success with copper needle thrombosis after frontotemporal craniotomy and with irradiation [12], but the risk–benefit ratio of such approaches is uncertain. The neovascular glaucoma of ocular ischemia may respond to panretinal photocoagulation (see Chap. 21) [5].

1. Débrun, G., Lacour, P., Vinuela, F., et al. Treatment of 54 traumatic carotid-cavernous fistulas. *J. Neurosurg.* 55:678–692, 1981.
   Débrun and co-workers review available techniques for treatment and discuss their results using balloon embolization.
2. Farley, M.K., Clark, R.D., Fallor, M.K., et al. Spontaneous carotid-cavernous fistula and the Ehlers-Danlos syndromes. *Ophthalmology* 90:1337–1342, 1983.
   Carotid-cavernous fistulae may be a manifestation of connective tissue disorders.
3. Grossman, R.I., Sergott, R.C., Goldberg, H.I., et al. Dural malformations with ophthalmic manifestations: Results of particulate embolization in seven patients. *A.J.N.R.* 6:809–813, 1985.
   Seven patients with symptoms of at least 3 months' duration were treated with polyvinyl alcohol embolization.
4. Grove, A.S. The dural shunt syndrome: Pathophysiology and clinical course. *Ophthalmology* 90:31–44, 1983.
   Grove offers the hypothesis that intracranial venous thrombosis underlies dural AV shunts.
5. Harris, M.J., Fine, S.L., Miller, N.R. Photocoagulation treatment of proliferative retinopathy secondary to a carotid-cavernous fistula. *Am. J. Ophthalmol.* 90:515–518, 1980.
   Disk neovascularization and rubeosis iridis from a spontaneous fistula successfully treated by photocoagulation.
6. Klein, R., Meyers, S.M., Smith, J.L., et al. Abnormal choroidal circulation: Association with arteriovenous fistula in the cavernous sinus area. *Arch. Ophthalmol.* 96:1370–1373, 1978.
   Central serous and choroidal detachments are rare manifestations of dural AV fistulae.
7. Kupersmith, M.J., Berenstein, A., Flamm, E., et al. Neuroophthalmologic abnormalities and intravascular therapy of traumatic carotid cavernous fistulas. *Ophthalmology* 93:906–912, 1986.
   Thirty of 33 cases of traumatic carotid-cavernous fistulae were caused by motor vehicle accidents. Excellent results were obtained by embolization techniques, although one patient required emergency removal of a balloon because of hemispheric neurologic dysfunction.

8. Leonard, T.K., Moseley, I.F., Sanders, M.D. Ophthalmoplegia in carotid cavernous sinus fistula. *Br. J. Ophthalmol.* 68:128–134, 1984.
   The authors conclude that both congestion of the orbit and sixth nerve palsies contribute to ophthalmoplegia with carotid-cavernous fistulas.
9. Merlis, A.L., Schaiberger, C.L., Adler, R. External carotid-cavernous fistula simulating unilateral Graves' ophthalmopathy. *J. Comput. Assist. Tomogr.* 6:1006–1009, 1982.
   An example of a difficult clinical presentation.
10. Modic, M.T., Berlin, A.J., Weinstein, M.A. The use of digital subtraction angiography in the evaluation of carotid cavernous sinus fistulas. *Ophthalmology* 89:441–444, 1982.
    While the presence of a fistula may be confirmed by intravenous digital subtraction angiography, selected conventional arterial angiography may be preferable both because the involved vessels are better defined and because of the possible therapeutic effect.
11. Newton, T.H., Hoyt, W.F. Dural arteriovenous shunts in the region of the cavernous sinus. *Neuroradiology* 1:71–81, 1970.
    This clinical series best defined the syndrome.
12. Nukui, H., Shibasaki, T., Kaneko, M., et al. Long-term observations in cases with spontaneous carotid-cavernous fistulas. *Surg. Neurol.* 21:543–552, 1984.
    A series from Japan.
13. Phelps, C.S., Thompson, H.S., Ossonig, K.C. The diagnosis and prognosis of atypical carotid-cavernous fistula (red-eye shunt syndrome). *Am. J. Ophthalmol.* 93:423–436, 1982.
    Clinical and ultrasonographic findings are emphasized.
14. Pollock, S., Miller, N.R. Central retinal vein occlusion complicating spontaneous carotid-cavernous fistula. *Arch. Ophthalmol.* 104:331, 1986.
    Despite spontaneous resolution of her fistula, this patient suffered permanent visual loss from a central retinal vein occlusion. (See also Brunette and Boghen's letter, Arch. Ophthalmol. 105:464–465, 1987.)
15. Rizzo, M., Bosch, E.P., Gross, C.E. Trigeminal sensory neuropathy due to dural external carotid cavernous sinus fistula. *Neurology* 32:89–91, 1982.
    Rizzo and colleagues encountered an unusual clinical presentation.
16. Sergott, R.C., Grossman, R.I., Savino, P.J., et al. The syndrome of paradoxical worsening of dural-cavernous arteriovenous malformations. *Ophthalmology* 94:205–212, 1987.
    In three cases, the sudden worsening apparently caused by superior ophthalmic vein thrombosis was followed by spontaneous improvement.
17. Viñuela, F., Fox, A.J., Débrun, G.M., et al. Spontaneous carotid-cavernous fistulas: Clinical, radiological, and therapeutic considerations; Experience with 20 cases. *J. Neurosurg.* 60:976–984, 1984.
    This series contains more severe cases of spontaneous fistulas, including two that resulted from rupture of giant intracavernous aneurysms.

13. ORBITAL VASCULAR MALFORMATIONS

Orbital vascular malformations may be arterial, venous, or arteriovenous (AV). Arterial malformations, consisting of aneurysms and anomalous vessels, are rarely clinically significant in the orbit and will not be considered further. Venous malformations characteristically produce an exophthalmos that appears or increases with elevated venous pressure, a type of dynamic proptosis. Coughing, crying, or bending forward results in fullness of the orbital tissues and protrusion of the eye. Experts are divided over whether this clinical picture is more common with *orbital varices* or *orbital lymphangiomas*.

In children, lymphangiomas present most often as proptosis, which may be stationary but is usually slowly progressive. Occasionally, hemorrhage into the tumor spontaneously or as a result of trauma leads to rapid progression. Associated vascular lesions occur elsewhere, especially in the roof of the mouth. Diagnosis is made by biopsy, which is warranted in the presence of an expanding orbital lesion.

Pathologically, lymphangiomas are benign tumors consisting of endothelium-lined channels that resemble blood vessels but are filled with proteinaceous material rather than blood. As with orbital capillary hemangiomas (see Chap. 9), the orbits may be enlarged on radiographs, a finding that helps to distinguish them from tumors with rapid onset such as rhabdomyosarcomas. Surgical excision, although difficult, is considered the treatment of choice in most cases.

Orbital varices present in much the same way, and the two entities overlap clinically. Venous varices slowly increase in size until bodily growth ceases during the late teens. Characteristic radiologic findings in venous varices are small, round calcifications known as *phleboliths*. Ultrasonography may reveal a dilated superior ophthalmic vein, and the demonstration of large venous spaces on orbital venography is diagnostic. Vision is seldom affected, and surgery is undertaken only if cosmetic considerations dictate intervention.

Orbital varices may be associated with varicosities elsewhere in the body, especially the scalp and frontal bone on the affected side. The occurrence of varicosities in the legs, cutaneous vascular nevi, and hypertrophy of involved tissues is the *Klippel-Trénaunay-Weber syndrome*.

Primary venous varices must be distinguished from venous dilation secondary to AV malformations. Cranial AV malformations can affect the eyes in several ways. Probably the most common ophthalmic manifestation of an AV malformation is the visual field defect that results from involvement of intracranial visual pathways. AV malformations located in or near the orbits cause proptosis that may be pulsatile and dilated conjunctival, episcleral, and retinal vessels.

Retinal AV malformations of various types may occur in isolation or with associated facial and intracranial malformations. This association between retinal and orbital AV malformations and intracranial AV malformations is known as the *Wyburn-Mason syndrome*. This syndrome should be distinguished from two other disorders also classified as phakomatoses (the Sturge-Weber and the von Hippel-Lindau syndromes), in which the vascular lesion is not an AV malformation. Some AV malformations appear to induce capillary proliferation, pathologically resembling capillary hemangiomas of infancy (see Chap. 14).

Management of AV malformations depends on their symptomatology and vascular supply. They may be difficult to approach surgically, and spontaneous thrombosis has been reported. Enlargement during pregnancy is also observed. Embolization alone or embolization plus surgery is now attempted in some centers. The embolized material sometimes excites a secondary foreign body reaction that is difficult to distinguish clinically from tumor recurrence.

1. Archer, D.B., Deutman, A., Ernest, J.T., et al. Arteriovenous communications of the retina. *Am. J. Ophthalmol.* 75:224–242, 1973.
   This paper classifies and illustrates the various types of retinal AV malformations.
2. Bullock, J.D., Bartley, G.B. Dynamic proptosis. *Am. J. Ophthalmol.* 102:104–110, 1986.
   A good discussion of the differential diagnosis in 26 patients with exophthalmos that varied spontaneously or could be induced. Two instances of orbital varices are included.
3. Flanagan, J.C. Vascular problems of the orbit. *Ophthalmology* 86:896–913, 1979.
   Flanagan reviews capillary hemangiomas, cavernous hemangiomas, and vascular malformations.
4. Forman, A.R., Luessenhop, A.J., Limaye, S.R. Ocular findings in patients with arteriovenous malformations of the head and neck. *Am. J. Ophthalmol.* 79:626–633, 1975.

A series of patients with various manifestations from one institution.

5. Hopen, G., Smith, J.L., Hoff, J.T., et al. The Wyburn-Mason syndrome: Concomitant chiasmal and fundus vascular malformations. *J. Clin. Neuro-ophthalmol.* 3:53–62, 1983.
   A case report with review of the syndrome.
6. Howard, G.M., Jakobiec, F.A., Michelsen, W.J. Orbital arteriovenous malformation with secondary capillary angiomatosis treated with silastic liquid. *Ophthalmology* 90:1136–1139, 1983.
   An AV malformation with secondary capillary angiomatosis was managed with embolization and surgery.
7. Iliff, W.J., Green, W.R. Orbital lymphangiomas. *Ophthalmology* 86:914–929, 1979.
   Iliff and Green draw upon their large experience to distinguish lymphangiomas from orbital varices.
8. Michelsen, W.J., Hilal, S.K., Stern, J. The management of arteriovenous malformations of the orbit. In F.A. Jakobiec (ed.), *Ocular and Adnexal Tumors.* Birmingham: Aesculapius Publishing Co., 1978. Pp. 782–786.
   Three cases are used to illustrate the diagnostic and therapeutic possibilities.
9. Moster, M.R., Kennerdell, J.S. B-scan ultrasonic evaluation of a dilated superior ophthalmic vein in orbital and retro-orbital arteriovenous anomalies. *J. Clin. Neuro-ophthalmol.* 3:105–108, 1983.
   Ultrasound proves useful in diagnosis.
10. Murali, R., Berenstein, A., Hirschfeld, A. Intraorbital arteriovenous malformation with spontaneous thrombosis. *Ann. Ophthalmol.* 13:457–459, 1981.
    An angiographically documented case where episodes of sudden worsening appeared to represent spontaneous thrombosis of an orbital AV malformation.
11. Rathbun, J.E., Hoyt, W.F., Beard, C. Surgical management of orbitofrontal varix in Klippel-Trénaunay-Weber syndrome. *Am. J. Ophthalmol.* 70:109–112, 1971.
    A case with orbital and systemic findings is successfully managed surgically.
12. Rootman, J., Hay, E., Graeb, D., et al. Orbital-adnexal lymphangiomas: A spectrum of hemodynamically isolated vascular hamartomas. *Ophthalmology* 93:1558–1570, 1986.
    The authors of this well-illustrated report distinguish three clinical types of lymphangiomas among their 13 patients: superficial, deep, and combined. Five of 10 patients with deep lymphangiomas presented with sudden proptosis from spontaneous retrobulbar hemorrhage, and 3 required orbitotomies for relief of optic nerve decompression.
13. Théron, J., Newton, T.H., and Hoyt, W.F. Unilateral retinocephalic vascular malformations. *Neuroradiology* 7:185–196, 1974.
    An excellent clinical and radiologic review.

14. ORBITAL CAPILLARY HEMANGIOMA

Vascular tumors are the most common orbital neoplasms, and the *capillary hemangioma* is the commonest orbital and adnexal tumor of childhood. Capillary hemangiomas present at birth or in early childhood as a mass or discolored area of skin. In most series there is a predominance of girls and low-birth-weight infants. Capillary hemangiomas are clinically distinct from *port-wine stain hemangiomas,* which are flat and often follow the distribution of the fifth cranial nerve (the *nevus flammeus* of the Sturge-Weber syndrome), and from *cavernous hemangiomas,* which most authorities agree are tumors of adulthood, presenting as slowly progressive proptosis with a discrete intraorbital mass.

Diagnosis
Anterior orbital and adnexal capillary hemangiomas are soft, compressible masses that enlarge when the child cries. When the overlying skin is discolored, they are called

strawberry nevi. Many are located in the superior medial quadrant of the orbit. Occasionally, similar hemangiomas are found elsewhere on the body. In one reported case extensive facial hemangiomas were accompanied by subglottic hemangiomas that led to respiratory distress and death [13]. A potential complication of extensive capillary hemangiomas is depletion of circulating platelets, the *Kasabach-Merritt syndrome.* This is rarely encountered with pure orbital and adnexal involvement.

Deep orbital capillary hemangiomas must be differentiated from other orbital tumors, especially rhabdomyosarcoma. In doubtful cases, arteriography demonstrates diagnostic features since capillary hemangiomas, as opposed to cavernous hemangiomas, have arterial feeders [1].

The natural history of capillary hemangiomas is a period of growth, usually lasting about six months, followed by quiescence, and then spontaneous involution. An estimated 75 percent have resolved by the time the patient is 7 years old. Unfortunately, despite this apparently benign course, the prognosis for vision in the adjacent eye is not good. As the tumor enlarges, the lid may become ptotic, leading to an occlusion amblyopia and to myopia. The deformation of the globe results in an astigmatism with the plus axis along the meridian of greatest compression, mimicking the effects of a tight corneoscleral suture after cataract extraction. This astigmatism tends to persist even when the tumor involutes. Myopia and high astigmatism produce anisometropic amblyopia. Both mechanical and sensory factors may contribute to the high incidence of strabismus in these children [7].

Less common complications of untreated capillary hemangiomas are ulceration and infection of the lid margin and severe exophthalmos with exposure keratitis. Cosmetic deformities may persist when the skin is extensively involved.

Treatment

The high incidence of visual loss gives an impetus to intervention despite the expectation that the tumor will eventually involute. Unfortunately, none of the current modalities is completely satisfactory. Biopsy appears to be a relatively safe procedure, and surgical removal is possible in some cases. Treatment with radon implants or high-dose irradiation has been abandoned in major centers because of the high incidence of radiation-associated side effects, but low-dose radiation with protection of the eye may still have a place. Other treatments include injection of sclerosing agents and local application of cryotherapy.

The therapy currently exciting the most interest is treatment with local or systemic corticosteroids. Systemic steroids seem to be most effective if they are begun early in the growth phase of the tumor. Older children or those with more discrete hemangiomas appear to respond less well. Alternate-day therapy may decrease the incidence of steroid-induced side effects, and the patient must be observed after a course of steroids for rebound growth.

Intralesional injections avoid the complications of systemic steroids, but are contraindicated in deep orbital tumors because of the risk of hemorrhage. A combination of a long-acting (triamcinolone) and a short-acting (betamethasone or dexamethasone) steroid is injected with a fine needle [3, 4]. This approach requires a brief period of general anesthesia, with its attendant risks. Involution of the hemangioma usually begins after several days, is obvious after a week, and reaches its maximum after two to three months, when the injection may be repeated. Steroid injections make tissues friable, with breakdown of the lid [12]. Periocular injection also carries a small risk of central retinal artery occlusion [9].

1. Dilenge, D. Arteriography in angiomas of the orbit. *Radiology* 113:355–361, 1974. *Arteriography is useful in the differential diagnosis and demonstrates that the angioma is more extensive than appreciated clinically.*
2. Haik, B.G., Jakobiec, F.A., Ellsworth, R.M., et al. Capillary hemangioma of the lids and orbit: An analysis of the clinical features and therapeutic results in 101 cases. *Ophthalmology* 86:760–792, 1979.

The authors of this, the largest series in the literature ("a landmark paper") detail the diagnosis, management, and complications of capillary hemangiomas.

3. Kushner, B.J. Intralesional corticosteroid injection for infantile adnexal hemangioma. *Am. J. Ophthalmol.* 93:496–506, 1982.

   Nine of 10 patients in this series responded to treatment. No direct complications occurred, but three of nine responders still developed amblyopia, and two developed strabismus.

4. Kushner, B.J. The treatment of periorbital infantile hemangioma with intralesional corticosteroid. *Plast. Reconstr. Surg.* 76:517–524, 1985.

   From an experience expanded to 25 patients, Kushner suggests alterations in technique and notes that 4 patients did not respond. An accompanying discussion by Edgerton points out complications (localized areas of necrosis and scarring) and argues that systemic steroids are equally effective and less risky.

5. Nelson, L.B., Melick, J.E., Harley, R.D. Intralesional corticosteroid injections for infantile hemangiomas of the eyelid. *Pediatrics* 74:241–245, 1984.

   These case reports confirm Kushner's observations.

6. Plesner-Rasmussen, H.-J., Marushak, D., Goldschmidt, E. Capillary haemangiomas of the eyelids and orbit: A review of 5 children. *Acta Ophthalmolog.* 61:645–654, 1983.

   A group of children in whom various modalities of treatment were used, with photographs before and after treatment.

7. Robb, R.M. Refractive errors associated with hemangiomas of the eyelids and orbit in infancy. *Am. J. Ophthalmol.* 83:52–58, 1977.

   Robb emphasizes the mechanisms of anisometropia and amblyopia.

8. Sasaki, G.H., Pang, C.Y., Wittliff, J.L. Pathogenesis and treatment of infant skin strawberry hemangiomas: Clinical and in vitro studies of hormonal effects. *Plast. Reconstr. Surg.* 73:359–370, 1984.

   This clinical and experimental study of systemic steroid treatment on various types of hemangiomas presents evidence that capillary hemangioma patients have abnormalities of estrogen metabolism.

9. Shorr, N., Seiff, S.R. Central retinal artery occlusion associated with periocular corticosteroid injection for juvenile hemangioma. *Ophthal. Surg.* 17:229–231, 1986.

   Despite ophthalmoscopic signs of a central retinal artery occlusion and a persistent relative afferent pupillary defect, this child retained good central vision.

10. Sklar, E.L., Quencer, R.M., Byrne, S.F., et al. Correlative study of the computed tomographic, ultrasonographic, and pathological characteristics of cavernous versus capillary hemangiomas of the orbit. *J. Clin. Neuro-ophthalmol.* 6:14–21, 1986.

    Capillary and cavernous hemangiomas may be differentiated by their enhancement characteristics.

11. Stigmar, G., Crawford, J.S., Ward, C.M., et al. Ophthalmic sequelae of infantile hemangiomas of the eyelids and orbit. *Am. J. Ophthalmol.* 85:806–813, 1978.

    Another series documenting the ophthalmic complications.

12. Sutula, F.C., Glover, A.T. Eyelid necrosis following intralesional corticosteroid injection for capillary hemangioma. *Ophthalmic Surg.* 18:103–105, 1987.

    Another complication of this therapy.

13. Yee, R.D., Hepler, R.S. Congenital hemangiomas of the skin with orbital and subglottic hemangiomas. *Am. J. Ophthalmol.* 75:876–879, 1973.

    This unusual case had a fatal outcome.

III. CORNEA AND SCLERA

John W. Gittinger, Jr.

15. KERATOCONUS

Keratoconus is a noninflammatory thinning and ectasia of the cornea that is usually bilateral and involves the inferior cornea. Most keratoconus has its onset in young adulthood and ceases progressing by the age of 40 years. In advanced cases the involved area takes the shape of a truncated cone, sometimes with scarring at the apex. The distortion of the normal corneal architecture produces an irregular astigmatism and reduces vision.

Keratoglobus refers to a related condition with ectasia of the entire cornea and increased corneal diameter. Keratoglobus, which is much less common than keratoconus, is most often congenital and seldom progresses. Since cases of both keratoglobus and keratoconus are found in some families, the conditions are thought to be different manifestations of the same basic pathophysiology. Another related disorder is *pellucid marginal degeneration,* in which the thinning and ectasia are confined to the inferior peripheral cornea. This is more common in orientals and may coexist with keratoconus in the same eye [8].

Posterior keratoconus is a congenital concavity in the deep corneal tissues that probably has no relation to true keratoconus; instead, it belongs in the spectrum of central corneal mesenchymal dysgeneses (Peters' anomaly and related disorders) [20], although a similar picture may be acquired following trauma [21].

Pathogenesis

The cause of keratoconus is uncertain. Some cases are hereditary, but the chance of a second family member being involved is estimated at less than 1 in 10 [10]. An abnormality of the corneal collagen is suspected, but no specific biochemical defect has been identified. Keratoconus occasionally develops in persons with the Ehlers-Danlos syndrome or osteogenesis imperfecta, suggesting that isolated cases represent a forme fruste of some connective tissue disorder. An association with mitral valve prolapse, which is considered a noninflammatory degeneration of the valve leaflets, has been suggested [1]. Epidemiologic studies in Olmsted County, Minnesota, demonstrated that persons with keratoconus have a normal survival rate relative to the general population, so if keratoconus is just one manifestation of a systemic disorder, this disorder does not affect life expectancy [9].

Keratoconus has also been associated with atopy and with vernal conjunctivitis [21]. In addition, children with disorders causing severe visual loss such as Leber's congenital amaurosis and the congenital rubella syndrome are prone to develop keratoconus. There is an increased incidence of keratoconus in Down's syndrome. Persons with chronic ocular allergies and visually impaired children, especially those who are also mentally retarded, tend to rub their eyes vigorously, and such manipulation has been suggested to cause their keratoconus. Supporting this hypothesis is a report of unilateral keratoconus in a man who repeatedly massaged one eye to control a cardiac arrhythmia [4].

Hard contact lenses wear has also been linked to keratoconus, where it is presumably the result of corneal warping and chronic hypoxia. Since many eyes with incipient keratoconus would be fitted with contact lenses, this association is difficult to prove, and its significance is uncertain [14].

Diagnosis

The initial manifestation of keratoconus is usually blurring or distortion of vision, with increasing irregular myopic astigmatism. The diagnosis is made by observing an abnormal retinoscopic reflex—with scissoring or an "oil droplet" visible in the inferior cornea—followed by keratoscopy and keratometry. The reflection of Placido's disk or an illuminated keratoscope on the cornea should be foreshortened inferiorly, although this is difficult for the inexperienced observer to see in early cases. The mires on the keratometer are often irregular, with steepening of the inferior corneal curvature. Increasing corneal curvature over time is considered by some authorities to be the most sensitive indicator of keratoconus [10].

When the cone is large, angulation of the lower lid on down gaze is apparent (Munson's sign). Many cones are partially surrounded by epithelial deposits of iron (Fleischer's ring). Corneal striae that disappear with pressure on the globe are visible on slit lamp examination.

Occasionally, especially in mentally retarded patients with poor vision, keratoconus is not recognized until there is an episode of acute corneal thickening and opacification caused by the rupture of Bowman's membrane *(corneal hydrops)*. Despite its dramatic appearance, corneal hydrops is not an ocular emergency. Most corneas with hydrops will clear spontaneously with time, although a few cases become chronic. Hydrops is relatively common in keratoconus associated with Down's syndrome and perhaps congenital rubella, but it is rare otherwise.

Treatment

Mild or moderate keratoconus is managed refractively; glasses or contact lenses are used as required to improve vision. Fitting of contact lenses in eyes with keratoconus is challenging [3, 17, 19]. Advanced keratoconus is an important indication for penetrating keratoplasty, with excellent long-term results [15, 18], although in one population keratoplasty was required in only about 20 percent of cases within 20 years of diagnosis [9]. A relatively new surgical procedure, epikeratophakia, is favored by some surgeons because of the less serious complications associated with this extraocular procedure [12]. Thermal keratoplasty has also been attempted, especially when more extensive surgery is contraindicated, but it seems to be declining in favor as newer techniques emerge.

1. Beardsley, T.L., Foulks, G.N. An association of keratoconus and mitral valve prolapse. *Ophthalmology* 89:35–37, 1982.
   Twelve of 32 patients with keratoconus had mitral valve prolapse by ultrasonography.
2. Boger, W.P. III, Petersen, R.A., Robb, R.M. Keratoconus and acute hydrops in mentally retarded patients with congenital rubella syndrome. *Am. J. Ophthalmol.* 91:231–233, 1981.
   Four patients with keratoconus and corneal hydrops all had a history of rubbing or poking their eyes.
3. Cohen, E.J., Parlato, C.J. Fitting polycon lenses in keratoconus. *Int. Ophthalmol. Clin.* 26(1):111–117, 1986.
   A series of 123 eyes were fitted with this type of gas-permeable, rigid lens.
4. Coyle, J.T. Keratoconus and eye rubbing. *Am. J. Ophthalmol.* 97:527–528, 1984.
   Unilateral keratoconus developed in a man who used ocular massage to abort attacks of tachycardia.
5. Flanders, M., Lapointe, M.L., Brownstein, S., et al. Keratoconus and Leber's congenital amaurosis: A clinicopathological correlation. *Can. J. Ophthalmol.* 19:310–314, 1984.
   Clinical and pathologic material from a 42-year-old man with Leber's congenital amaurosis and mental retardation.
6. Goodman, G.L., Peiffer, R.L. Jr., Werblin, T.P. Failed epikeratoplasty for keratoconus. *Cornea* 5:29–34, 1986.
   The clinical and pathologic description of a failed graft.
7. Ihalainen, A. Clinical and epidemiological features of keratoconus: Genetic and external factors in the pathogenesis of the disease. *Acta Ophthalmol.* 64 (Suppl. 178):1–64, 1986.
   This monograph concerns a Scandinavian population in whom keratoconus was more common in males than females, and in whom some cases appeared to have an autosomal dominant pattern of inheritance. Rapid progression during pregnancy was also observed.
8. Kayazawa, F., Nishimura, K., Kodama, Y., et al. Keratoconus with pellucid marginal corneal degeneration. *Arch. Ophthalmol.* 102:895–896, 1984.

Seventeen of 20 Japanese patients with pellucid marginal degeneration also had keratoconus. Why these should not be considered simply cases of keratoconus is not clear.

9. Kennedy, R.H., Bourne, W.M., Kyer, J.A. A 48-year clinical and epidemiologic study of keratoconus. *Am. J. Ophthalmol.* 101:267–273, 1986.
   The Mayo Clinic computers contain 64 cases of keratoconus in residents of Olmsted County up to 1982, an incidence of 2.0 per 100,000 per year and a prevalence of 54.5 per 100,000 population.

10. Krachmer, J.H., Feder, R.S., Belin, M.W. Keratoconus and related noninflammatory corneal thinning disorders. *Surv. Ophthalmol.* 28:293–322, 1984.
    An extensive review with 261 references.

11. Leibowitz, H.M. Keratoconus. In H.M. Leibowitz (ed.), *Corneal Disorders: Clinical Diagnosis and Management.* Philadelphia: Saunders, 1984. Pp. 100–120.
    This chapter provides excellent illustrations and a particularly good discussion of diagnosis.

12. McDonald, M.B., Kaufman, H.E., Durrie, D.S., et al. Epikeratophakia for keratoconus: The nationwide study. *Arch. Ophthalmol.* 104:1294–1300, 1986.
    The results of the first 177 epikeratophakia operations for keratoconus are encouraging.

13. Millodot, M., Owens, H. Sensitivity and fragility in keratoconus. *Acta Ophthalmol.* 61:908–917, 1983.
    The corneal sensitivity to touch was diminished, and the epithelial fragility was increased, in keratoconus.

14. Nauheim, J.S., Perry, H.D. A clinicopathologic study of contact-lens-related keratoconus. *Am. J. Ophthalmol.* 100:543–546, 1985.
    Keratoconus developed in a woman wearing contact lenses, eventually leading to keratoplasty. The word "related," rather than "caused," was used on purpose, as discussed in subsequent correspondence (Am. J. Ophthalmol. 101:390, 1986).

15. Paglen, P.G., Fine, M., Abbott, R.L., et al. The prognosis for keratoplasty in keratoconus. *Ophthalmology* 89:651–654, 1982.
    Ninety percent of 326 grafts for keratoconus performed by Fine and followed for a minimum of five years were clear, and another 3 percent were nebulous but retained 20/40 or better vision.

16. Pouliquen, Y. Doyne Lecture: Keratoconus. *Eye* 1:1–14, 1987.
    The first paper in the renamed Transactions of the Ophthalmological Societies of the United Kingdom is an overview of keratoconus with excellent color illustrations.

17. Raber, I.M. Fitting cellulose acetate butyrate lenses in keratoconus. *Int. Ophthalmol. Clin.* 26(1):91–99, 1986.
    Raber discusses fitting with another type of gas-permeable, rigid lens.

18. Renardel de Lavalette, J.G.C., Renardel de Lavalette, A., van Rij, G., et al. Long-term results of corneal transplantations in keratoconus patients. *Doc. Ophthalmol.* 59:93–97, 1985.
    The results of 86 corneal transplantations, including 19 lamellar keratoplasties, for keratoconus are reported.

19. Rosenthal, P. The Boston lens and the management of keratoconus. *Int. Ophthalmol. Clin.* 26(1):101–109, 1986.
    Rosenthal describes fitting with still another gas-permeable polymer, hard lens.

20. Streeten, B.W., Spitzker, K.H., Karpik, A.G. Posterior keratoconus associated with systemic abnormalities. *Arch. Ophthalmol.* 101:616–622, 1983.
    The clinical and pathologic findings of posterior keratoconus are described. The indications for keratoplasty in this case prompted a subsequent exchange of letters (Arch. Ophthalmol. 102:195, 1268–1270, 1984).

21. Tabbara, K.F., Butrus, S.I. Vernal conjunctivitis and keratoconus. *Am. J. Ophthalmol.* 95:704–705, 1983.
    These authors thought this was a new association, but it had been previously recognized (see Am. J. Ophthalmol. 96:555–556, 1983).

22. Williams, R. Acquired posterior keratoconus. *Br. J. Ophthalmol.* 71:16–17, 1987.
    Corneal changes resembling posterior keratoconus developed after penetrating trauma.

16. HERPES SIMPLEX KERATITIS

Infections by the herpes simplex virus, *Herpesvirus hominis,* are divided into primary and recurrent disease. Most people have had primary infections, and most primary infections go unrecognized, perhaps consisting of only a few skin vesicles on the face of a child between the ages of 6 months and 5 years. Many cases of follicular conjunctivitis are herpetic; these occasionally progress to epithelial keratitis and stromal disease more characteristic of recurrent infections. In neonates and others with incompetent immune systems, primary infections are life-threatening.

Pathogenesis
Herpes simplex has been divided into type I, usually involving the face, and type 2, usually affecting the genitals. This distinction is becoming less significant, however, as type 2 is increasingly being isolated from ocular infections. Perhaps of more importance is the strain of the virus. Some strains appear to be genetically more virulent, with increased incidence of recurrence and severity of disease [5].

The herpes simplex virus colonizes the trigeminal ganglion and then may travel back up the nerve to manifest as recurrent disease. Identifiable factors triggering such recurrences are trauma to the trigeminal ganglion or the eye, stress, immunosuppression, sunlight, and fever. While recurrent ocular disease may manifest as a blepharoconjunctivitis, the characteristic lesion is a *herpetic dendritic keratitis,* a branching corneal ulcer.

Diagnosis
Herpetic dendritic keratitis often presents as a foreign body sensation. Pain is less prominent than with other keratitides, making decreased corneal sensation useful in the differential diagnosis. *Herpes zoster ophthalmicus* (see Chap. 2) occasionally manifests as dendritic keratitis; zoster dendrites are usually thin and multiple. A dendritic keratitis may be the primary manifestation of herpes simplex infection, as when there is autoinoculation of virus from a herpetic whitlow, a localized infection of the fingertip.

A dendritic epithelial keratitis that does not heal may progress to a *geographic ulcer.* Even if treatment results in healing of a dendrite, the keratitis often recurs months or years later. Recurrent epithelial keratitis may progress to involve the stroma. Topical steroids accelerate this process and are contraindicated in herpetic blepharoconjunctivitis or epithelial keratitis. In some cases the denervation of the cornea leads to a *trophic epithelial keratitis,* or *metaherpetic ulcer.*

The progression from epithelial disease to stromal disease worsens the visual prognosis as the epithelium heals without scarring, whereas the stroma cannot. Clinically distinct types of stromal involvement include disciform keratitis, interstitial keratitis, limbal vaculitis, and necrotizing keratitis. All of these may lead to vascularization, scarring, stromal melting, and even corneal perforation.

Treatment
Antiviral agents are potentially effective in treating primary herpetic blepharoconjunctivitis, but they are seldom used because it is difficult clinically to distinguish herpetic infections from the other causes of follicular conjunctivitis. When there are herpetic vesicles on the lids, prophylactic antiviral agents are warranted even in the absence of corneal involvement. Initial management of dendritic keratitis consists of gentle debridement of the infected epithelium after application of topical cocaine anesthesia, antiviral agents, or both. The current antiviral agent of choice is 1% trifluridine solution (Viroptic) applied every 1 to 2 hours initially and then tapered to twice a day over 2 weeks. In most cases the ulcer will heal, and the trifluridine may then be rapidly tapered and discontinued to avoid hypersensitivity or epithelial toxicity. If the epithelium is not completely healed after 3 weeks, treatment with another antiviral agent should be instituted. Those currently approved for general use are idoxuridine (Stoxil) and vidarabine (Vira-A), with others (acyclovir, bromovinyldeoxyuridine) being the subject of cur-

rent clinical trials. Trifluridine has the theoretical advantage that it penetrates the eye and may have some effect on deep keratitis and uveitis.

Peripheral ulcers seem to be more resistant to treatment than central ulcers. If a trophic ulcer develops, a bandage contact lens is placed, and artificial tears and prophylactic antibiotics are added. Once healing has occurred, an ocular lubricant (bland ointment, artificial tears, Lacrisert) may prevent recurrent erosions. Steroids and antiviral agents slow the healing of a trophic ulcer.

Stromal melting may be treated with steroids, acetylcysteine (Mucomist), and cyanoacrylate glue. Acetylcysteine is not approved for ophthalmic use and cyanoacrylate glue is not available in the United States, but they are often recommended by opthalmologists who have considerable experience managing these difficult complications.

Deciding when to start topical corticosteroids and how much to use in herpetic stromal keratitis is one of the most difficult therapeutic decisions facing an ophthalmologist. In addition to the usual risks of glaucoma and cataract, there are the added possibilities of reactivating the epithelial keratitis, of making the cornea steroid-dependent, and of encouraging superinfection. Steroid dependency means that attempts to taper topical steroids increase the activity of the stromal keratitis. When stromal keratitis is improving spontaneously or is off the visual axis, some ophthalmologists withhold steroids. In any event, the lowest effective dosage should be used, and attempts at tapering must be monitored closely. When higher dosages of steroids are being applied, many ophthalmologists add prophylactic antiviral and antibacterial agents.

Most eyes with keratitis develop an associated uveitis. This is treated with cycloplegics and, if necessary and possible, steroids. Intraocular pressures must be monitored closely in the presence of uveitis to watch for a marked pressure rise attributable to trabeculitis. This usually responds to intensive applications of topical steroids. If, despite the best therapeutic efforts, the cornea opacifies, penetrating keratoplasty may be successful, especially if there is no extensive vascularization. There remains, however, a significant risk of recurrent keratitis in the graft.

1. Boisjoly, H.M., Pavan-Langston, D., Kenyon, K.R., et al. Superinfections in herpes simplex keratitis. *Am. J. Ophthalmol.* 96:354–361, 1983.
   A persistent epithelial defect, recurrent keratouveitis, and the use of topical steroids were found to be risk factors for bacterial and fungal superinfections in 15 cases of herpes simplex keratitis.
2. Collum, L.M.T., McGettrick, P., Akhtar, J., et al. Oral acyclovir (Zovirax) in herpes simplex dendritic corneal ulceration. *Br. J. Ophthalmol.* 70:435–438, 1986.
   Oral administration was as effective as topical application in this trial of acyclovir.
3. Easty, D.L. *Virus Disease of the Eye.* Chicago: Year Book, 1985.
   A monograph with several chapters on herpesvirus.
4. Eiferman, R.A., Adams, G., Stover, B., et al. Herpetic whitlow and keratitis. *Arch. Ophthalmol.* 97:1079–1081, 1979.
   Two cases of inadvertent ocular inoculation by young health workers.
5. Kaufman, H.E., Varnell, E.D., Centifanto, Y.M., et al. Effect of the herpes simplex virus genome on the response of infection to corticosteroids. *Am. J. Ophthalmol.* 100:114–118, 1985.
   One of a series of papers from the group studying the significance of viral strain on clinical disease.
6. Kono, R., Nakajima, A. *Herpes Virus and Virus Chemotherapy: Pharmacological and Clinical Approaches.* Amsterdam: Excerpta Medica, 1985.
   The proceedings of an international symposium; many brief papers indicate the directions of current research.
7. Maudgal, P.C., Vrijhem, J.C., Molemans, M., et al. Effect of topical acyclovir therapy on experimental herpes simplex keratouveitis. *Arch. Ophthalmol.* 103:1389–1392, 1985.
   This animal study suggests that topical trifluridine ointment suppresses keratouveitis.

8. Pavan-Langston, D., Boisjoly, H.M. Management for herpes simplex virus ocular infections. In R.W. Darrell (ed.), *Viral Diseases of the Eye*. Philadelphia: Lea & Febiger, 1985. Pp. 29–41.
   The senior author of this clinical review is an authority on the treatment of herpetic keratitis.
9. Smolin, G. Immunotherapy of herpetic infections. *Int. Ophthalmol. Clin.* 25(2):165–177, 1985.
   An overview of research into the treatment of herpetic infections by enhancing host immunity.
10. Wander, A.H. Herpes simplex and recurrent corneal disease. *Int. Ophthalmol. Clin.* 24(2):27–38, 1984.
   Another good clinical review with specific therapeutic suggestions.

17. ACANTHAMOEBA KERATITIS

Acanthamoeba is one genus of the free-living amoebae, which have been isolated from moist soil, bodies of water, and the human oral cavity and thus are ubiquitous. Once considered nonpathogenic, species of amoebae were recognized in the 1940s as the agent of an almost always fatal meningoencephalitis. This developed in otherwise healthy young persons who had been swimming in freshwater lakes and as an opportunistic infection in immunocompromised hosts. In the early 1970s, *Acanthamoeba* was identified as a cause of keratitis.

Pathogenesis
Acanthamoeba keratitis develops in persons with otherwise healthy eyes after they have been swimming in contaminated freshwater lakes, bathing in hot tubs, or wearing soft contact lenses. It may also develop following minor trauma, often caused by vegetable matter. The association with soft lenses may represent contamination of the distilled water used in the preparation of cleansing solution and left standing for prolonged periods. In a few instances, no predisposition has been recognized.

Diagnosis
The diagnosis is often delayed. Most patients are initially thought to have herpetic keratitis. *Mycobacterium* and fungal keratitis must also be considered in the differential diagnosis. *Acanthamoeba* keratitis is an indolent, relapsing, but progressive corneal infiltration that is recalcitrant to therapy with antibiotics and steroids. The corneal infiltrate may form into a characteristic ring [14]; hypopyon and hyphema sometimes develop. Other suggestive clinical features are epithelial breakdown and severe pain and chemosis out of proportion to the activity of the keratitis. One explanation for the severe pain is the presence of an associated scleritis, which in one case manifested as a posterior scleritis with disk edema [9].

The amoebae are not easy to culture, requiring inoculation onto nonnutrient agar plates covered with *Escherichia coli* or *Aerobacter aerogenes* and daily microscopic examination of the incubated plates for growth of amoebae. Even with the use of such techniques, the organisms have often been recognized only after pathologic examination of the enucleated eye or after removal of the host button at the time of keratoplasty performed for a presumed herpetic keratitis. Acanthamoebae may sometimes be observed on Giemsa-stained corneal scrapings as clear, nonstaining cystic structures. Air drying before fixation should be avoided as this destroys the fragile amoebae. Recently, techniques have been described that permit rapid identification of *Acanthamoeba* from corneal scrapings by fluorescent-antibody staining of formaldehyde-fixed scrapings [2] and by fluorescent microscopy of methanol-fixed scrapings treated with calcofluor white [10, 15].

Treatment

Even if the diagnosis is established, treatment remains difficult. *Acanthamoeba* is relatively resistant to most available chemotherapeutic agents. The amoebae exist in two forms; relatively fragile trophozoites and hardier cysts. Irradication of the trophozoites does not eliminate the infection as long as viable cysts persist. Cryotherapy appears to be ineffective in killing cysts [12]. Ketoconazole, miconazole, are used in combination with mydriatics and steroids, but with limited success. A medical "cure" has been reported in an English patient receiving dibromopropamidine ointment, propamidine isethionate drops, and neomycin drops, but even this patient required keratoplasty [16]. Dibromopropamidine and propamidine are not commercially available in the United States as of this writing.

Virtually all patients with *Acanthamoeba* keratitis are eventually treated by keratoplasty, and some have required multiple keratoplasties to preserve useful vision. The optimal timing of keratoplasty is debated. Some clinicians think that, since the infection is generally unresponsive to medical therapy, early surgery is warranted. Others prefer to wait until the infection is quiescent.

1. Cohen, E.P., Buchanan, H.W., Laughrea, P.A., et al. Diagnosis and management of *Acanthamoeba* keratitis. *Am. J. Ophthalmol.* 100:389–395, 1985.
   Acanthamoeba was identified histologically in four cases from the Wills Eye Hospital, two by retrospective review of corneal buttons. The authors believe that early keratoplasty is warranted.
2. Cohen, E.J., Parlato, C.J., Arentsen, J.J., et al. Medical and surgical treatment of *Acanthamoeba* keratitis. *Am. J. Ophthalmol.* 103:615–625, 1987.
   The Wills Eye Hospital group provide a therapeutic overview based on their experience with seven patients, all soft contact lens wearers, and a review of previously reported cases.
3. Epstein, R.J., Wilson, L.A., Vivesvara, G.S., et al. Rapid diagnosis of *Acanthamoeba* keratitis from corneal scrapings using indirect fluorescent antibody staining. *Arch. Ophthalmol.* 104:1318–1321, 1986.
   Giemsa staining and indirect fluorescent-antibody studies were used to identify Acanthamoeba.
4. Hirst, L.W., Green, W.R., Merz, W., et al. Management of acanthamoeba keratitis: A case report and review of the literature. *Ophthalmology* 91:1105–1111, 1984.
   A case report with tabular review of 11 previously reported patients.
5. Jones, D.B. *Acanthamoeba*—the ultimate opportunist? *Am. J. Ophthalmol.* 102:527–530, 1986.
   A review masquerading as an editorial. Jones asks that the Centers for Disease Control be contacted if the diagnosis is suspected.
6. Key, S.N. III, Green, W.R., Willaert, E., et al. Keratitis due to *Acanthamoeba castellani:* A clinicopathologic case report. *Arch. Ophthalmol.* 98:475–479, 1980.
   The diagnosis was made only at enucleation.
7. Ludwig, I.H., Meisler, D.M., Rutherford, I., et al. Susceptibility of *Acanthamoeba* to soft contact lens disinfection systems. *Invest. Ophthalmol. Vis. Sci.* 27:626–628, 1986.
   Heat disinfection is more effective in killing amoebae than cold disinfection.
8. Ma, P., Willaert, E., Juechter, K.B., et al. A case of keratitis due to *Acanthamoeba* in New York, New York, and features of 10 cases. *J. Infect. Dis.* 143:662–667, 1981.
   A case report and review from the infectious disease literature.
9. Mannis, M.J., Tamaru, R., Roth, A.M., et al. *Acanthamoeba* sclerokeratitis: Determining diagnostic criteria. *Arch. Ophthalmol.* 104:1313–1317, 1986.
   Sclerokeratitis was prominent in these two patients.
10. Marines, H.M., Osato, M.S., Font, R.L. The value of calcofluor white in the diagnosis of mycotic and *Acanthamoeba* infections of the eye and ocular adnexa. *Ophthalmology* 94:23–26, 1987.
    Calcofluor white was used retrospectively on formalin-fixed, paraffin-embedded tissues known to contain fungi and proved reliable.

11. Mathers, W., Stevens, G., Jr., Rodrigues, M., et al. Immunopathology and electron microscopy of *Acanthamoeba* keratitis. *Am. J. Ophthalmol.* 103:626–635, 1987.
    Pathologic studies offer insight into the mechanism of the keratitis.
12. Meisler, D.M., Ludwig, I.H., Rutherford, I., et al. Susceptibility of *Acanthamoeba* to cryotherapeutic method. *Arch. Ophthalmol.* 104:130–131, 1986.
    A freeze-thaw-refreeze cycle did not kill Acanthamoeba *cysts in vitro.*
13. Samples, J.R., Binder, P.S., Luibel, F.J., et al. *Acanthamoeba* keratitis possibly acquired from a hot tub. *Arch. Ophthalmol.* 102:707–710, 1984.
    This nicely illustrated case report implies that people who wear soft contact lenses should avoid hot tubs.
14. Theodore, F.H., Jakobiec, F.A., Juechter, K.G., et al. The diagnostic value of a ring infiltrate in acanthamoebic keratitis. *Ophthalmology* 92:1471–1479, 1985.
    The corneal ring infiltrate is considered the most characteristic diagnostic feature.
15. Wilhelus, K.R., Osato, M.S., Font, R.L., et al. Rapid diagnosis for *Acanthamoeba* keratitis using calcofluor white. *Arch. Ophthalmol.* 104:1309–1312, 1986.
    Calcofluor white, a chemofluorescent dye used as a fabric brightener, binds to the polysaccharide polymers of amoebic cysts, permitting them to be recognized.
16. Wright, P., Warhurst, D., Jones, B.R. Acanthamoeba keratitis successfully treated medically. *Br. J. Ophthalmol.* 69:778–782, 1985.
    The patient received dibromopropamidine, propamidine, and neomycin topically, and the infection was quiescent for about 1 year during treatment and 4 months off all medications. Success in this case means that no organisms were found in the corneal button from a keratoplasty performed 22 months after presentation.

18. SCLERITIS AND EPISCLERITIS

Inflammation of the episclera, sclera, and peripheral cornea form a clinical continuum. *Episcleritis,* although often recurrent, is generally benign. Two clinical types are recognized: *diffuse* or *simple episcleritis* and *nodular episcleritis. Scleritis,* on the other hand, is a threat to vision. Most scleritis is *anterior,* being subdivided into *diffuse, nodular,* and *necrotizing.* The noninflammatory form of necrotizing scleritis is often referred to as *scleromalacia perforans. Sclerokeratitis* is another variant of anterior scleritis related to *peripheral ulcerative keratitis* or *peripheral corneal melting. Posterior scleritis* is less common than anterior keratitis, may present in various ways, and is frequently difficult to diagnose.

Pathogenesis
Episcleritis is less often associated with systemic disease than is scleritis. A form of episcleritis has long been recognized in conjunction with acute gout, and two patients have recently been reported who also had familial Mediterranean fever [9]. By contrast, anterior scleritis is a relatively common manifestation of rheumatoid arthritis. The sclera is involved in the same way as the joint synovium by an immune-mediated microvasculitis. Scleritis may be a part of other collagen-vascular diseases and also develops in other granulomatoses, especially Wegener's but also syphilis and tuberculosis. Instances are also observed following ocular surgery, in the vasculitic process that is a complication of herpes zoster, in aspergillus infection [11], and in patients with inflammatory bowel disease [12].

Scleromalacia perforans develops—often in the eyes of elderly women with rheumatoid arthritis—because arterial occlusion causes scleral necrosis. A sequestrum is formed that then may slough, with perforation of the globe. The prognosis for vision in such eyes is poor.

Diagnosis
Episcleritis is frequently confused with conjunctivitis. In episcleritis there is no discharge and often little discomfort. Phenylephrine (2.5%) applied topically will blanch

onjunctival but not all episcleral vessels. Scleritis, by contrast, characteristically auses pain, which may be severe and spread to involve the entire face and jaw. Both piscleritis and scleritis are often bilateral. The involved tissue in scleritis is thickened, ark red or purple, and tender to palpation. An avascular, white or gray area in the enter of a focus of scleritis indicates necrosis and is a grave prognostic sign. Thinning f the sclera following acute inflammation leads to localized areas of ectasia.

The diagnosis of anterior scleritis is usually evident clinically, but Watson and co- vorkers [15] use anterior segment fluorescein angiography as a diagnostic tool. They istinguish an inflammatory necrotizing scleritis whose characteristic sign is venular cclusion from noninflammatory necrotizing scleritis or scleromalacia perforans in vhich there is total obliteration of the vasculature. In more benign forms of scleritis and n episcleritis, the blood circulates rapidly through dilated vessels.

Posterior scleritis is most easily diagnosed when it accompanies anterior scleritis. 'ain is variable; visual loss, sometimes simply an effect of increasing hyperopia, is the nost constant symptom. Funduscopic examination often reveals a mass that is some- imes associated with a serous detachment with cloudy subretinal fluid. The disk may e swollen, with radiating choroidal folds. The differential diagnosis of those fundos- opic findings includes intraocular tumor, and eyes have been inadvertently enucleated or posterior scleritis. The most useful diagnostic test is ultrasonography, which reveals hickening of the uveoscleral layers of the eye [6].

Treatment

Episcleritis is generally self-limited, lasts 10 days to 3 weeks, and requires no treat- nent, although topical steroids are sometimes used. Topical steroids are not effective in reating scleritis, and subconjunctival injections of corticosteroids are contraindicated ecause they predispose to scleral thinning and perforation. In the milder forms of scler- tis, nonsteroidal inflammatory agents such as oxyphenbutazone, indomethacin, and buprofen may shorten the course of the disease.

In more severe anterior scleritis, administration of systemic steroids may lead to ini- ial improvement and then become ineffective. When steroids are used, an initial high losage (60 mg or more daily) is reduced when the pain diminishes. Megadose pulse ste- oid therapy has been tried [7]. Some investigators caution against the use of systemic teroids in posterior scleritis, since in their patients such treatment did not seem to ffect the outcome [10].

Systemic immunosuppression with cytotoxic agents rather than corticosteroids may mprove both a scleritis and the prognosis for life [2]. Cyclophosphamide, methotrexate, nd azathioprine had fewer side effects than penicillamine. Cyclophosphamide seems to e particularly effective in the management of Wegener's granulomatosis [7]. The ability f topical cyclosporin therapy to suppress a necrotizing scleritis remains to be confirmed y other workers [3]. Surgical reinforcement of thinning sclera by autogenous perios- eum and other homografts and autografts may be beneficial in some patients [5].

1. Benson, W.E., Shields, J.A., Tasman, W., et al. Posterior scleritis: A cause of diag- nostic confusion. *Arch. Ophthalmol.* 97:1482–1486, 1979.
   All seven patients with both anterior and posterior scleritis in this series had a good visual prognosis.
2. Foster, C.S., Forstot, S.L., Wilson, L.A. Mortality rate in rheumatoid arthritis pa- tients developing necrotizing scleritis or peripheral ulcerative keratitis. *Opthalmol- ogy* 91:1253–1263, 1984.
   A nonrandomized clinical trial in 34 patients with rheumatoid arthritis found both improved survival rate and visual prognosis with cytotoxic immunosuppression as compared with steroidal and nonsteroidal anti-inflammatory therapy.
3. Hoffman, F., Wiederholt, M. Local treatment of necrotizing scleritis with cyclosporin A. *Cornea* 4:3–7, 1985–86.
   Topical treatment with a cytotoxic agent appeared to be effective when other measures failed in this 83-year-old woman with rheumatoid arthritis.

4. Kleiner, R.C., Raber, I.M., Passero, F.C. Scleritis, pericarditis, and aortic insuff ciency in a patient with rheumatoid arthritis. *Ophthalmology* 91:941–946, 1984.
   Scleritis was the first manifestation of this patient's systemic disease.
5. Koenig, S.B., Kaufman, H.E. The treatment of necrotizing scleritis with an autoge nous periosteal graft. *Ophthalmic Surg.* 14:1029–1032, 1983.
   Scleral defects were successfully repaired with periosteum in two patients.
6. Marushak, D. Uveal effusion attending scleritis posterior. A case report with A-sca and B-scan echograms. *Acta Ophthalmol.* 60:773–778, 1982.
   Ultrasound was used to diagnose and follow this patient with posterior scleritis.
7. Pavelka, K. Jr., Dostal, C., Rossman, P., et al. Wegener's granulomatosis with bilat eral necrotizing scleritis, polyarthritis and renal failure efficiently treated with im munosuppressive therapy. *Clin. Rheumatol.* 5:112–117, 1986.
   A case report of this therapy.
8. Rao, N.A., Marak, G.E., Hidayat, A.A. Necrotizing scleritis: A clinicopathologic stud of 41 cases. *Ophthalmology* 92:1542–1549, 1985.
   These 41 cases include patients with rheumatoid arthritis, Wegener's granulomatosis polychondritis, Goodpasture's syndrome, and infectious scleritis (zoster and pseudo monas), and 19 cases that were idiopathic.
9. Scharf, J., Meyer, E., Zonis, S. Episcleritis associated with familial Mediterranea fever. *Am. J. Ophthalmol.* 100:337–339, 1985.
   These two patients developed episcleritis during a period when their familial Medi terranean fever was inactive, and the significance of this association is uncertain.
10. Singh, G., Guthoff, R., Foster, C.S. Observations on long-term follow-up of posterio scleritis. *Am. J. Ophthalmol.* 101:570–575, 1986.
    Nine cases with various referring diagnoses were diagnosed as having posterior scler itis. In subsequent correspondence, Kalina and Mills argue that some of these coul better be classified as "acquired hyperopia with choroidal folds" (Am. J. Ophthalmol 102:671–672, 1986).
11. Stenson, S., Brookner, A., Rosenthal, S. Bilateral endogenous necrotizing scleriti due to *Aspergillus oryzae*. *Ann. Ophthalmol.* 14:67–72, 1982.
    A case report of an unusual infectious scleritis.
12. Tesar, P.J., Burgess, J.A., Goy, J.A.E., et al. Scleromalacia perforans in ulcerativ colitis. *Gastroenterology* 81:153–155, 1981.
    In this 36-year-old man, proctocolectomy was followed by immediate improvement i the scleritis.
13. Watson, P.G. The diagnosis and management of scleritis. *Ophthalmology* 87:716– 720, 1980.
    A brief but beautifully illustrated discussion of Watson's experience.
14. Watson, P.G. The nature and treatment of scleral inflammation. *Trans. Ophthalmol Soc. U.K.* 102:257–281, 1982.
    Watson provides a more extensive review.
15. Watson, P.G., Bovey, E. Anterior segment fluorescein angiography in the diagnosi of scleral inflammation. *Ophthalmology* 92:1–11, 1985.
    A presentation of the details in the interpretation of this study.
16. Watson, P.G., Young, R.D. Changes at the periphery of a lesion in necrotising scler itis: Anterior segment fluorescein angiography correlated with electron microscopy *Br. J. Ophthalmol.* 69:656–663, 1985.
    Pathologic correlation of Watson's anterior segment angiography findings.
17. Young, R.D., Watson, P.G. Microscopical studies of necrotising scleritis. I. Cellula aspects. II. Collagen degradation in the scleral stroma. *Br. J. Ophthalmol.* 68:778– 789, 1984.
    Two sequential papers present pathologic studies in eight surgical specimens from eyes with advanced necrotizing scleritis. Even though the etiologies differed, the chronic granulomatous changes were the same in all.

IV. ANTERIOR CHAMBER AND GLAUCOMA

John W. Gittinger, Jr.

19. ANGLE-CLOSURE GLAUCOMA

In open-angle glaucoma the aqueous has constant access to the trabecular meshwork; in *angle-closure glaucoma* this access is blocked by the peripheral iris. There are three ways that the iris may close the angle: by being forced forward by aqueous unable to get through the pupil *(pupillary block);* by obstructing the trabecular meshwork directly without pupillary block as the result of posterior pressure from the ciliary body, vitreous, or lens or because of anterior rotation and swelling of the ciliary body; or by adhesions called *peripheral anterior synechiae* forming between the peripheral iris and the angle structures. In many cases, more than one of these mechanisms is responsible for the block in aqueous reabsorption and the consequent elevation of intraocular pressure.

Pathogenesis
The primary importance of pupillary block in the majority of cases is demonstrated by the fact that an iridectomy, which allows free flow of aqueous between the anterior and posterior chambers, usually cures angle-closure glaucoma. Direct mechanical obstruction of the trabecular meshwork without pupillary block occurs only when the entire lens-iris diaphragm is pushed forward or when the peripheral iris has a specific anomaly, a configuration called *plateau iris.*

The most common type of primary angle-closure glaucoma arises from a more common bilateral anomaly of the entire anterior segment that has a shallow anterior chamber as its most obvious manifestation. The incidence of this anomaly differs in various human populations, being prevalent, for example, in Eskimos and Japanese and rare in blacks. In contrast to eyes predisposed to open-angle glaucoma, the eye at risk for angle-closure glaucoma has normal pressures, aqueous outflow facility, and optic disk cupping until the acute glaucoma develops.

The lens normally thickens with age, thus making the anterior chamber more shallow, and the pupil becomes smaller, increasing pupillary block. The extreme enlargement of the lens associated with cataract formation may precipitate angle closure even in eyes with initially deep chambers (see Chap. 26). A rapid change in lens size may also explain the sudden development of angle-closure glaucoma after hyperglycemia [18]. Lens-induced pupillary block is also a feature of ectopia lentis (see Chap. 25) and the Weill-Marchesani syndrome, in which lax zonules allow the lens to move forward into the pupil. The Weill-Marchesani syndrome is an important consideration in a child who presents with angle-closure glaucoma, since miotics may be contraindicated (see below) [22].

Peripheral anterior synechiae are sequelae of postsurgical flat chambers and attacks of angle closure from any mechanism. They also may be congenital, develop in association with inflammation or iris neovascularization, or appear in the course of the iridocorneal endothelial dystrophy syndromes (essential iris atrophy, Chandler's syndrome, and Cogan-Reese syndrome). Once enough peripheral anterior synechiae have formed, iridectomy alone will not control even what was initially a primary pupillary block angle-closure glaucoma.

Acute angle-closure attack is more likely to occur in older women. The most important proximal cause is pupillary mydriasis, which may be spontaneous, pharmacologic, or neurologic. Since sympathetic discharge causes mydriasis, angle closure may be related to emotional stress. All physicians should be aware of the possibility of precipitating angle closure in eyes with narrow angles by the use of topical cycloplegic mydriatics. Various systemic medications with anticholinergic activity have also been implicated, including transdermal scopolamine (for which it is unclear whether the action is systemic or local, i.e., an inadvertent transfer of the medication into the eye by a contaminated finger) and atropine or other drugs used preoperatively [5, 11]. Of course, the labeling of such drugs as contraindicated in patients with glaucoma is of little practical value, since few of the estimated one in 4,000 adult Americans at risk actually carry this diagnosis. Neurologic pupillary dilation—third nerve palsy and the mydriasis accompanying a transient ischemic attack—is among recently reported causes of acute angle-closure glaucoma [4, 21].

Direct mechanical obstruction of the angle without significant pupillary block occurs in eyes with the plateau iris configuration or eyes in which the iris-lens diaphragm shifts forward as the result of pressure from posterior ocular structures. This mechanism explains the high incidence of angle closure in eyes with the retinopathy of prematurity and also its occasional occurrence following scleral buckling procedures or panretinal photocoagulation complicated by choroidal effusion or hemorrhage. Of course, these are also procedures in which the pupil is dilated. Shifting forward of the vitreous is the likely explanation for acute angle-closure glaucoma following subretinal pigment epithelium hemorrhage in senile macular degeneration [9], in patients with acquired immune deficiency syndrome who have choroidal effusions [19], and in nonneovascular angle closure following occlusion of the central retinal vein [15].

Myopic eyes have deep anterior chambers and are at low risk for angle closure. Familial exceptions to this rule are encountered [10], and eyes with ectopia lentis are often highly myopic. In general, however, the more hyperopic the eye, the more likely it is that the angle will close. A subgroup with high hyperopia and small eyes *(nanophthalmos)* is at high risk for angle closure. This may be precipitated by spontaneous uveal effusions that are a consequence of thickened sclera obstructing venous drainage. Recognition of nanophthalmos is important since these eyes respond poorly to conventional medical and surgical therapy. Vortex vein decompression to improve venous drainage is an aggressive treatment for nanophthalmos with uveal effusion [1].

Another familial ocular structural abnormality that can lead to angle closure is peripheral iris or ciliary body cysts [20]. Puncturing these cysts with a laser (laser cystotomy) opens the angle. Pupillary block glaucoma may develop after intracapsular cataract extraction if the iridectomy is not patent—either partial thickness or blocked by vitreous. Similarly, pseudophakic eyes, especially those with certain types of anterior chamber lenses, are at risk for pupillary block.

Diagnosis

The diagnosis of acute angle-closure glaucoma is not difficult when the presentation is typical: a painful, red eye with markedly increased intraocular pressure accompanied by diaphoresis, nausea, and vomiting. Atypical presentations include chronic angle closure, which represents a relatively common diagnosis in a glaucoma referral practice, and acute angle closure without pain. The presence of a midposition, fixed pupil in an eye with reduced vision, especially in an elderly person, should suggest the possibility of unrecognized angle-closure glaucoma; tonometry and gonioscopy confirm the diagnosis.

Treatment

Treatment of patients with acute angle-closure attack consists of topical miotics and beta blockers, systemic carbonic anhydrase inhibitors, and hyperosmolar agents, and perhaps analgesics and antiemetics. Indentation of the central cornea with a gonioprism or other blunt instrument may open the angle peripherally and help break the acute attack; iridectomy is occasionally required. In some eyes, notably those with nanophthalmos or the Weill-Marchesani syndrome, miotics increase pupillary block and are contraindicated. Even when neither of these syndromes is present, strong miotics such as echothiophate may actually aggravate pupillary block, and, conversely, strong mydriatics, which widely dilate the pupil, may relieve it.

The primary surgical management of angle-closure glaucoma in which pupillary block is suspected remains iridectomy. Laser iridectomy (also called laser iridotomy) has replaced surgical iridectomy as the procedure of choice for most eyes. Prophylactic iridectomy in the fellow eye is usually indicated, as the underlying anatomic abnormality is almost always bilateral. When iridectomy alone does not deepen the anterior chamber and reduce intraocular pressure, other surgical procedures must be considered, since mechanisms besides pupillary block are active. When there are recently formed peripheral anterior synechiae, a chamber-deeping procedure with mechanical lysis of the synechiae, (a technique some call *goniosynechialysis*) may be warranted. In some eyes only a filtering procedure offers the possibility of intraocular pressure control.

1. Brockhurst, R.J. Vortex vein decompression for nanophthalmic uveal effusion. *Arch. Ophthalmol.* 98:1987–1990, 1980.
   A clinician who has helped define this entity describes a radical surgical approach.
2. Campbell, D.G., Vela, A. New concepts in angle-closure glaucoma. In *Symposium on the Laser in Ophthalmology and Glaucoma Update.* St. Louis: Mosby, 1985. Pp. 15–26.
   The major part of this paper is a discussion of the technique of goniosynechialysis.
3. Cashwell, L.F. Laser iridotomy for management of angle-closure glaucoma. *Southern Med. J.* 78:288–291, 1985.
   This personal series of 112 patients documents the indications, safety, and efficacy of laser iridectomy.
4. Coppeto, J.R., Monteiro, M.L.R. Angle-closure glaucoma and transient ischemic attacks. *Am. J. Ophthalmol.* 99:493, 1985.
   A brief description of this association.
5. Fazio, D.T., Bateman, J.B., Christensen, R.E. Acute angle-closure glaucoma associated with surgical anesthesia. *Arch. Ophthalmol.* 103:360–362, 1985.
   These and previous cases suggest that premedications are the important factors.
6. Ghose, S., Sachdev, M.S., Kumar, H. Bilateral nanophthalmos, pigmentary retinal dystrophy, and angle closure glaucoma—a new syndrome? *Br. J. Ophthalmol.* 69:624–628, 1985.
   This unusual case may add retinal pigmentary degeneration to the abnormalities characteristic of nanophthalmic eyes.
7. Gieser, D.K., Wilensky, J.T. Laser iridectomy in the management of chronic angle-closure glaucoma. *Am. J. Ophthalmol.* 98:446–450, 1984.
   Further indications and experience with this procedure.
8. Greenstein, S.H., Abramson, D.H., Pitts, W.R. III. Systemic atropine and glaucoma. *Bull. N.Y. Acad. Med.* 60:961–968, 1984.
   This position paper makes some good points but adds little new information.
9. Grewal, K.S., Sharp, D., Yoshizumi, M.O. Acute angle-closure glaucoma due to senile macular degeneration treated by argon laser photocoagulation. *Ann. Ophthalmol.* 16:935–938, 1984.
   The authors propose that hemorrhage shifted the vitreous forward, precipitating the angle-closure attack.
10. Hagan, J.C. III, Lederer, C.M. Jr. Primary angle closure glaucoma in a myopic kinship. *Arch. Ophthalmol.* 103:363–365, 1985.
    Even myopia does not protect against angle closure in some families.
11. Hamill, M.B., Suelflow, J.A., Smith, J.A. Transdermal scopolamine delivery systems (TRANSDERM-V) and acute angle-closure glaucoma. *Ann. Ophthalmol.* 15:1011–1012, 1983.
    When pupillary dilation precipitates angle closure, look behind the ears.
12. Kramer, P., Ritch, R. The treatment of acute angle-closure glaucoma revisited. *Ann. Ophthalmol.* 16:1101–1103, 1984.
    An editorial outlines various considerations in management.
13. Mapstone, R. Acute shallowing of the anterior chamber. *Br. J. Ophthalmol.* 65:446–451, 1981.
    Mapstone is the principal proponent of the pilocarpine-phenylephrine provocative test.
14. Markowitz, S.N., Morin, J.D. The ratio of lens thickness to axial length for biometric standardization in angle-closure glaucoma. *Am. J. Ophthalmol.* 99:400–402, 1985.
    One in a series of papers by these authors on biometric considerations in angle-closure glaucoma.
15. Mendelsohn, A.D., Jampol, L.M., Shoch, D. Secondary angle-closure glaucoma after central retinal vein occlusion. *Am. J. Ophthalmol.* 100:581–585, 1985.
    In this case report, a secondary glaucoma not related to rubeosis iridis following occlusion of the central retinal vein appeared to respond to treatment with topical steroids and timolol.
16. Pollard, A.F. Lensectomy for secondary angle-closure glaucoma in advanced cicatricial retrolental fibroplasia. *Ophthalmology* 91:395–398, 1984.

Pollard suggests an approach to management of angle closure in retinopathy of pre maturity.

17. Smith, J., Shivitz, I. Angle-closure glaucoma in adults with cicatricial retinopathy of prematurity. *Arch. Ophthalmol.* 102:371–372, 1984.
    Angle closure is also a late complication in this entity.

18. Sorokanich, S., Wand, M., Nix, H.R. Angle closure glaucoma and acute hyperglyce mia. *Arch. Ophthalmol.* 101:1434, 1986.
    Acute lens swelling precipitated angle closure.

19. Ullman, S., Wilson, R.P., Schwartz, L. Bilateral angle-closure glaucoma in associa tion with the acquired immune deficiency syndrome. *Am. J. Ophthalmol.* 101:419– 424, 1986.
    In two homosexual men with AIDS, angle closure developed as the result of ciliocho roidal effusions. One patient required surgical drainage of suprachoroidal fluid.

20. Vela, A., Rieser, J.C., Campbell, D.G. The heredity and treatment of angle-closure glaucoma secondary to iris and ciliary body cysts. *Ophthalmology* 91:332–337, 1983
    Another familial, treatable cause of angle-closure glaucoma.

21. Wilson, W.B., Barmatz, H.E. Acute angle-closure glaucoma secondary to an aneu rysm of the posterior communicating artery. *Am. J. Ophthalmol.* 89:868–870, 1980
    Anything that causes pupillary dilation can cause angle closure.

22. Wright, K.W., Chrousos, G.A. Weill-Marchesani syndrome with bilateral angle-clo sure glaucoma. *J. Pediatr. Ophthalmol. Strab.* 22:129–132, 1985.
    This type of angle closure, which occurs in children with anomalous eyes, is worsened by miotic treatment.

20. LOW-TENSION GLAUCOMA

The diagnosis of low-tension glaucoma is attached to eyes with characteristic glaucomatous cupping and visual field defects but consistently normal intraocular pressures. The more that is known about such eyes, the fewer seem to meet these criteria; low-tension glaucoma remains a diagnosis of exclusion.

Diagnosis

The largest number of eyes to be excluded actually have primary open-angle glaucoma, but the intraocular pressure is not elevated at the time of measurement. One reason for this is the diurnal variation in intraocular pressure. Most authorities will not accept the diagnosis of low-tension glaucoma unless intraocular pressure is normal (less than 20 to 24 mm Hg) on multiple determinations at different times of the day. Ideally, a diurnal curve is obtained by performing applanation tonometry every 2 to 4 hours around the clock.

The eye may also have had elevated intraocular pressures in the past; for example, during a period of topical steroid use. A group of elderly patients with "burnt out" primary open-angle or pigmentary glaucoma has been described. The ability of their eyes to secrete aqueous has apparently decreased with age, compensating for reduced outflow. Another cause of normal intraocular pressure in an eye with cupping and field loss is effective treatment. While a prior filtering procedure in the eye of a patient providing a poor history will be evident to the examiner, evidence of a laser trabeculoplasty usually is not seen. Occasionally, a patient with undiscovered glaucoma is serendipitously on a medication for another problem, such as a systemic beta blocker for hypertension, that also reduces intraocular pressure.

Any cause of a large cup-disk ratio may be confused with low-tension glaucoma, including congenital disk anomalies. Such disk colobomas and pits often have associated nerve fiber bundle visual field defects, making the distinction even more difficult. Other optic neuropathies may mimic the cupping and, to a lesser degree, the visual field changes of chronic open-angle glaucoma. Excavation of the optic disk is not specific to glaucoma, but is found in some eyes with compressive optic neuropathy or hereditary optic neuropathy, and as a sequela of retrobulbar neuritis and ischemic optic neuropathy. The major ophthalmoscopic clue that distinguishes true glaucomatous optic atrophy from other causes of optic atrophy with disk excavation is the extent of the disk pallor. In glaucomatous optic atrophy the residual neural rim retains its normal pink color, whereas in neurologic optic atrophy with cupping, the pallor extends beyond the excavation. This criterion is not completely reliable and will not distinguish glaucomatous disks from those with developmental defects mimicking glaucomatous cupping, in which the neural rim may also be normal.

The distinction between low-tension glaucoma and compressive optic neuropathy can usually be made on the basis of the visual acuity and fields. Compressive optic neuropathy characteristically reduces visual acuity, with visual fields demonstrating central scotomata or bitemporal field defects. A case has been reported in which cupping and field loss that suggested ischemic optic neuropathy or low-tension glaucoma proved to be optic nerve compression by a carotid-ophthalmic aneurysm that was not detected by computed tomography [14]. In retrospect, the only clues to the nature of the process were the history of gradual progression and the reduction in acuity to 20/50, the former ruling out ischemic optic neuropathy and the latter being atypical militating against low-tension glaucoma. The large majority of patients referred to neuroophthalmologists to rule out compressive lesions have findings that distinguish between compression and glaucoma or ischemic optic neuropathy.

Pathogenesis

The relationship between low-tension glaucoma and ischemic optic neuropathy is uncertain. One theory of field loss and cupping in primary open-angle glaucoma is that they represent disk infarction caused by an imbalance between the vascular supply of the disk tissues and the intraocular pressure. Small disk hemorrhages in eyes with glaucoma and ocular hypertension that then evolve nerve fiber bundle defects and increased cupping may imply a vascular etiology. An alternative mechanical explanation is that the disk substance collapses and causes secondary bleeding. Disk hemorrhages appear in eyes with low-tension glaucoma, and there could be perfusion abnormalities in these disks that predispose them to ischemia, even with normal intraocular pressure. There is at present, however, no clear evidence that low-tension glaucoma is caused by intercurrent vascular disease, including carotid occlusion. There is some suggestion of a link between low-tension glaucoma and migraine, a disease complex characterized by vasospasm and ischemia [13].

Glaucoma-like cupping is observed as a sequela of the anterior ischemic optic neuropathy associated with giant cell arteritis. Such cases are not likely to be called low-tension glaucoma because of the history of sudden, severe visual loss with disk swelling. Arteritic ischemic optic neuropathy produces pathologic cupping more often than does the more common nonarteritic ischemic optic neuropathy. This may be both because the ischemia is usually more severe with arteritic ischemic optic neuropathy and because the disks that are affected are structurally different. In nonarteritic ischemic optic neuropathy, the disk is anomalous, with a decreased cup–disk ratio (see Chap. 52). This anatomic variation predisposes the eyes to the ischemic event. By contrast, there is no known relationship between disk structure and arteritis. Thus, the disk affected by arteritic ischemic optic neuropathy probably had a larger cup–disk ratio to begin with.

Another possible cause of disk ischemia implicated in the pathogenesis of low-tension glaucoma is systemic hypotension. In some series of patients who fulfilled the criteria for low-tension glaucoma, a history of blood loss or hypotension was elicited in a large minority. These patients were thought to have a *shock-induced optic neuropathy*. A prospective study of 20 patients who had survived shock, however, failed to identify any with glaucomatous cupping or field loss [7]. A related question, whether patients with hypertension or those with chronic hypotension are more likely to develop low-tension glaucoma, remains unresolved.

Treatment

Once other diagnoses have been excluded, the major problem that remains is the management of eyes with low-tension glaucoma. A distinction should be made between nonprogressive and progressive low-tension glaucoma. Those patients who have a history of blood loss, for example, are likely to have stable visual deficits, and no treatment is warranted. When progressive cupping and field loss are documented, the approach is similar to that in ordinary glaucoma; that is, the pressure is lowered by medical or surgical means until visual field loss ceases. Most patients with progressive low-tension glaucoma are older, with borderline but still normal intraocular pressure and outflow facility. This suggests that their disks are simply more vulnerable to damage by a given level of intraocular pressure than are normal disks. Filtering procedures may be required to achieve the low levels of intraocular pressure that such disks can tolerate.

1. Abedin, S., Simmons, R.J., Grant, W.M. Progressive low-tension glaucoma: Treatment to stop glaucomatous cupping and field loss when these progress despite normal intraocular pressure. *Ophthalmology* 89:1–6, 1982.
   This case series supports the proposition that, if visual field loss and cupping progress despite "normal" intraocular pressure, the pressure should be lowered further. When the pressure was brought below 12 mm Hg by a filtering procedure, progressive visual loss ceased.
2. Caprioli, J., Spaeth, G.L. Comparison of the optic nerve head in high- and low-tension glaucoma. *Arch. Ophthalmol.* 103:1145–1149, 1985.
   Eyes with low-tension glaucoma have thinner neural rims than eyes with high-tension glaucoma with similar degrees of visual field loss, suggesting two distinct mechanisms for the optic disk damage. Another possible explanation is that eyes with low-tension glaucoma are not detected unless the cup is large.
3. Caprioli, J., Spaeth, G.L. Comparison of visual field defects in the low-tension glaucomas with those of the high-tension glaucomas. *Am. J. Ophthalmol.* 97:730–737, 1984.
   The two mechanisms mentioned in the previous paper may be barotrauma and ischemia. The significance of the visual field findings reported here has been challenged (see Am. J. Ophthalmol. 98:823–825, 1984, and King and co-workers below).
4. Corbett, J.J., Phelps, C.D., Eslinger, P., et al. The neurologic evaluation of patients with low-tension glaucoma. *Invest. Ophthalmol. Vis. Sci.* 26:1101–1104, 1985.
   No evidence of intercurrent neurologic disease except for migraine was found among 27 patients with low-tension glaucoma.
5. Drance, S.M. Low-tension glaucoma: Enigma and opportunity. *Arch. Ophthalmol.* 103:1131–1133, 1985.
   An editorial analysis of the status of low-tension glaucoma by a prominent worker on the subject.
6. Epstein, D.L. Progressive low-tension glaucoma. In D.L. Epstein (ed.), *Chandler and Grant's Glaucoma*. Philadelphia: Lea & Febiger, 1986. Pp. 181–190.
   Epstein's chapter emphasizes the definition and management of progressive low-tension glaucoma.
7. Jampol, L.M., Board, R.J., Maumenee, A.E. Systemic hypotension and glaucomatous changes. *Am. J. Ophthalmol.* 85:154–159, 1978.
   Seventeen patients with one or more episodes of shock were examined, and none had glaucomatous field loss or cupping.
8. King, D., Drance, S.M., Douglas, G., et al. Comparison of visual field defects in normal-tension glaucoma and high-tension glaucoma. *Am. J. Ophthalmol.* 101:204–207, 1986.
   Another study of the visual field defects in these two entities finds little difference between the patterns of visual field loss at the comparable stages of disk excavation.
9. Kitazawa, Y., Shirato, S., Yamamoto, T. Optic disc hemorrhage in low-tension glaucoma. *Ophthalmology* 93:853–857, 1986.
   Recurrent disk hemorrhages were common in one group of patients with low-tension glaucoma.
10. Kupersmith, M.J., Krohn, D. Cupping of the optic disc with compressive lesions of the anterior visual pathway. *Ann. Ophthalmol.* 16:948–953, 1984.
    Sixteen of 250 patients with compression of the anterior visual pathways had abnor-

mal cupping, but this could be distinguished from glaucoma by visual acuity and fields.

11. Levene, R.Z. Low tension glaucoma: A critical review and new material. *Surv. Ophthalmol.* 24:621–664, 1980.
   In an extensive review, Levene attempts to define characteristics that separate low-tension glaucoma from chronic open-angle glaucoma.
12. Lichter, P.R., Henderson, J.W. Optic nerve infarction. *Am. J. Ophthalmol.* 85:302–310, 1978.
   The authors prefer to separate their three patients with sudden visual loss, cupping or hemorrhages in the inferotemporal disk, and superior arcuate field defects from other cases of low-tension glaucoma.
13. Phelps, C.D., Corbett, J.J. Migraine and low-tension glaucoma: A case-control study. *Invest. Ophthalmol. Vis. Sci.* 26:1105–1108, 1985.
   A companion article to reference 2 above, with additional evidence that the association with migraine is significant.
14. Portney, G.L., Roth, A.M. Optic cupping caused by an intracranial aneurysm. *Am. J. Ophthalmol.* 84:98–103, 1977.
   A 51-year-old woman with reduced acuity, an inferior altitudinal visual field defect, and pathologic cupping died after a carotid-ophthalmic aneurysm bled, and the optic nerves were studied pathologically.
15. Schwartz, A.L., Perman, K.I., Whitten, M. Argon laser trabeculoplasty in progressive low-tension glaucoma. *Ann. Ophthalmol.* 16:560–566, 1984.
   Further evidence that techniques used to reduce pressure in high-tension glaucoma are applicable to progressive low-tension glaucoma.
16. Sebag, J., Thomas, J.V., Epstein, D.L., et al. Optic disc cupping in arteritic anterior ischemic optic neuropathy resembles glaucomatous cupping. *Ophthalmology* 93:357–361, 1986.
   Five cases are presented that support the title's proposition.
17. Sugar, H.S. Low tension glaucoma: A practical approach. *Ann. Ophthalmol.* 11:1155–1171, 1979.
   A seasoned clinician offers guidelines for management of low-tension glaucoma.

21. NEOVASCULAR GLAUCOMA

The adjective "neovascular" has largely replaced the older term "hemorrhagic" to describe the glaucoma that develops in eyes with anterior segment or iris neovascularization, also called rubeosis iridis. *Neovascular glaucoma* is a type of secondary glaucoma. The underlying stimulus for the formation of new vessels is most often ischemia, and the majority of eyes that develop neovascular glaucoma already have either diabetic retinopathy or an occluded central retinal vein. Intraocular tumor growth also stimulates neovascularization.

Pathogenesis
There is increasing evidence that ischemic and neoplastic tissues elaborate angiogenic factors that promote new vessel growth. The precise nature of these vasoproliferative substances, however, has not been defined. Any process that causes ischemia of ocular tissues, including inflammation, may stimulate neovascularization. In addition, neovascular glaucoma develops in some eyes harboring choroidal or iris melanomas [19], metastatic carcinomas, reticulum-cell sarcomas, and retinoblastomas.

The natural history of neovascular glaucoma has been clinically observed and experimentally reproduced. In the initial stages, new vessels form at the pupillary border and in the angle. As these vessels then spread over the iris, their thin walls expose the redness of the blood they contain; thus, the description *rubeosis iridis*. Gonioscopy often reveals small vessels growing from the iris across the trabecular meshwork. If the ischemic stimulus is sufficient, fibrovascular tissue eventually seals the angle, forming peripheral anterior synechiae. At some point aqueous outflow is so compromised that intraocular pressure rises, often to high levels, and the patient experiences symptoms similar to those of an attack of angle-closure glaucoma: severe pain and reduced vision.

Diagnosis

The differential diagnosis in a case of acute neovascular glaucoma includes angle-closure glaucoma and uveitis, which also engorge iris vessels. Full anterior chamber depth in the fellow eye argues against a primary angle-closure mechanism; the distinction from uveitis may have to await observation of the response to treatment. Virtually all patients with neovascular glaucoma from diabetes have a history of the disease, and most, but not all, have had prior visual problems from diabetic retinopathy. Diabetics are the major group likely to develop bilateral neovascular glaucoma.

The pathogenic role of angiogenic factors may be indirectly demonstrated by the neovascular glaucoma that often follows vitrectomy in diabetics. Iris neovascularization is more likely after lensectomy than when the lens is left in place [17]. Also, clinicians have long believed that intracapsular cataract extraction in diabetics promotes iris neovascularization [1]. Neovascularization of the iris is less frequent following extracapsular cataract extraction with an intact posterior capsule [16]. In an animal model, leaving an intact capsule decreases the incidence of neovascularization [14]. The lens capsule apparently acts as a barrier to diffusion of an angiogenic factor into the anterior segment. Interruption of this barrier by secondary laser capsulotomy may lead to neovascularization [22].

Neovascular glaucoma characteristically develops about 3 months after an ischemic central retinal vein occlusion. Even if the diagnosis has not been made previously by ophthalmoscopy, the patient will probably give a history of painless decrease in vision. When the fundus cannot be visualized as the result of corneal edema, ultrasonography should be performed to rule out either intraocular tumor or complete retinal detachment, which also serve as precursors to neovascular glaucoma.

When there is no definite predisposition or when inflammation is prominent, carotid vascular disease should be considered as a cause of ocular ischemia. The *ocular ischemic syndrome* from poor perfusion may also be a feature of some carotid-cavernous fistulas (see Chap. 12) (especially when the fistula was treated by carotid ligation) and of giant cell arteritis. Neovascular glaucoma develops after 25 to 45 percent of central retinal vein occlusions, but follows less than 5 percent of central retinal artery occlusions. Hence, an ischemic eye should be suspected when neovascularization follows central retinal artery occlusion. In the ocular ischemic syndrome, ophthalmodynametric pressures are extremely low, and there are often diffuse, midperipheral, punctate retinal hemorrhages *(carotid occlusion retinopathy)* [4–6]. Digital subtraction or conventional angiography is required to confirm the diagnosis and plan treatment.

Treatment

Management of neovascular glaucoma is difficult. Miotics are contraindicated since they increase the pain and have little effect on intraocular pressure. Carbonic anhydrase inhibitors and beta blockers seldom control pressures for long. Conventional filtering operations fail because fibrovascular growth closes the fistula, but modified procedures with draining valves and laser coagulation of neovascular tissues are sometimes effective [13, 18]. Atropine and topical corticosteroids may relieve pain in an eye with no visual potential; retrobulbar alcohol injection is sometimes required. Cyclocryotherapy is another alternative in a painful eye; however, eyes so treated seldom retain useful vision even if their pressure normalizes.

Because of the poor response of fully developed neovascular glaucoma to any treatment, the emergence of panretinal photocoagulation as an effective prophylaxis in some cases constitutes a major breakthrough. Ablation of the ischemic retina by photocoagulation or cryotherapy may even decrease the ischemic stimulus sufficiently to involute established neovascularization, with normalization of the intraocular pressure if a sufficient amount of the angle remains open. After a recent ischemic central retinal vein occlusion in which fluorescein angiography demonstrates extensive capillary nonperfusion, panretinal photocoagulation lowers the incidence of neovascular glaucoma. Similarly, prophylactic photocoagulation may be indicated after intracapsular cataract extraction or vitrectomy with lensectomy in diabetics. When the early stages of angle neovascularization are recognized at gonioscopy, direct photocoagulation of the new vessels *(goniophotocoagulation)* inhibits synechia formation temporarily, but does not treat the underlying ischemia. Goniophotocoagulation is also recommended before filtering surgery [20] and as a temporizing measure in the period immediately after panretinal photocoagulation.

Neovascular glaucoma as the result of carotid disease is a special case, since large arteries rather than small vessels are involved, and vascular surgery has the potential to reverse the ischemia. When the angle is closed by peripheral anterior synechiae, restoring the ocular circulation often worsens the glaucoma. The ischemic ciliary body is producing less aqueous, and the restoration of normal perfusion in an eye with severely impaired outflow increases the intraocular pressure. On the other hand, there are now a few cases in which carotid endarterectomy or bypass surgery has improved an ischemic eye [11, 12]. If this etiology is recognized before the angle changes are irreversible, such vigorous treatment may occasionally be rewarded.

1. Aiello, L.M., Wand, M., Liang, G. Neovascular glaucoma and vitreous hemorrhage following cataract surgery in patients with diabetes mellitus. *Ophthalmology* 90:814–820, 1983.
   In this series of 154 patients, intracapsular cataract extraction was associated with an increased risk of developing iris neovascularization.
2. Apple, D.J., Craythorn, J.M., Olson, R.J. Anterior segment complications and neovascular glaucoma following implantation of a posterior chamber intraocular lens. *Ophthalmology* 91:403–419, 1984.
   Neovascular glaucoma leading to enucleation is attributed to a posterior chamber intraocular lens with one haptic in the ciliary sulcus. No other predisposition was identified, but details of the evaluation for carotid disease are not given.
3. Brodell, L.P., Olk, R.J., Arribas, N.P., et al. Neovascular glaucoma: A retrospective analysis of treatment with peripheral panretinal cryotherapy. *Ophthalmic. Surg.* 18:200–206, 1987.
   In this series of 31 eyes, retinal cryotherapy alone or with limited cyclocryotherapy was successful in some patients with neovascular glaucoma and cloudy media.
4. Brown, G.C., Magargal, L.E., Schachat, A., et al. Neovascular glaucoma: Etiologic considerations. *Ophthalmology* 91:315–320, 1984.
   Twenty-seven of 208 patients with neovascular glaucoma evaluated at the Retinal Vascular Unit at Wills Eye Hospital had carotid occlusive disease, a higher percentage than has been recognized in other series.
5. Carter, J.E. Chronic ocular ischemia and carotid vascular disease. *Stroke* 16:721–728, 1985.
   This review includes a tabulation of 30 cases of chronic ocular ischemia and discusses therapeutic options from a neurologic as well as ophthalmologic viewpoint.
6. Coppeto, J.R., Wand, M., Bear, L., et al. Neovascular glaucoma and carotid artery obstructive disease. *Am. J. Ophthalmol.* 99:567–570, 1985.
   Two case reports exemplify the characteristics of this clinical entity.
7. Effron, L., Zakov, A.N., Tomsak, R.L. Neovascular glaucoma as a complication of the Wyburn-Mason syndrome. *J. Clin. Neuro-ophthalmol.* 5:95–98, 1985.
   This well-illustrated case report describes a new association.
8. Ehrenberg, M., McCuen, B.W. II, Schindler, R.H., et al. Rubeosis iridis: Preoperative iris fluorescein angiography and periocular steroids. *Ophthalmology* 91:321–325, 1984.
   Periocular steroids may have decreased the severity of postvitrectomy neovascularization.

9. Gartner, S., Henkind, P. Neovascularization of the iris (rubeosis iridis). *Surv. Ophthalmol.* 22:291–312, 1978.
   A review that lists reported etiologies and discusses pathophysiology.
10. Gu, X.Q., Fry, G.L., Lata, G.F., et al. Ocular neovascularization: Tissue culture studies. *Arch. Ophthalmol.* 103:111–117, 1985.
    An in vitro bioassay detects vasoproliferative activity in the aqueous, vitreous, and intraocular fluid (what remains in the eye after lensectomy and vitrectomy) of eyes with neovascularization.
11. Hauch, T.L., Busuttil, R.W., Yoshizumi, M.O. A report of iris neovascularization: An indication for carotid endarterectomy. *Surgery* 95:358–362, 1984.
    Vitreous hemorrhages led to the recognition of early neovascularization of the angle and bilateral carotid stenosis. The neovascularization was treated with goniophotocoagulation and regressed after carotid endarterectomy.
12. Kiser, W.D., Gonder, J., Magaragal, L.E., et al. Recovery of vision following treatment of the ocular ischemic syndrome. *Ann. Ophthalmol.* 15:305–310, 1983.
    Evaluation of a patient with steroid-unresponsive uveitis revealed iris neovascularization and carotid occlusive retinopathy. After cyclocryotherapy and peripheral retinal cryoablation, a temporal artery-middle cerebral artery bypass was performed with regression of neovascularization and restoration of good vision.
13. L'Esperance, F.A. Jr., Mittle, R.N., James, W.A. Jr. Carbon dioxide laser trabeculostomy for the treatment of neovascular glaucoma. *Ophthalmology* 90:821–829, 1983.
    These surgeons report success with a filtering procedure utilizing a laser knife.
14. Moffat, K., Blumenkranz, M.S., Hernandez, E. The lens capsule and rubeosis iridis: An angiographic study. *Can. J. Ophthalmol.* 19:130–133, 1984.
    Preservation of an intact anterior capsule reduced the incidence of iris neovascularization after pars plana lensectomy, vitrectomy, and iatrogenic retinal detachment in rabbit eyes.
15. Packer, A.J., Tse, D.T., Gu, X.Q., et al. Hematoporphyrin photoradiation therapy for iris neovascularization: A preliminary report. *Arch. Ophthalmol.* 102:1193–1197, 1984.
    A newer technique that may be both treatment and cause of neovascularization (see Arch. Ophthalmol. 102:839–842, 1984).
16. Poliner, L.S., Christianson, D.J., Escoffery, R.F., et al. Neovascular glaucoma after intracapsular and extracapsular cataract extraction in diabetic patients. *Am. J. Ophthalmol.* 100:637–643, 1985.
    In this retrospective study, neovascular glaucoma was significantly less common after extracapsular surgery than after intracapsular surgery in diabetics.
17. Rice, T.A., Michels, R.G., Maguire, M.G., et al. The effect of lensectomy on the incidence of iris neovascularization and neovascular glaucoma after vitrectomy for diabetic retinopathy. *Am. J. Ophthalmol.* 95:1–11, 1983.
    Removal of the lens increased the incidence of postvitrectomy neovascular glaucoma.
18. Schocket, S.S., Nirankari, V.S., Lakhanpal, V., et al. Anterior chamber tube shunt to an encircling band in the treatment of neovascular glaucoma and other refractory glaucomas: A long-term study. *Ophthalmology* 92:553–562, 1985.
    Another group reports success with a modified filtering procedure.
19. Shields, M.B., Proia, A.D. Neovascular glaucoma associated with an iris melanoma: A clinicopathologic report. *Arch. Ophthalmol.* 105:672–674, 1987.
    Neovascular glaucoma in an eye with an iris melanoma is most likely the effect of release of an angiogenic factor.
20. Simmons, R.J., Depperman, S.R., Kueker, D.K. The role of goniophotocoagulation in neovascularization of the anterior chamber angle. *Ophthalmology* 87:79–82, 1980.
    The indications for this procedure are reviewed.
21. Wand, M. Neovascular glaucoma. In R. Ritch and M.B. Shields (eds.), *The Secondary Glaucomas.* St. Louis: Mosby, 1982. Pp. 162–193.
    An extensive review with over 200 references.
22. Weinreb, R.N., Wasserstrom, J.P., Parker, W. Neovascular glaucoma following neodymium-YAG laser posterior capsulotomy. *Arch. Ophthalmol.* 104:730–731, 1986.
    Three cases in which posterior capsulotomy in diabetics was followed by neovascular glaucoma.

22. PRIMARY CONGENITAL GLAUCOMA

Glaucoma in early childhood is usually the consequence of maldevelopment of the eye. Various descriptions and classifications of these so-called developmental glaucomas have been offered. When the anomalies are largely confined to the angle structures, the resulting glaucoma is termed *primary congenital* (or *infantile*) *glaucoma*. Older terminology refers to the enlargement of the corneal diameter characteristic of this glaucoma: buphthalmos (literally, "ox eye") or hydrophthalmos. In one modern classification, this type of glaucoma is considered to represent *trabeculodysgenesis* [6].

Pathogenesis

The pathogenesis of primary infantile glaucoma is incompletely understood. However, it appears to represent either a maturation arrest or a maldevelopment of the trabecular meshwork and associated angle structures. This is often familial, with a genetically heterogeneous inheritance pattern. Isolated trabeculodysgenesis or primary congenital glaucoma is distinguished from those developmental glaucomas in which other anomalies predominate. These include the glaucomas associated with aniridia, Lowe's syndrome, and the phakomatoses, which are considered secondary infantile glaucomas.

Diagnosis

Primary congenital glaucoma presents with photophobia, epiphora, and blepharospasm in otherwise normal children. All these symptoms are effects of corneal edema. Examination reveals corneal enlargement and sometimes clouding. The cornea of normal infants is less than 10.5 mm in diameter; thus, a corneal diameter of 12 mm or greater suggests congenital glaucoma. Another cause of a large corneal diameter is congenital megalocornea, usually inherited as a sex-linked recessive. Megalocornea is also encountered in some families in which other members have congenital glaucoma; thus, it may also represent a forme fruste of primary congenital glaucoma. Other causes of corneal clouding include birth trauma and various corneal dystrophies and metabolic disorders. The combination of a corneal diameter of 12 mm or greater and tears in Descemet's membrane (sometimes called Haab's striae) is virtually pathognomonic for glaucoma.

Since the initial clinical evaluation is often inconclusive, an examination under anesthesia is usually undertaken. This includes accurate measurement of the corneal diameters, inspection of the disks, gonioscopy, and determination of the intraocular pressures. A-scan ultrasonography, if available, may be performed. Unfortunately, the utility of intraocular pressure measurement in this situation is limited because general anesthesia lowers intraocular pressure. When the level of anesthesia is light, as during induction or with ketamine, the pressure obtained may be more representative.

Disk cupping is less an indicator of permanent damage than in adults. Cupping may increase rapidly in immature eyes with elevated pressures and then decrease when the pressure returns to normal. This variability in cupping is probably a consequence of the flexibility of the lamina cribrosa in these eyes [13].

If the presence of glaucoma can be established from other criteria, gonioscopy is important in determining the type of glaucoma. If corneal edema is present, visualization of the angle is difficult unless the epithelium is removed, either with a blade or with a cotton swab soaked in alcohol. The angle in primary congenital glaucoma is open, with a deep anterior chamber, and may be indistinguishable from normal. In some eyes, abnormalities are recognizable, especially a subtle translucency overlying the trabecular meshwork. At one time this was thought to represent a membrane and was named Barkan's membrane after its describer; however, no discrete structure has been identified histologically. Rather, the trabecular meshwork appears immature and thickened.

Experienced clinicians emphasize that the recognition of congenital glaucoma may be difficult and may require repeated examinations under anesthesia. Once the diagnosis has been made, the definitive treatment is surgical. Medications may be indicated in the preoperative and postoperative periods, especially if corneal edema is prominent or the eye must be protected before further surgery. Systemic carbonic anhydrase inhibitors reliably lower intraocular pressure. Topical medications are less effective than in adult glaucoma, but some children respond to beta blockers.

Treatment

The classic operation for primary congenital glaucoma, *goniotomy,* is still considered the initial procedure of choice by many ophthalmologists. Goniotomy is performed by inserting a fine knife through the peripheral cornea into the anterior chamber and then, under gonioscopic guidance, incising the most superficial layers of the trabecular meshwork just below Schwalbe's line over about one-fourth of the angle. The disadvantage of goniotomy is that it is technically demanding, and an experienced surgeon and a skilled assistant are required. Corneal clouding makes accurate visualization of angle structures difficult. Some surgeons report close to 100 percent success in pressure control when surgery is performed when the patient is between the ages of 1 month and 2 years, although two goniotomies may be required. The major complications of goniotomy are due to the anesthesia, leading Shaffer and Hoskins to recommend bilateral surgery during one anesthesia [14]. Goniotomy is less successful in older children.

An alternative to goniotomy, also used when the angle cannot be well visualized and when two goniotomies have failed to control intraocular pressure, is *trabeculotomy,* usually performed ab externo. In trabeculotomy, a thin wire threaded into Schlemm's canal through a limbal incision is rotated into the anterior chamber through the trabecular meshwork. The surgery involved is more extensive than with goniotomy, increasing the risk of complications. Hyphemas often develop; however, most resolve spontaneously.

Filtering procedures—trabeculectomy and thermal sclerostomy—are usually reserved for eyes when goniotomy and trabeculotomy have failed. When the cornea is cloudy, a few surgeons prefer a primary filtering procedure to a trabeculotomy [3]. The low success rate of conventional filtering procedures in young patients has led to the use of draining implants [10].

The prognosis for vision in an eye with untreated primary congenital glaucoma is nil. Even when intraocular pressure can be controlled by surgery, the visual prognosis is guarded. When the eye enlarges, it becomes highly myopic, with the accompanying predisposition to retinal detachment and vulnerability to trauma. The cornea may be scarred or highly astigmatic, and many eyes become amblyopic. Intraocular pressure control is not necessarily permanent, and congenital glaucoma patients must be followed for the rest of their lives.

1. Beauchamp, G.R., Lubeck, D., Knepper, P.A. Glycoconjugates, cellular differentiation, and congenital glaucoma. *J. Pediatr. Ophthalmol. Strab.* 22:149–155, 1985.
   These initial histologic and biochemical studies on the development of the mouse trabecular meshwork promise a better understanding of congenital glaucoma.
2. Cadera, W., Pachtman, M.A., Cantor, L.B., et al. Congenital glaucoma with corneal cloudiness treated by thermal sclerostomy. *Can. J. Ophthalmol.* 20:98–100, 1985.
   In this series of nine patients with congenital glaucoma and corneal clouding, a primary filtering procedure was performed.
3. DeLuise, V.P., Anderson, D.R. Primary infantile glaucoma (congenital glaucoma). *Surv. Ophthalmol.* 28:1–19, 1983.
   This comprehensive review with 146 references is perhaps the best single source of information now available.
4. Demerais, F. Further analysis of familial transmission of congenital glaucoma. *Am. J. Hum. Genet.* 35:1156–1160, 1983.
   Statistical analysis of a large group of cases suggests genetic heterogeneity.
5. Hoskins, H.D. Jr., Hetherington, J. Jr., Magee, S.D., et al. Clinical experience with timolol in childhood glaucoma. *Arch. Ophthalmol.* 103:1163–1165, 1985.
   Timolol was effective in 31 of 40 patients with childhood glaucoma. Previous studies are tabulated.
6. Hoskins, H.D. Jr., Shaffer, R.N., Hetherington, J. Anatomical classification of the developmental glaucomas. *Arch. Ophthalmol.* 102:1331–1336, 1984.

The anomalies causing primary developmental glaucoma are grouped into three major categories: trabeculodysgenesis (which includes primary congenital glaucoma), iridodysgenesis, and corneodysgenesis.

7. Jerndal, T. Congenital glaucoma due to dominant goniodysgenesis. A new concept of the heredity of glaucoma. *Am. J. Hum. Genet.* 35:645–651, 1983.
   Although most families have followed an autosomal recessive inheritance, Jerndal presents an autosomal dominant pedigree of what he prefers to call dysgenic glaucoma.

8. Kiskis, A.A., Markowitz, S.N., Morin, J.D. Corneal diameter and axial length in congenital glaucoma. *Can. J. Ophthalmol.* 20:93–97, 1985.
   Ultrasonographic measurement of axial length was less sensitive than corneal diameter measurements in the detection of congenital glaucoma.

9. Luntz, M.H., Schenker, H.I. Congenital, infantile and juvenile glaucoma. In M.H. Luntz, R. Harrison, and H.I. Schenker (eds.), *Glaucoma Surgery.* Baltimore: Williams & Wilkins, 1984. Pp. 3–39.
   This monograph provides a well-illustrated description of one technique of trabeculotomy.

10. Molteno, A.C.B., Ancker, E., Van Biljon, G. Surgical technique for advanced juvenile glaucoma. *Arch. Ophthalmol.* 102:51–57, 1984.
    A two-stage placement of a draining implant was used in 83 eyes with only four failures.

11. Morgan, K.S., Black, B., Ellis, F.D., et al. Treatment of congenital glaucoma. *Am. J. Ophthalmol.* 92:799–803, 1981.
    These clinicians review the results in their consecutive series of 39 patients.

12. Morin, J.D. Primary infantile glaucoma: Influence of age at onset. *Can. J. Ophthalmol.* 18:233–234, 1983.
    When corneal enlargement or enlargement and clouding are actually present at birth, the prognosis of the glaucoma is worse than when the signs occur later.

13. Quigley, H.A. Childhood glaucoma: Results with trabeculotomy and study of reversible cupping. *Ophthalmology* 89:219–226, 1982.
    Quigley presents the results of 28 trabeculotomy ab externo operations and notes that reversal of cupping was encountered only during the first year of life.

14. Seidman, D.J., Nelson, L.B., Calhoun, J.H., et al. Signs and symptoms in the presentation of primary infantile glaucoma. *Pediatrics* 77:399–404, 1986.
    In 24 children presenting to the Wills Eye Hospital, corneal enlargement and clouding were often recognized before the classic triad of epiphora, photophobia, and blepharospasm, and 21 percent never had these signs.

15. Shaffer, R.N., Hoskins, H.D. Goniotomy in the treatment of isolated trabeculodysgenesis (primary congenital [infantile] developmental glaucoma). *Trans. Ophthalmol. Soc. U.K.* 103:581–585, 1983.
    These surgeons obtained good initial results with goniotomy but encountered a number of late complications.

16. Tawara, A., Inomata, H. Developmental immaturity of the trabecular meshwork in congenital glaucoma. *Am. J. Ophthalmol.* 92:508–525, 1981.
    The trabecular meshwork removed by trabeculectomy was studied in nine eyes. Thickened subcanalicular tissue was present in all specimens, and Schlemm's canal was absent in one.

17. Weinberger, D., Cohen, S., Wissenkorn, I., et al. Combined congenital glaucoma, pigmentary glaucoma, and high myopia in an infant. *J. Pediatr. Ophthalmol. Strab.* 22:147–148, 1985.
    Pigment in the angle and transillumination defects in the iris were found in a case of congenital glaucoma.

18. Wright, J.D. Jr., Robb, R.M., Kueker, D.K., et al. Congenital glaucoma unresponsive to conventional therapy: A clinicopathological case presentation. *J. Pediatr. Ophthalmol. Strab.* 20:172–179, 1983.
    A histopathologic study of the eyes of a child who died at age 3 months while under treatment for congenital glaucoma reveals various anterior segment anomalies.

23. TRAUMATIC HYPHEMA

Blood in the anterior chamber is termed *hyphema.* Hyphemas are graded according to the level of the blood when the head has been upright long enough to allow the cells to settle out of the aqueous. According to one classification, a grade I hyphema fills less than one-third of the chamber; grade II, one-third to one-half; and grade III, one-half or more [18]. If red cells are visible in the aqueous on slit lamp examination but there is no hyphema level, this is a *microhyphema.*

Pathogenesis
Hyphemas are encountered after surgery or penetrating injury and when there are fragile vessels in the anterior segment, as with anomalies, neovascularization, and tumors. By far the most common cause of hyphema, however, is blunt trauma to a previously normal eye. The force of the blow deforms and displaces the structures of the anterior eye, tearing vessels of the ciliary body or iris. A permanent change in the gonioscopic anatomy of the angle, the *angle recession,* is found in most eyes with a history of hyphema. A small percentage of such eyes eventually develop a secondary open-angle glaucoma, especially if the angle recession is large.

Treatment
Despite the frequency of hyphemas, the details of their appropriate management remain controversial. Unless there is intercurrent injury, the visual prognosis is good if the blood clears spontaneously. Rebleeding, which occurs 1 to 5 days after the initial injury in 6 to 38 percent of eyes, markedly worsens the prognosis. The problem of hyphema treatment is twofold: how to decrease the incidence of rebleeding and how to manage the rebleed if it happens.

Initial evaluation of an eye with hyphema should include measurement of visual acuity and intraocular pressure. An eye with a complete hyphema but with normal or low intraocular pressure has probably ruptured, and surgical exploration to repair the globe may be indicated. If the patient is black, a screening test for sickle cell trait should be performed. If the patient is on anticoagulants or aspirin, these medications should be stopped.

The traditional management of traumatic hyphema was hospitalization, bed rest with bilateral patching, and sedation as needed. Many ophthalmologists now modify this regimen in various ways. Patients who are hospitalized with patching and shielding of the traumatized eye, but without sedation or bed rest, appear to suffer no increased risk of rebleeding. There are studies to indicate that smaller hyphemas have a better prognosis, and some ophthalmologists do not admit patients with small hyphemas if they are in social situations where limited activities at home are possible, and the patient is able to return for daily reexaminations. Others believe that, since the risk of rebleeding exists even with small hyphemas, hospitalization permits better control of activity and facilitates reexamination.

In the large literature on hyphema, a variety of medications have been advocated to prevent rebleeding. These claims are difficult to evaluate because they are often contradictory. Cycloplegics, for example, are reported both to decrease and increase the chance of rebleeding. Systemic corticosteroid treatment is thought by some to decrease the incidence of secondary hemorrhage; however, no controlled, prospective study is available to support this proposition. Currently, the only drug successfully subjected to such study is aminocaproic acid, an antifibrinolytic agent [8–10]. Administration of this drug orally in dosages of either 50 or 100 mg/kg up to a maximum dosage of 5 gm every 4 hours (30 gm/day) has been demonstrated to reduce the incidence of rebleeding significantly. The side effects include nausea and vomiting, systemic hypotension, and light-headedness; thus, treated patients should be hospitalized. Also, this drug should not be administered to pregnant women or to patients with certain coagulation abnormalities.

The management of hyphema in blacks with sickle cell trait or in other patients with hemoglobinopathies is more difficult. These eyes, apparently sensitive to even moderate rises in intraocular pressure, are predisposed to develop optic atrophy or retinal infarction. Sickled cells in the anterior chamber clog aqueous outflow channels and cause the pressure to rise, and the treatment of elevated pressures with hyperosmolar agents or carbonic anhydrase inhibitors may induce further sickling by hemoconcentration or changes in the aqueous pH. Because of the role of hypoxia in sickling, administration of supplemental oxygen or even hyperbaric oxygen has been attempted.

The major complications of traumatic hyphema are glaucomatous optic atrophy, retinal vascular occlusion, and corneal blood staining. All three relate to increased intraocular pressure. Intraocular pressure is in turn a function of the amount of blood in the anterior chamber. The serious prognosis of rebleeds is largely because most rebleeds produce complete hyphemas. The blood in a complete hyphema in an eye with increased intraocular pressure often is very dark, an appearance known as a "black-ball" or "eightball" hyphema. In a very real sense, when this is present, both the doctor and the patient are behind the proverbial eight ball.

Treatment of a large hyphema causing elevated intraocular pressure initially consists of lowering the pressure and waiting for the blood to reabsorb. If some combination of topical and systemic antiglaucoma medications does not control the pressure, then surgical intervention becomes necessary. The precise timing of such surgery is debated. Various intraocular pressure criteria for surgery have been proposed; e.g., greater than 40 mm Hg for over 24 hours, greater than 50 mm Hg for 4 days, greater than 35 mm Hg for 6 days, or greater than 25 mm Hg for 6 days. Surgery also may be indicated to prevent peripheral anterior synechiae if a total hyphema has persisted for 5 days or a diffuse hyphema has persisted for 9 days. If sickle cell trait is present, intraocular pressure should probably not be allowed to remain above 24 mm Hg for any consecutive 24-hour period [6].

Surgical intervention is usually performed under general anesthesia. The simplest technique is anterior chamber paracentesis followed by refilling of the chamber with balanced salt solution [2]. Irrigation and aspiration by using a two-needle technique, a single irrigation-aspiration needle, or automated irrigation-aspiration devices is also possible. Occasionally, a firm, retracted clot resistant to these techniques requires a limbal incision with expression of the clot (which may be large and have an hourglass shape because of blood in the posterior chamber). Viscoelastic material may be used to force blood out of the eye [1]. An alternative to removal of blood from the anterior chamber is to perform a surgical iridectomy alone [11]. The success of simple iridectomy suggests that relief of the pupillary block produced by the blood clot lowers the intraocular pressure and thus allows time for reabsorption. A trabeculectomy may also function long enough for the hyphema to resolve.

1. Bartholomew, R.S. Viscoelastic evacuation of traumatic hyphema. *Br. J. Ophthalmol.* 71:27–28, 1987.
   Bartholomew's technique involves two incisions, with introduction of viscoelastic material through one to expel blood through the other.
2. Belcher, D.D., Brown, S.V.L., Simmons, R.J. Anterior chamber washout for traumatic hyphema. *Ophthalmic Surg.* 16:475–479, 1985.
   A series of 13 patients successfully treated by anterior chamber paracentesis includes 9 patients with postoperative hyphemas.
3. Beyer, T.L., Hirst, L.W. Corneal blood staining at low pressures. *Arch. Ophthalmol.* 103:654–655, 1985.
   Two corneas developed blood staining without a documented intraocular pressure rise.
4. Cassel, G.H., Jeffers, J.B., Jaeger, E.A. Wills Eye Hospital traumatic hyphema study. *Ophthalmic Surg.* 16:441–443, 1985.

A consecutive series of 100 cases confirms the well-known observation that trauma is more common in young men, but fails to identify specific risk factors that predict rebleeding.

5. Deutch, T.A., Feller, D.B. *Paton and Goldberg's Management of Ocular Injuries.* Philadelphia: Saunders, 1985. Pp. 188–198.
   The authors of this useful monograph favor hospitalization and atropinization as the initial management.

6. Deutch, T.A., Weinreb, R.N., Goldberg, M.F. Indications for surgical management of hyphema in patients with sickle cell trait. *Arch. Ophthalmol.* 102:566–569, 1984.
   A series of 22 hyphemas in blacks with sickle cell trait suggests that even primary hyphemas in these patients often require surgery if the pressure cannot be controlled within the first day.

7. Ganley, J.P., Geiger, J.M., Clement, J.R., et al. Aspirin and recurrent hyphema after blunt ocular trauma. *Am. J. Ophthalmol.* 96:797–801, 1983.
   Aspirin-induced platelet aggregation abnormalities predispose hyphemic eyes to rebleeding, and transfusion with fresh platelets may be indicated.

8. Kutner, B., Fourman, S., Brein, K., et al. Aminocaproic acid reduces the risk of secondary hemorrhage in patients with traumatic hyphema. *Arch. Ophthalmol.* 105:206–208, 1987.
   Another prospective, randomized, double-masked study of 34 patients demonstrates that aminocaproic acid reduces rebleeding.

9. McGetrick, J.J., Jampol, L.M., Goldberg, M.F., Frenkel, M., et al. Aminocaproic acid decreases secondary hemorrhage after traumatic hyphema. *Arch. Ophthalmol.* 101:1031–1033, 1983.
   The first prospective, double-blind, controlled study to demonstrate a significantly decreased incidence of rebleeding when aminocaproic acid is administered (see also the exchange of letters in Arch. Ophthalmol. *102:818–821, 1984).*

10. Palmer, D.J., Goldberg, M.F., Frenkel, M., et al. A comparison of two dose regimens of epsilon aminocaproic acid in the prevention and management of secondary traumatic hyphemas. *Ophthalmology* 93:102–108, 1986.
    Half of the original dosage, 50 mg/kg every 4 hours up to a maximum of 30 gm/day, reduced both rebleeding and side effects of dizziness, hypotension, and syncope.

11. Parrish, R., Bernardino, V. Jr. Iridectomy in the surgical management of eight-ball hyphema. *Arch. Ophthalmol.* 100:435–437, 1982.
    Improvement of complete hyphemas after peripheral iridectomies suggests that pupillary block is important, which also may explain why postoperative hyphemas when an iridectomy is present are usually benign.

12. Romano, P.E. Pro steroids for systemic antifibrinolytic treatment for traumatic hyphema. *J. Pediatr. Ophthalmol. Strab.* 23:92–95, 1986.
    This paper rehashes the steroids versus aminocaproic acid controversy. A companion paper by Crouch summarizes his approach to management.

13. Spoor, T.C., Hammer, M., Belloso, H. Traumatic hyphema: Failure of steroids to alter its course. A double-blind prospective study. *Arch. Ophthalmol.* 96:116–119, 1980.
    This negative prospective study has failed to convince proponents of steroids (see Romano's letter, Arch. Ophthalmol. *102:189–190, 1984).*

14. Thomas, M.A., Parrish, R.K. II, Feuer, W.J. Rebleeding after traumatic hyphema. *Arch. Ophthalmol.* 104:206–210, 1986.
    A series of 156 patients admitted for management of traumatic hyphema is analyzed; 16 percent rebled during hospitalization. The group of patients who rebled before hospitalization is also identified.

15. Wallyn, C.R., Jampol, L.M., Goldberg, M.F., et al. The use of hyperbaric oxygen therapy in the treatment of sickle cell hyphema. *Invest. Ophthalmol. Vis. Sci.* 26:1155–1158, 1985.
    An animal study of this potential therapy.

16. Wax, M.B., Ridley, M.E., Magargal, L.E. Reversal of retinal and optic disc ischemia in a patient with sickle cell trait and glaucoma secondary to traumatic hyphema. *Ophthalmology* 89:845–851, 1982.

This case report emphasizes the difficulties in the management of even primary hyphemas in patients with sickle cell trait.

17. Weiss, J.S., Parrish, R.K., Anderson, D.R. Surgical treatment of traumatic hyphema. *Ophthalmic Surg.* 14:343–345, 1983.

Seventy-five percent of patients with total hyphema eventually required surgery. The prognosis was better if this surgery was performed before 8 days had passed after development of the hyphema.

18. Wilson, F.M. II. Traumatic hyphema: Pathogenesis and management. *Ophthalmology* 87:910–919, 1980.

Wilson summarizes the information available at the end of the 1970s and offers an informed perspective on a number of controversies.

V. LENS

John W. Gittinger, Jr.

24. CONGENITAL CATARACTS

The evaluation and treatment of cataracts is more difficult in children than in adults. The immature visual system is vulnerable to deprivation amblyopia (see Chap. 27). In addition, visual acuity is difficult to quantitate in infants, and a cataract may be just one manifestation of more diffuse developmental abnormalities. Even the determination whether a cataract is indeed congenital is often uncertain, as many presumably congenital lens opacities are not discovered until the child is older. Pediatric cataracts are separable into several groups in terms of their etiology, visual prognosis, and appropriate management.

Pathogenesis
Most congenital cataracts with identifiable causes are hereditofamilial. Congenital cataracts that result from intrauterine infections such as rubella, rubeola, cytomegalovirus, herpes, toxoplasmosis, and syphilis constitute another large fraction. There are also a number of metabolic disorders (e.g., galactosemia, hypoglycemia, hypocalcemia), chromosomal disorders, and systemic syndromes with cataracts as one manifestation [15]. Associated malformations include persistent hyperplastic primary vitreous and posterior lenticonus or lentiglobus. Trauma and intraocular tumors sometimes induce congenital cataracts.

Diagnosis
Of equal importance to etiology in terms of the eventual visual prognosis are the density of the cataract and whether it is unilateral or bilateral. Many bilateral congenital cataracts are discrete opacities that are not very dense and that therefore allow formed images during visual development. With such cataracts, early surgery is probably contraindicated, as the initial operation creates an amblyogenic disparity between the two eyes. Surgery can be delayed until the early teens in a child with 20/50 to 20/70 acuity bilaterally without compromising function.

Treatment
Dense bilateral congenital cataracts should be removed within the first 8 weeks of life, before the deprivation of formed vision leads to nystagmus. Once nystagmus has become established, the prognosis for vision is poor. In one protocol, the two eyes are operated on within 48 hours of each other, with bilateral total occlusion maintained during the interoperative period [5]. Even when surgery is performed early in life, many children with bilateral dense cataracts evolve esotropias and never develop binocularity.

An eye with a purely unilateral cataract is less likely to achieve good acuity than eyes with partial bilateral cataracts. If there is to be any chance for useful vision, surgery must be undertaken within the first few months of life, followed by a vigorous antiamblyopia regimen. In most centers this consists of early fitting of an aphakic contact lens followed by occlusion of the good eye. The eyes of infants are difficult to fit, and their refraction changes rapidly with growth, requiring multiple refittings and re-refractions. Despite the best efforts of the physician and parents, the probability of success is so low that some pediatric ophthalmologists consider the risks of surgery and the emotional and financial trauma to the child and family greater than the potential benefits. Others argue that even if the acuity of the operated eye remains poor, it could have some useful peripheral vision, might be less likely to become strabismic, and has a better cosmetic appearance after surgery.

The question as to whether a unilateral cataract is truly congenital also bears on prognosis. Eyes with posterior lentiglobus appear to evolve cataracts over time, and their visual potential is better than eyes that have never had any formed vision. Certainly, eyes with traumatic cataracts are more likely to achieve good vision than those with developmental or congenital cataracts [6]. Unfortunately, some series lump all children with cataracts together, which makes interpretation of data difficult.

Because of the poor visual prognosis in eyes with unilateral congenital cataracts when conventional therapies are used, intraocular lens implantation has been attempted. Hiles, the major advocate of this approach in the United States, has reported a large series in which 17 percent of this approach in the United States, has reported a large series in which 17 percent of "infantile"—meaning detected any time from birth until the eighth birthday—cataractous eyes had acuities in the 20/20 to 20/40 range [8]. Most of the good acuities were achieved in children who received their implants after the age of 3 years, a result that would be surprising if these were unilateral, dense cataracts present from birth. This result suggests that a number of acquired cataracts, with correspondingly better prognosis, were included.

Of the series treated conventionally with contact lens correction, the best results are those of Beller and co-workers [1], in which seven of eight children achieved acuity in the 20/20 to 20/40 range. All these children had surgery before 2 months of age. Hiles has compared his results using conventional techniques with those obtained by lens implantation and believes that the two groups are similar [7]. A study from Israel in which lens implantation was performed between 3 and 25 months of age describes good results [2]. Despite the higher incidence of surgical complications, intraocular lens implantation remains a reasonable option for children with uniocular cataracts in whom contact lens fitting will be impossible.

An alternative surgical procedure that is less invasive than lens implantation is epikeratophakia. Children receiving these superficial corneal grafts had not yet reached an age at which visual acuity measurements are possible as of the initial report, so the visual results are not yet directly comparable with those of other approaches [12].

The surgical removal of congenital cataracts may be accomplished by using an irrigation-aspiration technique to perform a planned extracapsular extraction. In one surgical variant, the capsule is then stripped from the hyaloid face to produce a completed extracapsular extraction [4]. An alternative, currently considered the procedure of choice in many centers, is lensectomy with anterior vitrectomy using either a limbal or a pars plana approach. The material in an axial cataract may be very hard, and care must be taken to keep it out of the vitreous, where it may cause prolonged inflammation. Inflammation was also a significant problem in children with rubella embryopathy when two-stage extracapsular procedures were used, since active virus remained in the lens for a prolonged period after birth. Current single-stage operations prevent the immunologic exposure of the virus that incites this inflammation.

As has been aptly stated, the easiest part of the management of congenital cataracts is the surgery itself [6]. Especially with early surgery, considerable and prolonged efforts must be expended to assure formed vision and prevent deprivation amblyopia.

1. Beller, R., Hoyt, C.S., Marg, E., et al. Good visual function after neonatal surgery for congenital monocular cataracts. *Am. J. Ophthalmol.* 91:559–565, 1981.
   These authors report the best visual results ever obtained in eyes with congenital monocular cataracts using a regimen of early surgery, fitting of contacts lenses, and patching beginning within four postoperative days.
2. BenEzra, D., Paez, J.H. Congenital cataract and intraocular lens. *Am. J. Ophthalmol.* 96:311–314, 1983.
   In this group of six children who underwent implantation of intraocular lenses for monocular congenital cataracts, two achieved visual acuities of 20/40 (compared with 20/20 in the normal eye) and none had operative complications.
3. Birch, E.E., Stager, D.R., Wright, W.W. Grating acuity development after early surgery for congenital unilateral cataract. *Arch. Ophthalmol.* 104:1783–1787, 1986.
   Sixteen children who had cataract surgery in one eye before the age of 9 weeks had grating acuities determined by a preferential looking technique. The visual acuity was within the normal range up to the age of 1 year, but lagged during the next 3 years despite optical correction and amblyopia therapy.
4. Escapini, H. Intracapsular extraction of congenital cataract: Technique in two successive stages. *Am. J. Ophthalmol.* 66:683–687, 1968.
   Irrigation and aspiration are followed by removal of the capsule after enzymatic zonulysis.

5. Gelbart, S.S., Hoyt, C.S., Jastrebski, G., et al. Long-term visual results in bilateral congenital cataracts. *Am. J. Ophthalmol.* 93:615–621, 1982.
In these 24 infants operated on for bilateral congenital cataracts, good visual results were correlated with early surgery, short intervals between operations on the two eyes, bilateral occlusion in these intervals, and aggressive postoperative management of the refractive consequences of aphakia.

6. Helveston, E.M., Saunders, R.A., Ellis, F.D. Unilateral cataracts in children. *Ophthalmic Surg.* 11:102–108, 1980.
Fifty-eight children who had undergone cataract surgery at Indiana University had visual results that depended largely on their age at the onset of the cataract. The authors provide a critical review of the management of congenital cataracts.

7. Hiles, D.A. Visual acuities of monocular IOL and non-IOL aphakic children. *Ophthalmology* 87:1296–1300, 1981.
Hiles finds comparable results with contact lenses and intraocular lenses. Not unexpectedly, visual prognosis was better with acquired than with congenital (infantile) cataracts.

8. Hiles, D.A. Intraocular lens implantation in children with monocular cataracts 1974–1983. *Ophthalmology* 91:1231–1237, 1984.
Two hundred twenty-five intraocular lens implants in children, the largest reported series from the United States.

9. Jain, I.S., Pillai, P., Gangwar, D.N., et al. Congenital cataract: Management and results. *J. Pediatr. Ophthalmol. Strab.* 20:243–246, 1983.
This series from India, consisting largely of bilateral cataracts, details the complications in 146 eyes.

10. Kushner, B.J. Visual results after surgery for monocular juvenile cataracts of undetermined onset. *Am. J. Ophthalmol.* 102:468–472, 1986.
The visual results of surgery on monocular cataracts discovered in patients between the age of 1 and 5¼ were 20/50 or better when the eye was not microphthalmic (14 of 17 cases).

11. Lewis, T.L., Maurer, D., Brent, H.P. Effects on perceptual development of visual deprivation during infancy. *Br. J. Ophthalmol.* 70:214–220, 1986.
Asymmetrical optokinetic nystagmus and depression of the nasal field were among the sensory abnormalities detected in children with unilateral congenital cataract.

12. Migdal, C. Congenital cataracts—management and visual results (Cape Town 1956–1976). *J. Pediatr. Ophthalmol. Strab.* 18:13–21, 1981.
Migdal's experience with 123 cases is summarized. A significant proportion of the patients had mental retardation, which complicated management.

13. Morgan, K.S., Werblin, T.P., Asbell, P.A., et al. The use of epikeratophakia grafts in pediatric monocular aphakia. *J. Pediatr. Ophthalmol. Strab.* 18:23–29, 1981.
The initial results of a new and promising technique.

14. Morgan, K.S., Karcioglu, Z.A. Secondary cataracts in infants after lensectomies. *J. Pediatr. Ophthalmol. Strab.* 24:45–48, 1987.
In three cases of congenital cataracts removed by using extracapsular technique, postoperative opacities from growth of lens epithelium developed in spite of posterior capsulotomies and anterior vitrectomies.

15. Nelson, L.B. Diagnosis and management of cataracts in infancy and childhood. *Ophthalmic Surg.* 15:688–697, 1984.
Nelson reviews the literature, citing 170 references and tabulating the possible etiologies of cataracts in infancy and childhood.

16. Parks, M.M. Visual results in aphakic children. *Am. J. Ophthalmol.* 94:441–449, 1982.
An overview of the experience of a respected pediatric ophthalmologist.

17. Rogers, G.L., Tishler, C.L., Tsou, B.H., et al. Visual acuities in infants with congenital cataracts operated on prior to 6 months of age. *Arch. Ophthalmol.* 99:999–1003, 1981.
Seven infants with bilateral dense cataracts had surgery. All four children operated on before 10 weeks of age (range, 2–8 weeks) had vision measured as better than 6/60; the three children with surgery after this age (range, 12–32 weeks) had vision measured under 6/480.

25. ECTOPIA LENTIS

Displacement of the crystalline lens is called *subluxation* when the lens remains behind the pupil and *luxation* or *dislocation* when all the zonular attachments are broken and the lens falls free into the vitreous or is propelled forward into the anterior chamber. The description *ectopia lentis* is applied to any abnormality of lens position.

Pathogenesis
Ectopia lentis may be an isolated, heritable defect or it may occur in association with various systemic disorders, notably, Marfan's syndrome, homocystinuria, and Weill-Marchesani syndrome. Less important are hyperlysinemia, sulfite oxidase deficiency, Ehlers-Danlos syndrome, and various disorders in which the relationship between the lens dislocation and the primary process is unclear (see Table 25-1).

Familial simple ectopia lentis appears to be inherited as an autosomal dominant [1]. The onset of lens displacement is difficult to document, but may be recognized in early childhood. In some families, there is also correctopia or distortion of the pupil *(ectopia lentis et pupillae)* or accompanying blepharoptosis and high myopia.

Trauma is also an important cause of lens dislocation. At one time syphilis was thought to predispose patients to traumatic dislocation, but the incidence of positive serologies is about the same in a control population. Many patients with traumatic dislocations will have other injuries that limit the visual prognosis.

Diagnosis

Marfan's Syndrome
Marfan's syndrome is an autosomal dominant disorder; however, no specific metabolic defect has been defined. The possibility that familial ectopia lentis is a forme fruste of Marfan's syndrome has been raised, but this seems unlikely since the major clinical manifestations of Marfan's syndrome other than subluxed lenses (aortic dilatation, severe kyphoscoliosis, and deformity of the anterior thorax) have not been recognized in other members of these families.

In the subluxation observed with Marfan's syndrome, the lens moves superiorly or superotemporally and the zonules remain attached. Surprisingly, accommodation is normal for age. The eye is often highly myopic, with an increased incidence of retinal detachment and glaucoma. In a large series from an ophthalmology department, only 60 percent of patients with a putative diagnosis of Marfan's syndrome had subluxed lenses, and the ocular findings did not correlate well with the cardiovascular and skeletal manifestations [6].

Homocystinuria
The second large group of patients with a systemic disorder manifesting as ectopia lentis have a subtype of homocystinuria characterized by a defect in cystathionine beta-synthase [7]. The eyes are initially normal and then evolve lens subluxation that is virtually always downward. (A small percentage of Marfan's lenses sublux downward; conversely, upward dislocation in homocystinuria is distinctly rare.) By the age of 8 years, about half the children with homocystinuria have ectopia lentis. Overall, about 90 percent of homocystinurics develop lens displacement. Unlike the situation in Marfan's syndrome, the zonules break and may be seen on slit lamp biomicroscopy as a mat on the lens surface. The dislocated lens may cause pupillary block and be forced into the anterior chamber by aqueous pressure.

Another important consideration in homocystinuria is the increased incidence of thromboembolic events, including retinal vascular occlusions, which are thought to be the result of abnormal platelet function. Fatal thrombosis has developed following general anesthesia for ocular surgery, and it is important to screen any child or young adult with ectopia lentis for homocystinuria [4]. The cyanide-nitroprusside (also called sodium nitroprusside) test is performed by mixing 5 ml of urine from the patient with 2 ml of 5% sodium cyanide. After 10 minutes, two to four drops of sodium nitroprusside will

Table 25-1. Causes of ectopia lentis

Relatively common causes
  Trauma
  Familial
  Marfan's syndrome
  Homocystinuria
  Weill-Marchesani syndrome (dystrophia mesodermalis congenita hyperelastica)
Relatively uncommon causes (or significance uncertain)
  Alport's syndrome (hereditary nephritis and nerve deafness)
  Aniridia
  Crouzon's disease (craniofacial dysostosis)
  Ehlers-Danlos syndrome (fibrodysplasia hyperelastica)
  Klinefelter's syndrome
  Pfandler's syndrome
  Rieger's syndrome
  Treacher Collins syndrome (mandibulofacial dysostosis)

produce a bright red color if there is homocysteine or cystine in the urine. This screening test is not specific for homocystinuria, and amino acid analysis or enzymatic assay is necessary to establish the metabolic defect unequivocally.

The correct diagnosis is important because some children with homocystinuria respond to administration of pyridoxine (vitamin B_6). Early treatment, which may also include methionine dietary restriction, appears to decrease the incidence of lens dislocation and other complications including mental retardation and seizures. Other therapies directed at the thromboembolic complications are being attempted in pyridoxine-unresponsive patients.

Weill-Marchesani Syndrome
The third major disorder associated with ectopia lentis is the Weill-Marchesani syndrome [11]. Microspherophakia is characteristic, and the anterior chambers are shallow. Angle-closure glaucoma worsened by miotic therapy is a major complication of the Weill-Marchesani syndrome (see Chap. 19), and prophylactic laser iridectomies to prevent pupillary block have been recommended.

Treatment
The management of ectopia lentis is controversial. Most patients do not require surgery since they achieve good vision with either a phakic or an aphakic correction in place [9]. Mydriatics or photocoagulation have been used to enlarge the pupil or cause it to peak and thus increase the aphakic pupillary zone [5]. In children, anisometropic amblyopia is probably the most common cause of reduced vision. There are only a few indications for removal of a clear lens, and most posteriorly dislocated lenses may remain in place even if they are cataractous. Occasionally, a hypermature dislocated lens is responsible for phacolytic glaucoma (see Chap. 26) and must be removed. A lens in the anterior chamber should be treated because of the elevated intraocular pressure and the damage to the corneal endothelium caused by lens touch. The lens may be removed, or alternatively, a laser iridectomy is followed by miotic therapy.

Historically, the outcome in cataract extraction with subluxed or dislocated lenses has been limited by the high incidence of complications related to vitreous loss. Current surgical techniques for the removal of displaced lenses are more successful. When the lens is subluxed and becomes cataractous in an older patient, a modification of the intracapsular technique, including anterior vitrectomy if necessary, may be sufficient [14]. Subluxed cataracts in younger patients have been successfully managed by using an extracapsular technique without lens implantation [12]. Posteriorly dislocated lenses that are soft can be removed by pars plana lensectomy. When the lens is hard, a combination of pars plana technique and corneal section with lens extraction may be required [10].

1. Casper, D.S., Simon, J.W., Nelson, L.B., et al. Familial simple ectopia lentis: A case study. *J. Pediatr. Ophthalmol. Strab.* 22:227–230, 1985.
   Describes a family with nine members affected in three generations.
2. David, R., MacBeath, L., Jenkins, T. Aniridia associated with micro-cornea and subluxated lenses. *Br. J. Ophthalmol.* 62:118–121, 1978.
   Studies four family members from an African tribe.
3. Gillum, W.N., Anderson, R.L. Dominantly inherited blepharoptosis, high myopia, and ectopia lentis. *Arch. Ophthalmol.* 100:282–284, 1982.
   A mother and her two daughters had similar findings.
4. Hayasaka, S., Asano, Y., Tateda, H., et al. Lens subluxation in homocystinuria: A case report. *Acta Ophthalmol.* 62:425–431, 1984.
   The lens of a 6-year-old girl with homocystinuria and recurrent pupillary block glaucoma was extracted under general anesthesia after administration of pyridoxine and dextran to prevent thrombosis.
5. Lamba, P.A., Kuman, D.S., Arora, A. Xenon arc photocoagulation for treatment of subluxation of lens. *Br. J. Ophthalmol.* 69:291–293, 1985.
   Repositioning of the pupil with photocoagulation yielded good visual results in two cases.
6. Maumenee, I.H. The eye in the Marfan syndrome. *Trans. Am. Ophthalmol. Soc.* 79:684–733, 1981.
   An extensive analysis of a large series of patients.
7. Mudd, S.H., Skovby, F., Levy, H.L., et al. The natural history of homocystinuria due to cystathionine beta-synthase deficiency. *Am. J. Hum. Genet.* 37:1–31, 1985.
   A compilation of data on 629 patients with homocystinuria supports the effectiveness of early treatment with pyridoxine.
8. Nelson, L.B., Maumenee, I.H. Ectopia lentis. In W.A. Renie (ed.), *Goldberg's Genetic and Metabolic Eye Disease* (2nd ed.). Boston: Little, Brown, 1986. Pp. 389–410.
   An excellent review with over 200 references.
9. Nelson, L.B., Szymyd, S.M. Aphakic correction in ectopia lentis. *Ann. Ophthalmol.* 17:445–447, 1985.
   The prescription of an aphakic correction with atropine mydriasis improved visual function in two patients.
10. Peyman, G.A., Rauchand, M., Goldberg, M.F., et al. Management of subluxated and dislocated lenses with the vitreophage. *Br. J. Ophthalmol.* 63:771–778, 1979.
    This paper describes the use of pars plana vitrectomy instrumentation in surgery of posteriorly dislocated lenses.
11. Ritch, R., Wand, M. Treatment of the Weill-Marchesani syndrome. *Ann. Ophthalmol.* 13:665–667, 1981.
    An editorial discussing the specific problems related to this syndrome.
12. Seetner, A.A., Crawford, J.S. Surgical correction of lens dislocation in children. *Am. J. Ophthalmol.* 91:106–110, 1981.
    This paper describes the application of the irrigation-aspiration extracapsular technique to subluxed lenses in young persons.
13. Toczolowski, J.R. The use of sodium hyaluronate (Hyalcon) for the removal of severely subluxated lenses. *Ophthalmic Surg.* 18:214–216, 1987.
    Dense viscoelastic material is used to float a dislocated lens anteriorly.
14. Zaidman, G.W. The surgical management of dislocated traumatic cataracts. *Am. J. Ophthalmol.* 99:583–585, 1985.
    A personal series of seven cases in adults in whom good results were obtained by using modified intracapsular techniques.
15. Zuckerman, D., Lahav, M. A simple method for delivery of a subluxed lens. *Am. J. Ophthalmol.* 102:537–538, 1986.
    A maneuver to simplify delivery of a subluxed lens.

26. LENS-INDUCED GLAUCOMA AND INFLAMMATION

The terminology applied to lens-induced inflammations and glaucoma is confusing. *Phakomorphic glaucoma* refers to the secondary angle-closure glaucoma caused by an intumescent lens. The description *phacolytic glaucoma* denotes an acute, secondary open-angle glaucoma caused by leakage of lens protein from a cataractous lens. Alternative descriptions are *phacogenic* or *phacogenetic glaucoma*.

The description *phacoanaphylactic endophthalmitis* refers to an acute, severe anterior segment inflammation following cataract surgery, trauma, or, occasionally, spontaneous lens rupture. Lesser degrees of inflammation are sometimes called *phacotoxic uveitis*.

Pathogenesis

Lens-Induced Glaucoma
There are two major mechanisms by which the lens causes glaucoma. The first is pupillary block. An intumescent lens shallows the anterior chamber to produce angle-closure glaucoma, or a dislocated lens becomes trapped in the pupil and propelled forward into the anterior chamber by aqueous production (see Chap. 25). A dislocated lens also allows the vitreous face to come forward into the pupil and cause an "aphakic" pupillary block glaucoma.

The second basis for lens-induced glaucoma is release of lens protein from the capsular bag into the aqueous. This may occur spontaneously in the natural history of a cataract (usually when it has become hypermature) or result from trauma or surgery. Both the lens protein itself and the inflammatory reaction it incites may contribute to the pressure rise. The clinical picture is similar to that of an acute angle-closure or neovascular glaucoma (see Chaps. 19 and 21), with pain and markedly increased intraocular pressure in one eye. When the corneal edema is cleared with glycerin, however, gonioscopy reveals open angles without neovascularization. While the anterior chamber cellular reaction is not marked, flare from soluble proteins suspended in the aqueous is intense. Characteristically, white flocculent chunks of lens material circulate in the aqueous. Precipitates on the lens surface, thought to represent macrophages responding to proteins leaking through the capsule, are more common than keratitic precipitates. In some eyes an actual rupture in the capsule of the cataractous lens can be identified.

The macrophage cellular response is thought to be mediated through T lymphocytes. Circumstantial evidence suggests that a phacolytic reaction is more likely to occur in eyes of persons with a previous disturbance of their cell-mediated immune system. Clinical and experimental studies, however, support the proposition that the aqueous outflow channels in the trabecular meshwork are obstructed primarily by the large lens proteins, not by the macrophages [4, 5]. Aging of the lens may be required for these high-molecular-weight proteins to develop, as phacolytic glaucoma is rare in children or young adults.

Aqueous outflow obstruction is probably also the cause of the increased intraocular pressure that sometimes follows extracapsular cataract extraction or traumatic rupture of the lens. This has been termed *lens-particle glaucoma*. Instances of delayed lens-particle glaucoma following extracapsular surgery appear to result from dissolution of residual lens material, such as that contained in a Soemmering's ring cataract. A similar mechanism may explain some of the intraocular pressure rises seen after Nd-YAG laser posterior capsulotomy [12].

Lens-Induced Inflammation
The term *phacoanaphylaxis* is traditionally used for lens-induced inflammation, although the immune mechanisms involved are not those of true anaphylaxis. The immunologic basis for phacoanaphylactic inflammation appears to be a humoral response to lens protein. The lens proteins in the normal eye are semisequestered; that is, they are present only in low concentrations outside the lens. Exposure of the aqueous to large amounts of lens protein excites, in some persons, an autoimmune disorder that is antibody mediated and complement dependent. This disorder can be reproduced experimen-

tally. Subcutaneous injection of lens protein in an emulsion with Freund adjuvant followed by Ziegler knife injury to the lens results in a granulomatous endophthalmitis in mice, the percentage of which depends on the size of the antigen challenge [8].

Diagnosis

Lens-induced Glaucoma
The diagnosis of phacolytic glaucoma can be confirmed by evaluation of aqueous aspirates. Cells concentrated by passage of the aqueous through a Millipore filter are stained. After staining, cytologic examination by phase-contrast microscopy or light microscopy often enables macrophages to be identified [6]. Available assays for the high-molecular-weight proteins in the aqueous have not been widely utilized [5].

Lens-induced Inflammation
Phacoanaphylactic endophthalmitis may develop during the immediate postoperative period in any age group. The uveitis is granulomatous and must be distinguished from postoperative infection. In contrast to phacolytic glaucoma, the predominant inflammatory cell is usually the polymorphonuclear leukocyte. However, the granulomatous inflammation contains other cell types, including macrophages.

Phacoanaphylactic reactions are sometimes sympathetic; that is, they develop in the second eye after initial sensitization by capsule rupture or extracapsular cataract extraction. This etiology should always be considered with uveitis in the cataractous fellow eye of a unilateral aphakic eye. The tendency toward bilaterality is also an important consideration in the management of traumatic cataracts and in the choice of surgical technique in the second eye of a patient with a history of inflammation following extracapsular surgery. Early removal of traumatic cataracts may be warranted, and intracapsular cataract extraction has less chance of provoking a sympathizing reaction.

Treatment

Lens-induced pupillary block glaucoma often responds to laser iridectomy [13]. Despite their differences, the ideal therapy for both phacolytic glaucoma and phacoanaphylactic uveitis is the same: removal of the remaining lens material. In the instance of lens-particle glaucoma or phacotoxic uveitis, medical treatment may be successful, but the more severe cases in this spectrum are resistant. Most ophthalmologists proceed with surgery when a hypermature lens causes phacolytic glaucoma, and dramatic visual improvement may result even when, preoperatively, the eye has only light perception with poor projection. Phacolytic glaucoma is one of the remaining indications for intracapsular cataract extraction, although careful extracapsular surgery is still possible.

The situation in phacoanaphylactic uveitis is different. The possibility of phacoanaphylaxis is often not even considered, and the inflammation is attributed to the trauma, to infection, or to a "toxic lens syndrome" provoked by the implant [1, 9, 11]. In most reported cases, the correct diagnosis has been made only by pathologic examination of the enucleated eye. The recent transition from intracapsular surgery to extracapsular surgery has increased the likelihood of this complication and should encourage earlier recognition and treatment.

1. Apple, D.J., Mamalis, N., Steinmetz, R.L., et al. Phacoanaphylactic endophthalmitis associated with extracapsular cataract extraction and posterior chamber intraocular lens. *Arch. Ophthalmol.* 102:1528–1532, 1984.
   Postoperative inflammation that was initially responsive to steroids eventually led to removal of the intraocular lens 6 months after its insertion with the diagnosis of toxic lens syndrome. This did not save the eye, which on pathology examination demonstrated a granulomatous reaction centering about residual lens material.
2. Brinkman, C.J.J., Broekhuyse, R.M. Cell mediated immunity in relation to cataract and cataract surgery. *Br. J. Ophthalmol.* 63:301–305, 1979.
   Sensitization of peripheral lymphocytes to lens protein was present in some patients with cataracts. The sensitization increased with extracapsular cataract extraction and was absent in normal eyes and after intracapsular cataract extraction.

3. Epstein, D.L. Diagnosis and management of lens-induced glaucoma. *Ophthalmology* 89:227–230, 1982.
   A brief clinical review by an authority.
4. Epstein, D.L., Jedziniak, J.A., Grant, W.M. Obstruction of aqueous outflow by lens particles and by heavy-molecular-weight soluble lens proteins. *Invest. Ophthalmol. Vis. Sci.* 17:272–277, 1978.
   Both lens particles and soluble lens proteins can obstruct aqueous outflow in enucleated human eyes.
5. Epstein, D.L., Jedziniak, J.A., Grant, W.M. Identification of heavy-molecular-weight soluble protein in aqueous humor in human phacolytic glaucoma. *Invest. Ophthalmol. Vis. Sci.* 17:398–402, 1978.
   High-molecular-weight proteins were identified by agarose gel chromatography in the aqueous of six eyes with phacolytic glaucoma. Hypermature cataracts had a 14-fold increase in these proteins over the level in immature cataracts.
6. Goldberg, M.F. Cytological diagnosis of phacolytic glaucoma utilizing Millipore filtration of the aqueous. *Br. J. Ophthalmol.* 52:847–853, 1967.
   Goldberg describes the use of Papanicolaou staining of filtered aqueous in diagnosis.
7. Khalil, M.K., Lorenzetti, D.W. Lens-induced inflammations. *Can. J. Ophthalmol.* 21:96–102, 1986.
   This series includes two cases in which the clinical picture was that of phacoanaphylactic endophthalmitis, but the cellular reaction consisted largely of macrophages. These are termed phacolytic endophthalmitis.
8. Marak, G.E. Jr., Font, R.L., Alepa, F.P. Immunopathogenicity of lens crystallins in the production of experimental lens-induced granulomatous endophthalmitis. *Ophthalmol. Res.* 10:30–35, 1978.
   Experimental lens-induced granulomatous endophthalmitis is the animal model for phacoanaphylactic endophthalmitis.
9. McMahon, M.S., Weiss, J.S., Riedel, K.G., et al. Clinically unsuspected phacoanaphylaxis after extracapsular cataract extraction with intraocular lens implantation. *Br. J. Ophthalmol.* 69:836–840, 1985.
   Severe postoperative inflammation thought to represent infection was discovered after enucleation to be phacoanaphylactic endophthalmitis.
10. Müller-Hermelink, H.K. Recent topics in the pathology of uveitis. In E. Kraus-Mackiw and G.R. O'Connor (eds.), *Uveitis: Pathophysiology and Therapy.* New York: Thieme-Stratton, 1983. Pp. 152–197.
    Müller-Hermelink distinguishes six pathologic types of lens-induced reactions.
11. Perlman, E.M., Albert, D.M. Clinically unsuspected phacoanaphylaxis after ocular trauma. *Arch. Ophthalmol.* 95:244–246, 1977.
    Three eyes with posttraumatic cataract and chronic inflammation were found to have phacoanaphylaxis when examined pathologically.
12. Richter, C.U., Arzeno, G., Pappas, H.R., et al. Intraocular pressure elevation following Nd:YAG laser posterior capsulotomy. *Ophthalmology* 92:636–640, 1985.
    Capsulotomy produced a mean pressure increase of 13 mm Hg in 21 eyes, with a corresponding reduction in outflow facility.
13. Ritch, R. Glaucoma secondary to lens intumescence and dislocation. In R. Ritch and M. B. Shields, (eds.), *The Secondary Glaucomas.* St. Louis: Mosby, 1982. Pp. 131–149.
    A review with 93 references.

VI. STRABISMUS AND AMBLYOPIA

John W. Gittinger, Jr.

Amblyopia is unilateral or bilateral reduction in vision with no recognizable ocular abnormalities. An eye is said to be amblyopic when its visual acuity is reduced despite adequate optical correction in the absence of any apparent structural cause. Amblyopia as strictly defined is the result of physiologic processes active only in the immature visual system. In a looser sense, the term amblyopia is also sometimes attached to a group of optic neuropathies in which ophthalmoscopic findings are not prominent—*toxic, tobacco-alcohol,* or *nutritional amblyopia*—and is also applied to functional visual loss (see Ch. 65). In addition, the description "functional amblyopia" may be used to distinguish the component of physiologic amblyopia that is reversible by treatment (in contrast to "organic amblyopia").

Pathogenesis
Classification of amblyopia is difficult because the underlying physiology is not completely understood. One major mechanism for amblyopia is *deprivation,* the failure to present a formed visual image to the retina during a critical period in development. Another mechanism is *suppression,* the active turning off of visual input from one eye, probably at the cortical level. The commonest causes of amblyopia are strabismus and anisometropia. In strabismic amblyopia, suppression is more important; in anisometropia, deprivation predominates. Both mechanisms are sometimes active in the same eye, and it may be difficult to define their relative contributions.

Deprivation is the primary cause of amblyopia in eyes in which a medial opacity is present in early childhood, such as with unilateral ptosis or cataract. On the other hand, an eye with a cataract often has other associated developmental abnormalities that limit its potential visual acuity. Similarly, there is a "chicken-egg" problem with strabismic amblyopia (Does the visual abnormality cause the strabismus or does the strabismus cause the decreased vision?). The observation that amblyopia is not commonly found with large-angle, congenital esotropias unless they are operated on and made into small-angle esotropias supports the importance of suppression. Bilateral amblyopia is less common than unilateral amblyopia; however, bilateral amblyopia occurs when there are large refractive errors *(ametropic amblyopia)* or bilateral medial opacities, and thus it is a type of deprivation amblyopia. Rarely, reversible unilateral amblyopia is encountered in the absence of any known cause [14].

Diagnosis
Recognition of amblyopia in young children is important, since treatment is more successful when it is begun at an early age. In the strabismic child, amblyopia is usually detected by fixation behavior [18]. Free alternation of fixation between the two eyes implies equal vision. When the child objects to having one eye covered or fails to take up or hold fixation with the other, amblyopia is likely. Other methods of measuring visual acuity in young children, such as the visual evoked potential and preferential looking techniques, have yet to prove their value in detection of amblyopia [5, 6, 9].

Screening for amblyopia with subjective tests is usually possible when a child reaches the age of 3 or 4 years. Care must be taken in the interpretation of acuities obtained by presentation of single optotypes, since amblyopic eyes characteristically have better responses with individual symbols than with lines, an effect called the *crowding phenomenon.* Tests for stereopsis, such as the random-dot stereogram, have theoretical advantages over standard optotypes and are under evaluation in screening programs [12].

Treatment
Once amblyopia has been identified, treatment should be undertaken as soon as possible. In refractive amblyopia, an appropriate correction is prescribed. There is some evidence that unilateral high myopia causing anisometropic amblyopia should be managed by spectacle correction rather than with a contact lens to minimize anisoconia.

The standard treatment for amblyopia in the United States is occlusion of the nonamblyopic eye with an opaque adhesive patch. (In Europe the application of neutral-density "Einschleich" filters to glasses is also considered a form of occlusion [8].) In young children there is a risk of inducing a deprivation amblyopia of the good eye by occlusion, and the patching regimen must be monitored closely. For this reason, many clinicians avoid full-time occlusion in children under the age of 1 year. Part-time occlusion may also be indicated for older children, who often refuse to wear a patch because of the visual or social handicap this presents.

Part-time occlusion is often augmented by some visual activity that encourages use of the amblyopic eye. There has been considerable interest in a type of part-time occlusion in which rotating grating patterns, thought to represent an optimal stimulus, are presented to the amblyopic eye by a therapist for periods as brief as 7 minutes a week, with no other occlusion [10]. This probably represents only a variant of the so-called minimal occlusion therapy, the important factors being known compliance and concentration on a visually complicated task, rather than the nature of the grating pattern [4]. In some controlled series, this technique has not been as successful as occlusion in equalizing visual acuity [8]. At present, minimal occlusion is best considered a secondary alternative, along with penalization (see below), when full-time occlusion is not possible.

Penalization of the nonamblyopic eye may be warranted when the child or parents are unable to cooperate or the child is allergic or sensitive to the adhesive on the occluder. Various methods of penalization are used, depending on the refractive state of the eyes [13]. Penalization for near use, for example, involves atropinization and full correction for distance of the normal eye, while the amblyopic eye is overcorrected by 1 to 3 diopters to encourage its use for near work.

Treatment is continued until the visual acuity is equal to that of the nonamblyopic eye or until the vision in the amblyopic eye has not improved for 3 months. Once amblyopia has been successfully treated, the acuity must be monitored until the visual system is mature—about age 9 or 10 years—to be sure amblyopia does not recur. Recurrence is more likely when the initial visual acuity was low [3].

The treatment of amblyopia in older children and adults is difficult. Older children tend to be less compliant, but improvement is still possible with the use of occlusion [11]. Mild degrees of amblyopia are more likely to respond than is severe amblyopia. A special class of patients are those adults who have lost vision in their nonamblyopic eye [13]. In monocular adult amblyopes, pleoptic therapy, involving the stimulation of the fovea with special ophthalmoscopes, may be warranted. Pleoptics, which is tedious and expensive, is seldom used in the United States for childhood amblyopia.

Another special class of patients is the group with organic lesions. Some children with structural ocular abnormalities and reduced vision may have a combination of organic visual loss and amblyopia, and thus have a potential for improvement [7]. This possibility is suggested by a better acuity for letters than for lines or by a minimal decrease in acuity when a neutral density filter is interposed, both characteristics of amblyopic sight. A trial of occlusion is then warranted even in the presence of ocular disease.

1. Cadera, W., Pachtman, M.A., Ellis, F.D., et al. Depth of strabismic amblyopia determined with neutral density filters. *Am. J. Ophthalmol.* 95:763–766, 1983.
   The depth of amblyopia is quantitated by using neutral-density filters and fixation behavior.
2. Campos, E.C., Gulli, R. Lack of alternation in patients treated for strabismic amblyopia. *Am. J. Ophthalmol.* 99:63–65, 1985.
   Even when equal visual acuity was obtained, about one-half of patients with strabismic amblyopia fail to alternate. Alternation is not a reliable measure of visual acuity in treated amblyopes.
3. Ching, F.C., Parks, M.M., Friendly, D.S., et al. Practical management of amblyopia. *J. Pediatr. Ophthalmol. Strab.* 23:12–16, 1986.
   In a series of 116 patients treated with either full-time or part (half)-time occlusion before the age of 5 years, equal acuity was achieved in 82 percent. Those with poor vision initially were likely to regress and required part-time maintenance occlusion.
4. Fricker, S.J., Kuperwaser, M.C., Stromberg, A.E., et al. Stripe therapy for amblyopia with a modified television game. *Arch. Ophthalmol.* 99:1596–1599, 1981.

The presence or absence of stripes (equivalent to gratings) in a television game played with the nonamblyopic eye occluded made no difference in the visual result. Good vision was achieved in many patients by using eight to twelve 20-minute sessions at weekly intervals.

5. Friendly, D.W., Weiss, I.P., Barnet, A.B., et al. Pattern-reversal visual-evoked potentials in the diagnosis of amblyopia in children. *Am. J. Ophthalmol.* 102:329–339, 1986.
   In a series of 27 children with anisometropic amblyopia and four normal children, there were five false-negatives and one false-positive.

6. Hoyt, C.S., Jastrzebski, G.B., Marg, E. Amblyopia and congenital esotropia: Visually evoked potential measurements. *Arch. Ophthalmol.* 102:58–61, 1984.
   Amblyopia was uncommon in congenital esotropia until after surgery. These clinicians find visual evoked potentials to be useful in the evaluation of amblyopia.

7. Kushner, B.J. Functional amblyopia associated with abnormalities of the optic nerve. *Arch. Ophthalmol.* 102:683–685, 1984.
   Seven patients with optic nerve abnormalities responded to occlusion therapy.

8. Lennerstrand, G., Samuelsson, B. Amblyopia in 4-year-old children treated with grating stimulation and full-time occlusion: A comparative study. *Br. J. Ophthalmol.* 67:181–190, 1983.
   During the initial treatment period, minimal occlusion and grating stimulation were as effective as full-time occlusion or occlusion with neutral-density filters. The acuity was only obtained after longer-term occlusion in strabismic amblyopia.

9. Mayer, D.L., Fulton, A.B. Preferential looking grating acuities of infants at risk of amblyopia. *Trans. Ophthalmol. Soc. U.K.* 104:903–911, 1985.
   There were minimal differences between acuities in esotropic patients with a strong fixation preference as determined by preferential looking. This may be the result of a different neural basis for acuity in strabismic amblyopia.

10. Nyman, K.G., Singh, G., Rydberg, A., et al. Controlled study comparing CAM treatment with occlusion therapy. *Br. J. Ophthalmol.* 67:178–180, 1983.
    The results of total occlusion or neutral-density filter occlusion did not differ from those obtained with CAM (a grating stimulator) therapy.

11. Oliver, M., Neumann, R., Chaimovitch, Y., et al. Compliance and results of treatment for amblyopia in children more than 8 years old. *Am. J. Ophthalmol.* 102:340–345, 1986.
    The difference in the outcome of occlusion therapy in older children seems largely to be the result of poorer compliance. A compliant older child should be treated.

12. Ruttum, M.S., Bence, S.M., Alcorn, D. Stereopsis testing in a preschool vision screening program. *J. Pediatr. Ophthalmol. Strab.* 23:298–302, 1986.
    Stereoscopic testing at a threshold of 600 seconds of arc was used in conjunction with acuity testing in over 6000 children.

13. Vereecken, E.P., Brabant, P. Prognosis for vision in amblyopia after the loss of the good eye. *Arch. Ophthalmol.* 102:220–224, 1984.
    In a series of 144 cases collected by a questionnaire, 41 patients had improved vision with treatment. Pleoptics seemed beneficial.

14. von Noorden, G.K. Idiopathic amblyopia. *Am. J. Ophthalmol.* 100:214–217, 1985.
    Two cases in which no causative factors were identified.

15. von Noorden, G.K., Attiah, F. Alternating penalization in the prevention of amblyopia recurrence. *Am. J. Ophthalmol.* 102:473–475, 1986.
    Alternate-day penalization is effective prophylaxis against recurrence in patients who have already received occlusion therapy for amblyopia.

16. von Noorden, G.K., Avilla, C., Sidikaro, Y., et al. Latent nystagmus and strabismic amblyopia. *Am. J. Ophthalmol.* 103:87–89, 1987.
    Conventional occlusion therapy of amblyopia was successful in 11 of 12 patients with latent nystagmus.

17. Watson, P.G., Sanac, A.S., Pickering, M.S. A comparison of various methods of treatment of amblyopia: A block study. *Trans. Ophthalmol. Soc. U.K.* 104:319–328, 1985.
    In a comparison of conventional occlusion, minimal occlusion, and CAM (grating stimulation) therapy all were equally effective initially, but some patients benefited from another form of therapy.

18. Werner, D.B., Scott, W.E. Amblyopia case reports—bilateral hypermetropic ametropic amblyopia. *J. Pediatr. Ophthalmol. Strab.* 22:203–205, 1985.
   Six patients with bilateral hypermetropia and amblyopia responded to spectacle correction.
19. Wright, K.W., Edelman, P.M., Walonker, F., et al. Reliability of fixation preference testing in diagnosing amblyopia. *Arch. Ophthalmol.* 104:549–553, 1986.
   Fixation preference was reliable for deviations larger than 10 diopters. A 10-prism diopter test is described for use with smaller deviations and straight eyes.

28. CONGENITAL ESOTROPIA

Any esotropia noted during the first 6 months of life has been classified as congenital, although few deviations are established when the neonate first opens his eyes. The typical features of *congenital esotropia* are virtually never present at birth [11]. Examination of neonates reveals more who are exotropic than esotropic. In addition, disconjugate eye movements and even transient supranuclear disturbances are noted. Otherwise normal neonates with transient skew deviations may evolve the classic findings of congenital esotropia by 6 months of age (see Chap. 57, reference 5). Alternative terminologies to congenital esotropia are *infantile esotropia, essential infantile esotropia, congenital-infantile esotropia,* and *connatal esotropia.*

Pathogenesis
The incidence of congenital esotropia is as high as 1 percent of the population. Within this large group delimited by only one finding, there are several different etiologic groups. Although most congenital esotropias are assumed to be nonaccommodative, occasional instances of accommodative esotropia presenting early in life are encountered (see Chap. 29). Another identifiable cause is the *nystagmus blockage syndrome,* a compensatory esotropia that develops in a child with congenital nystagmus that damps on convergence [15]. This mechanism may also explain cases of unilateral esotropia following enucleation of one eye in early infancy [4]. Abducting nystagmus is common enough in congenital esotropia to have been designated the *Ciancia syndrome* [14]. Sixth nerve palsies must be included in the differential diagnosis, but are rare in infancy.

Diagnosis
Despite this potential heterogeneity, most children with congenital esotropias have a surprisingly consistent clinical picture. The deviation is large, usually 50 prism diopters or more. Amblyopia is relatively uncommon as compared with its incidence in acquired esotropias. The child often uses an alternation strategy known as *cross fixation,* looking to the right with the left eye and vice versa. The resulting lack of abduction may be misinterpreted as bilateral sixth nerve palsies, but vanishes with patching of one eye. Many children with congenital esotropia eventually develop inferior oblique overaction, producing a vertical component to their deviation. Also associated are *latent nystagmus* and the peculiar eye movement abnormality known as *dissociated vertical divergence* (or dissociated vertical deviation or alternating circumduction), both of which are rarely features of other types of strabismus.

Treatment
The initial evaluation of a child with congenital esotropia, as of any child with strabismus, should include a cycloplegic refraction and dilated fundus examination. Once ophthalmic pathology and an accommodative component have been identified or excluded, and any amblyopia has been treated (see Chap. 27), the important considerations are the timing and type of corrective surgery.

Unlike accommodative esotropia, in which there is a reasonable presumption that normal binocular function has been present at least for a short time, most congenital esotropia precludes the establishment of binocularity. There is still debate as to whether the esotropia develops because of an inherent inability to fuse or whether the abnormal binocular function is the result of misalignment of the eyes during a critical period in visual system development. If the former hypothesis is correct, then it should make little difference at what age the eyes are aligned. If the latter obtains, then early surgery could be more successful.

The case for delaying surgery can be summarized as follows. Some children with esotropia have variable deviations that may spontaneously improve with time. (This is certainly true of congenital esotropia in children with congenital encephalopathies, and even advocates of early surgery avoid intervention in such cases.) Also, the accuracy of the measurement of the deviation and the ability of the child to cooperate with postoperative orthoptics or glasses increases with age. The eye grows considerably during the first 2 years of life, and the effects of early surgery may be unpredictable. This in turn potentially exposes the child to repeated operations and anesthesias, which constitute the major risk of strabismus surgery. Since true binocular vision will never be achieved, the best potential result being a so-called monofixation syndrome, delaying surgery is reasonable. Only the most extraordinary case ever achieves bifixation [12].

The alternative arguments favoring early surgery are that the sensory results are better when the eyes are aligned in infancy and that complicating factors, such as dissociated vertical divergence, latent nystagmus, and inferior oblique overaction, are less likely to have developed. Leaving the eyes deviated for too long may also allow conjunctival shortening and contracture of the medial rectus muscles, making surgery technically more difficult. Early surgery has potential psychosocial advantages for the child and family.

The data available are far from conclusive. Successful surgical alignment is usually defined as less than 10 prism diopters of residual deviation. In one series, fusion (defined here as the ability to see the Worth four-dot test) was present in 11 of 12 patients whose eyes were aligned before the age of 9 months and in only 14 of 26 whose eyes were aligned between the ages of 10 and 24 months [17]. In another series, 62 of 66 patients whose eyes were aligned before the age of 12 months had (Worth) fusion, as did 22 of 24 patients whose eyes were aligned between the ages of 13 months and 24 months. Only 5 of 16 patients whose eyes were aligned after the age of 2 years achieved fusion [5]. Thus, in one group the age of 9 months appears to be critical, whereas in the other group 24 months is the watershed. In still another series, no child with congenital esotropia operated on before the age of 12 months achieved stereopsis, whereas some who had later surgery did [3].

Once the decision to operate has been made, the procedure performed is usually either symmetrical recessions of the medial rectus muscles or a medial rectus recession and a lateral rectus resection on one eye. Because of the high incidence of undercorrections and the advantages of achieving alignment after one operation, attempts are being made to increase the effectiveness of the initial surgery. These include larger recessions, beyond the 5 mm once considered the maximum recession possible without crippling the medial rectus, and augmentation of medial rectus recessions by en bloc recession of the conjunctiva [1, 16]. If inferior oblique overaction is present, these muscles are often simultaneously weakened. A few surgeons operate on three (usually both medial recti and one lateral rectus) or even four horizontal muscles initially when the deviation is very large and the child is older.

---

1. Barsoum-Homsy, M. Medial rectus insertion site in congenital esotropia. *Can. J. Ophthalmol.* 16:181–186, 1981.
   The mean distance of the insertion site of the medial rectus from the limbus in eyes with congenital esotropia was 4.5 mm in this series, suggesting that large recessions are possible without putting the insertion behind the equator.
2. Bateman, J.B., Parks, M.M., Wheeler, N. Discriminant analysis of congenital esotropia surgery: Predictor variables for short- and long-term outcomes. *Ophthalmology* 90:1146–1153, 1983.

A smaller preoperative deviation and earlier surgery were associated with the eventual development of some degree of stereopsis.

3. Helveston, E.M., Ellis, F.D., Schott, J., et al. Surgical treatment for congenital esotropia. *Am. J. Ophthalmol.* 96:218–228, 1983.
   In this retrospective series of 133 early-onset esotropias (not all noted before the age of 6 months), those congenital esotropes who had surgery before the age of 12 months did not develop steropsis, whereas some who had surgery after this age did. The authors offer a theory to explain this unexpected result.

4. Helveston, E.M., Pinchoff, B., Ellis, F.D., et al. Unilateral esotropia after enucleation in infancy. *Am. J. Ophthalmol.* 100:96–99, 1985.
   Five children had their remaining eye move into adduction after an enucleation during infancy. Various etiologic factors are considered.

5. Ing, M.R. Early surgical alignment for congenital esotropia. *Ophthalmology* 90:132–135, 1983.
   A compilation of 162 patients suggests that some binocularity is achieved more often when the eyes are aligned before 2 years of age.

6. Kraft, S.P., Scott, W.E. Surgery for congenital esotropia—an age comparison study. *J. Pediatr. Ophthalmol. Strab.* 21:57–68, 1984.
   This overlong and somewhat turgid paper analyzes the results in 79 patients managed at the University of Iowa.

7. Kushner, B.J. A randomized comparison of surgical procedures for infantile esotropia. *Am. J. Ophthalmol.* 98:50–61, 1984.
   In the hands of these surgeons, a standard recession of 10.5 mm from the limbus was more effective than a graded recession of up to 6 mm from the insertion.

8. Lang, J. The optimum time for surgical alignment in congenital esotropia. *J. Pediatr. Ophthalmol. Strab.* 21:74–77, 1984.
   A position paper, to be contrasted with Ing's views in the same journal issue.

9. Lee, D.A., Dyer, J.A. Bilateral medial rectus muscle recession and lateral rectus muscle resection in the treatment of congenital esotropia. *Am. J. Ophthalmol.* 95:528–535, 1983.
   These surgeons report good results from performing the initial surgery on from four to six muscles: 4.5- to 5-mm recession of the medial rectus and 4- to 8-mm resection of the lateral rectus in both eyes, combined with inferior oblique weakening if there was overaction.

10. Mohindra, I., Zwaan, J., Held, R., et al. Development of acuity and stereopsis in infants with esotropia. *Ophthalmology* 92:691–697, 1985.
    An attempt to use preferential looking techniques to measure stereopsis in young esotropes.

11. Nixon, R.B., Helveston, E.M., Miller, K., et al. Incidence of strabismus in neonates. *Am. J. Ophthalmol.* 100:798–801, 1985.
    None of 1,219 alert neonates had the findings of congenital esotropia.

12. Parks, M.M. Congenital esotropia with a bifixation result: Report of a case. *Doc. Ophthalmol.* 58:109–114, 1984.
    Parks describes the only patient he has encountered in whom surgery resulted in normal binocular vision and reviews the concept of a monofixation syndrome.

13. Szmyd, S.M., Nelson, L.B., Calhoun, J.H., et al. Large bimedial rectus recessions in congenital esotropia. *Br. J. Ophthalmol.* 69:271–274, 1985.
    Ninety-one percent of 45 patients with congenital esotropia who underwent bilateral medial ("bimedial") rectus recessions of 6 or 7 mm had deviations of 10 prism diopters or less 6 weeks after surgery. Several subsequently evolved accommodative esotropias.

14. von Noorden, G.K. Infantile esotropia: A continuing riddle. *Am. Orthoptic J.* 34:52–62, 1984.
    This lecture concentrates on the sensory outcome in patients with congenital esotropia, with "subnormal binocular vision" considered an optimal result.

15. von Noorden, G.K., Wong, S.Y. Surgical results in nystagmus blockage syndrome. *Ophthalmology* 93:1028–1031, 1986.
    Sixty-four consecutive cases of nystagmus blockage syndrome were managed surgically. The results were less predictable than those in essential infantile esotropia.

16. Willshaw, H.E., Mashhoudi, N., Powell, S. Augmented medial rectus recession in the management of esotropia. *Br. J. Ophthalmol.* 70:840–843, 1986.
    In a case-controlled series, these authors obtained better results when bilateral medial rectus recessions were augmented by recessions of conjunctiva and Tenon's capsule.
17. Zak, T.A., Morin, J.D. Early surgery for infantile esotropia: Results and influence of age upon results. *Can. J. Ophthalmol.* 17:213–218, 1982.
    An analysis of the results in 105 patients who underwent their surgery between 5 and 24 months of age.

29. ACCOMMODATIVE ESOTROPIA

The child who presents with an esotropia should first have a dilated fundus examination and cycloplegic refraction. Atropine, which takes about 6 hours to produce maximum cycloplegia and thus is usually instilled a day or more in advance, is still considered the standard by some, but many pediatric ophthalmologists feel that cyclopentolate produces adequate cycloplegia about an hour after instillation, thus allowing the initial evaluation to be completed within the scope of a single office visit. If there are 2 diopters or more of hyperopia, then spectacle correction is prescribed. When the child returns wearing these glasses, the residual deviation is measured both at 20 feet ("distance") and at 14 inches ("near") using an accommodative target.

There are several possibilities at this juncture:

1. The deviation is only reduced, both at distance and near. This child has a *partially accommodative esotropia.*
2. The child is fusing at distance but remains esotropic at near. If the addition of further plus lenses eliminates the deviation at near, this is a *nonrefractive accommodative esotropia.* If a deviation persists despite plus lenses, this is an accommodative esotropia with nonaccommodative convergence excess.
3. The child fuses both at distance and near and therefore has a *refractive accommodative esotropia.*
4. The deviation is unchanged and represents an *acquired nonaccommodative esotropia.*

Of course, if the child initially presented fusing at distance without correction but had an esotropia at near, the alternatives in No. 2 above also apply.

Pathogenesis

An accommodative component is common in esotropias because convergence is neurologically linked to accommodation in the near synkinesis and may be part of many types of esotropias, including those associated with Brown's and Duane's syndromes. The accommodative component is the result of at least two factors: the hyperopic eye must accommodate to see clearly, and the ratio of accommodation to accommodation-induced convergence varies. In refractive accommodative esotropia, the retinal blur produced by hyperopia is causative. When this is eliminated by an appopriate plus lens, the deviation disappears. In nonrefractive accommodative esotropia, a major part of the problem is an inappropriately large amount of convergence induced by a given amount of accommodation. This is quantitated as the accommodative convergence-to-accommodation ratio—the *AC/A ratio,* which may be measured in various ways [11]. The AC/A ratio ranges from 3 to 5 in normal persons, but averages around 7 in children with nonrefractive accommodative esotropia and may exceed 10.

If the degree of hyperopia and the AC/A ratio were the only considerations, then accommodative esotropias would be easy to explain. All high hyperopes would be esotropes, and all low hyperopes with high AC/A ratios would have nonrefractive accommodative esotropias. That this is not the case indicates that other, poorly understood factors are at work. The effect of some of these factors is expressed in the fusional divergence amplitude, a measure of the ability of the eyes to maintain fusion despite an underlying esodeviation.

Diagnosis
The typical patient presenting with an accommodative esotropia is a child aged 2 or 3 years, but onset may occur in the first year of life or be delayed until adulthood. The esotropia is frequently intermittent at first. By the time the child is evaluated, one eye is often amblyopic. The deviation is greater at near than at distance and is usually smaller than 40 prism diopters. Cycloplegic refraction yields a moderate hyperopia, averaging around 3 diopters.

Treatment
Management of accommodative esotropia depends on its type. A purely refractive accommodative esotropia will respond to correction alone. Surgery is usually required if the residual deviation after correction of a partially accommodative esotropia exceeds 10 prism diopters. Any coexistant amblyopia should be treated prior to surgery (see Chap. 27).

A nonrefractive accommodative esotropia may be controlled by medical treatment that changes the AC/A ratio pharmacologically or by bifocal correction that allows fusion at both distance and near. The so-called "irreversible" cholinesterase inhibitors such as echothiophate (Phospholine Iodide) or diisopropyl fluorophosphate administered topically decrease the AC/A ratio in accommodative esotropia. Such miotic therapy is less popular now than it once was because of the required duration of the treatment and the side effects of these drugs. These side effects include formation of iris cysts at the pupillary border, cholinergic crises with abdominal pain and diarrhea mimicking an acute surgical abdomen, depression of systemic cholinesterase levels with increased sensitivity to succinylcholine administration during induction of general anesthesia, and cataract formation. Nevertheless, miotic therapy may be substituted for glasses for periods when wearing glasses may be difficult or inappropriate, e.g., before the child has accepted glasses or during an active summer by the swimming pool. Miotic therapy is sometimes used as a diagnostic test to determine whether an accommodative component is present.

The mainstay of the treatment of nonrefractive accommodative esotropia is bifocals, which optically reduce the effect of the increased AC/A ratio for near work. The indications for bifocals are control of the deviation as measured at 20 feet with a full hyperopic correction (to 10 diopters or less of esotropia) and a similar reduction of the remaining esodeviation at 14 inches with plus lenses. Some authorities prescribe a full bifocal add initially (+ 2.50, + 3.00, or + 3.50 diopters), while others prefer to give the least plus lens that will reduce the near deviation in hopes of stimulating the fusional mechanisms of the patient. An executive type of bifocal is preferred, with the bifocal segment set higher than is standard with adults. Some ophthalmologists report success with progressive-addition bifocal lenses, which eliminate the cosmetic stigma of the bifocal line and may encourage fusion at intermediate distances. These lenses are both more difficult to fit and more expensive than executive bifocals [3, 9].

The prognosis for fusion even with appropriate treatment is variable. Some children tolerate reduction in the strength of their bifocal add and are weaned off bifocals by the time they are 9 or 10 years old. With the decreasing hyperopia that is characteristic of the growth spurt, they may eventually require no glasses and have good fusion. In contrast to this ideal result, some children experience a deterioration in their fusion while wearing bifocals and eventually require surgery. This subgroup tends to have lower (although in the normal range) AC/A ratios at the beginning of treatment. Another subgroup is never able to maintain fusion without bifocals. Continued wearing of bifocals may be unacceptable to a teenager and constitutes a relative indication for surgery. This is another situation in which progressive-addition bifocals may be prescribed.

1. Baker, J.D., Parks, M.M. Early-onset accommodative esotropia. *Am. J. Ophthalmol.* 90:11–18, 1980.
   A series of 21 patients in whom esotropia with an accommodative component had its onset before the age of 1 year.
2. Hiatt, R.L. Medical management of accommodative esotropia. *J. Pediatr. Ophthalmol. Strab.* 20:199–201, 1983.
   In this position paper Hiatt favors atropine refractions and considers miotics a supplement to, rather than a replacement for, glasses.
3. Jacob, J.L., Beaulieu, Y., Brunet, E. Progressive-addition lenses in the management of exotropia with a high accommodation/convergence ratio. *Can. J. Ophthalmol.* 15:166–169, 1980.
   These authors found progressive-addition lenses to be an acceptable substitute for conventional executive bifocals in the management of accommodative esotropia. Subsequently, Bixenman (Can. J. Ophthalmol. 16:163–164, 1981) called attention to some problems with the terminology and interpretation of data in this paper.
4. Pratt-Johnson, J.A., Tillson, G. The management of esotropia with high AC/A ratio (convergence excess). *J. Pediatr. Ophthalmol. Strab.* 22:238–242, 1985.
   Of 99 patients in this retrospective series, 86 achieved some fusion, but only 5 had central fusion. The use of bifocals, while apparently harmless, did not seem to improve the eventual sensory outcome.
5. Raab, E.L. Etiologic factors in accommodative esodeviation. *Trans. Am. Ophthalmol. Soc.* 80:657–694, 1982.
   This A.O.S. thesis provides an extensive review of the author's observations.
6. Raab, E.L. Hypermetropia in accommodative esodeviation. *J. Pediatr. Ophthalmol. Strab.* 21:194–197, 1984.
   Study of 68 children with accommodative esotropia revealed no dramatic increase in hyperopia over time.
7. Raab, E.L. Consecutive accommodative exotropia. *J. Pediatr. Ophthalmol. Strab.* 22:58–59, 1985.
   An accommodative esotropia may develop after surgery for an exodeviation.
8. Raab, E.L., Spierer, A. Persisting accommodative esotropia. *Arch. Ophthalmol.* 104:1777–1779, 1986.
   More than half of a group of 202 patients had persistence of their accommodative esotropia after the age of 10 years. No specific factors predicted resolution or persistence.
9. Smith, J.B. Progressive-addition lenses in the treatment of accommodative esotropia. *Am. J. Ophthalmol.* 99:56–62, 1985.
   Thirty-two more patients managed with progressive-addition lenses.
10. Swan, K.C. Accommodative esotropia: Long range follow-up. *Ophthalmology* 90:1141–1145, 1983.
    A series of 39 adult patients who continue to have problems related to their accommodative esotropias.
11. von Noorden, G.K. *Burian-von Noorden's Binocular Vision and Ocular Motility: Theory and Management of Strabismus* (2nd ed.). St. Louis: Mosby, 1980. Pp. 91–99.
    The pages cited contain a description of the various methods of determining the AC/A ratio.
12. von Noorden, G.K., Morris, J., Edelman, P. Efficacy of bifocals in the treatment of accommodative esotropia. *Am. J. Ophthalmol.* 85:830–834, 1978.
    Of 84 patients, 31 could have their bifocal segments decreased or eliminated, 39 were dependent on bifocals and some of them required surgery in their early teens, and 14 had deterioration of binocular function while wearing bifocals.

VII. RETINA AND VITREOUS

George K. Asdourian

Accumulation of extracellular fluid in the outer plexiform layer of the macula leads, as the consequence of the longitudinal orientation of the nerve fibers, to the formation of cystic spaces, an entity clinically known as *cystoid macular edema* (CME). CME is not a disease as such, but rather represents the end result of a variety of disorders that disrupt the blood-retinal barriers. CME has been linked with disease processes in the vitreous, retina, and choroid; surgery may also cause CME. Table 30-1 lists some of the reported associations of CME.

Pathogenesis
The normally functioning retina is kept free of extracellular fluid by a system known as the blood-retinal barrier. The two components of this system are an inner barrier and an outer barrier. The inner barrier is located at the level of the retinal vascular endothelium, where the tight junctions of the endothelial cells prevent the passage of serum and macromolecules into the sensory retina. The outer barrier is located at the level of the retinal pigment epithelium (RPE), where the tight zonula occludens between individual RPE cells prevents the passage of serum and macromolecules from the choriocapillaris of the choroid into the sensory retina. Thus, the constituents of the extracellular space in the retina are precisely regulated by the combined activity of the retinal vascular endothelium and the RPE.

If for any reason the blood-retinal barriers are disrupted, macromolecules and serum from the retinal or choroidal vasculature pass into the sensory retina, producing retinal edema. Edema fluid may accumulate in various layers of the neuroretina. The site is determined by the source of the fluid (from either the inner or outer blood-retinal barrier), by the extent of damage to the barrier, by the duration of the edema, and by the arrangement of cells in the neuroretina. With widespread areas of leakage, diffuse retinal edema results. If the leakage is from focal damage, localized edema develops, e.g., CME.

Diagnosis
Clinically, the edematous retina appears thickened, opalescent, and featureless. Irregular fundal light reflexes are thought to represent displacement of the inner limiting membrane. CME is readily diagnosed by Hruby or fundus contact lens biomicroscopy and may be confirmed with fluorescein angiography, which usually localizes the disruption of the blood-retinal barrier. The angiogram may also reveal the disease entity responsible for the macular edema. If the breakdown is at the level of the retinal capillary endothelium, then angiography demonstrates retinal capillaries that leak in the early dye transit. In the late frames of the angiogram, fluorescein has accumulated in the cystic spaces, forming the classic rosette pattern. If the blood-retinal barrier is disrupted at the level of the RPE, however, as it is in association with choroidal tumors or neovascularization, there will be early leakage of dye from the choriocapillaris into the sensory retina. Although breakdown of the inner blood-retinal barrier is more common, disruption of the outer barrier is being recognized with increasing frequency.

The CME that follows cataract extraction has been most extensively studied. Aphakic cystoid macular edema (ACME) was first distinguished as a clinical entity by Irvine [5] in 1953, and its clinical and angiographic features were elaborated by Gass and Norton in 1966 [3]. ACME is commonly referred to as the *Irvine-Gass syndrome*. ACME is the most common cause of visual loss following uneventful intracapsular cataract surgery, with a reported incidence of subclinical edema (angiographic edema) as high as 60 to 77 percent and an incidence of visually significant ACME between 2 and 10 percent. Most ACME resolves spontaneously, and the prevalence of chronic visual loss is in the 1 to 3 percent range. The placement of an iris-supported lens worsens the prognosis of ACME.

Extracapsular techniques have decreased the incidence of ACME. Uncomplicated ex-

Table 30-1. Causes of CME

Vitreous
Preretinal membranes
Inflammations—vitritis, chronic cyclitis

Retina and optic disk
Retinal vascular disease—diabetic retinopathy, branch and central retinal vein occlusion, retinal telangiectasia, retinal macroaneurysms, retinal vasculitis
Retinal tumors
Radiation retinopathy
Hereditary disease—retinitis pigmentosa, dominant CME
Papillitis

Choroid
Tumors—malignant melanoma, hemangioma, metastatic tumors
Subretinal choroidal neovascularization
Choroidal inflammation—chorioretinitis, posterior uveitis

Drugs
Epinephrine
Nicotinic acid

Ophthalmic surgery
Cataract extraction
Retinal detachment surgery
Filtering procedures
Vitrectomy
Cryotherapy
Photocoagulation

tracapsular cataract extraction with or without intraocular lens placement is associated with a lower rate of ACME than is intracapsular cataract extraction as long as the posterior capsule remains intact. If the posterior capsule ruptures or a primary capsulotomy is performed, this advantage may be lost. The effect of late laser capsulotomy is unknown. Secondary lens implantation, especially after intracapsular surgery, increases the risk of ACME. The incidence may be higher when the secondary implant is done within 1 year of the initial surgery and when there is vitreous loss.

The pathogenesis of ACME is uncertain. Hypotony, phototoxicity produced by the coaxial illumination of the operating microscope, vitreous traction on the macula, intraocular inflammation, and ultraviolet (UV) radiation exposure following cataract extraction have all been implicated. A form of ACME is associated with administration of epinephrine for aphakic glaucoma.

Treatment
The best management of CME varies with the cause. When there is underlying vascular disease, as in diabetic retinopathy or branch retinal vein occlusion, photocoagulation of leaking capillaries, microaneurysms, and ischemic retina may be helpful. Photocoagulation of leaking perifoveal capillaries not related to an underlying vasculopathy or to the macular RPE has not proved useful. There is no known effective treatment for CME associated with dystrophies such as retinitis pigmentosa.

Treatment may be directed at specific etiologic factors. When epinephrine is implicated, the drug is withdrawn. Vitrectomy is of value in selected patients in whom ACME is apparently the result of vitreous incarcerated in the surgical wound. The value of vitrectomy in the absence of obvious vitreous traction is unknown. Since inflammation may have a role in the pathogenesis of CME, topical and systemic steroids and prostaglandin synthesis inhibitors have been used, but there has been no randomized prospective study demonstrating their effectiveness.

Anti-inflammatory drugs have also been used preoperatively in hopes of decreasing the incidence of CME. Systemic steroids do not appear to be an effective prophylaxis, but prostaglandin synthesis inhibitors may have a role. Studies to date, however, have demonstrated only a transient improvement of visual acuity.

The role of UV radiation is under investigation at the present time. Filtration of UV light following cataract extraction may reduce the incidence of ACME [8].

1. Cunha-Vaz, J.G., Travassos, A. Breakdown of the blood-retinal barriers and cystoid macular edema. *Surv. Ophthalmol.* 28:485–492, 1984.
   A comprehensive discussion of the blood-retinal barriers and their role in CME.
2. The First International Cystoid Macular Edema Symposium. Special supplement. *Surv. Ophthalmol.* 28:431–619, 1984.
   The proceedings of the symposium with extensive bibliography.
3. Gass, J.D.M., Norton, E.W.D. Cystoid macular edema and papilledema following cataract extraction. A fluorescein funduscopic and angiographic study. *Arch. Ophthalmol.* 76:646–661, 1966.
4. Irvine, A.R. Cystoid maculopathy. Review. *Surv. Ophthalmol.* 21:1–17, 1976.
   A review of etiology and treatment of CME.
5. Irvine, S.R. A newly defined vitreous syndrome following cataract surgery: Interpreted according to recent concepts of the structure of the vitreous. *Am. J. Ophthalmol.* 36:599–619, 1953.
   An original observation by the author suggesting that post-cataract vitreal changes may be associated with macular changes.
6. Jampol, L.M. Pharmacologic therapy of aphakic cystoid macular edema. A review. *Ophthalmology* 89:891–897, 1982.
   A review of different pharmacologic agents used to treat CME.
7. Jampol, L.M., Kraff, M.C., Sanders, D.R., et al. Near-UV radiation from the operating microscope and pseudophakic cystoid macular edema. *Arch. Ophthalmol.* 103:28–30, 1985.
   In this randomized prospective study, it was shown that the presence or absence of a UV-blocking filter on the operating microscope made no difference on the incidence of angiographic CME or on the final visual outcome of patients undergoing extracapsular cataract surgery with posterior chamber lens implantation.
8. Kraff, M.C., Sanders, D.R., Jampol, L.M., et al. Effect of an ultraviolet-filtering intraocular lens on cystoid macular edema. *Ophthalmology* 92:366–369, 1985.
   In a prospective double-masked study, patients receiving ultraviolet-filtering intraocular lens had a statistically significant lower incidence of angiographic CME, although visual acuity was not affected significantly in patients having ultraviolet-filtering or nonfiltering intraocular lenses.
9. Kramer, S.G. Cystoid macular edema after aphakic penetrating keratoplasty. *Ophthalmology* 88:782–787, 1981.
   Anterior vitrectomy during aphakic penetrating keratoplasty may contribute to the development of CME.
10. The Miami Study Group. Cystoid macular edema in aphakic and pseudophakic eyes. *Am. J. Ophthalmol.* 88:45–48, 1979.
    The fluorescein angiographic incidence of CME compared in patients with intracapsular cataract extraction with and without an implant and patients with extracapsular cataract extraction with an implant.
11. Tso, M.O.M. Pathology of cystoid macular edema. *Ophthalmology* 89:902–915, 1982.
    The histopathology of different types of cystoid maculopathies is presented. Different layers of the retina may harbor the edema fluid. Disruption of the blood-retinal barriers is the pathogenic event leading to macular edema.
12. Vine, A.K. Advances in treating cystoid macular edema. *Int. Ophthalmol. Clin.* 21(3):157–165, 1981.
    A review of different medical and surgical modalities of treatment used for CME.

31. CENTRAL SEROUS CHORIORETINOPATHY

Central serous chorioretinopathy (formerly known as *central serous retinopathy*) is a localized detachment of the central sensory retina that is not associated with retinal or subretinal hemorrhages, exudates, or vasculopathy.

Pathogenesis
Central serous chorioretinopathy predominately affects young men. The etiology is unknown, but there is often a history of emotional stress. Only about 10 percent of cases are bilateral, but there is often evidence of previous, asymptomatic disease in the fellow eye consisting of small areas of hypopigmentation or hyperpigmentation of the retinal pigment epithelium.

Diagnosis
The presenting symptom is blurred or reduced central vision associated with metamorphopsia, micropsia, or a positive central scotoma. The visual acuity ranges from 20/20 to 20/100. Reduced acuity can often be improved by the addition of a plus sphere that focuses the image on the elevated macular retina. Even when acuity is normal, many patients complain of distorted or hazy vision. A small, relatively central scotoma may be detected on Amsler grid testing.

The anterior segment is normal; specifically, there is no evidence of inflammation. Ophthalmoscopy reveals a serous elevation of the sensory retina. The macula is characteristically involved, but extramacular detachments are observed, and in rare instances a total exudative detachment may be present (see Chap. 34). This serous detachment is best appreciated by contact lens slit lamp biomicroscopy. Multiple yellow dots, thought to represent proteinaceous precipitates, are often seen on the undersurface of the retina, especially in long-standing detachments. Occasionally, a small retinal pigment epithelial detachment or area of atrophy may be seen under the serous retinal detachment.

In central serous chorioretinopathy, serous fluid leaks from the choriocapillaris through a small defect in the retinal pigment epithelium into the subretinal space. The nature of the defect in the retinal pigment epithelium is not precisely known, but it is thought to involve the junctional complexes of adjacent retinal pigment epithelial cells—the zonula occludens, which controls the outer blood-retinal barrier (see Chap. 30).

The location of this disruption is best demonstrated by fluorescein angiography. Typically, early frames show a pinpoint leak. In the midphases of the angiogram, the leak enlarges. The dye pools under the detached retina, but never completely fills the entire subretinal space. The fluorescein leak has several typical appearances. The most common of these is the "ink blot," in which an early pinpoint leak enlarges with fuzzy margins. Another variation is the "smoke stack" or "mushroom" leak, in which the pinpoint leak expands and ascends through the subretinal fluid while expanding laterally. When there is an associated retinal pigment epithelial detachment, this fills first with fluorescein, and then the fluorescein leaks into the subretinal space. These different appearances have no prognostic significance. When no leak is demonstrated, this suggests that a spontaneous seal has formed. When this happens, the subretinal fluid will reabsorb with improvement of visual acuity within a month.

Treatment
Central serous chorioretinopathy characteristically runs a benign course. In the majority of patients, the leak seals spontaneously, and visual acuity returns to normal. In about 80 percent of cases, recovery occurs within 3 months of onset; in another 20 percent, symptoms persist for more than 6 months. It is in this latter group that the few patients with permanent reduction in acuity—usually in the 20/50 to 20/100 range—are found. Such patients often have their leaks close to the fovea.

Laser photocoagulation of leaks shortens the duration of the sensory detachment, but does not appear to improve the visual prognosis. Photocoagulation has rare but significant complications (foveal burns, preretinal fibrosis, and subretinal neovascular membrane formation, and hemorrhage) that are especially likely to occur when parafoveal leaks are treated. Many conservative ophthalmologists photocoagulate only those leaks remote from the fovea that have persisted for 3 months or longer.

1. Cassel, G.H., Brown, G.C., Annesley, W.H. Central serous chorioretinopathy: A seasonal variation? *Br. J. Ophthalmol.* 68:724–726, 1984.
   No definite seasonal variation was found in the incidence of central serous chorioretinopathy.
2. Frederick, A.R. Jr. Multifocal and recurrent (serous) choroidopathy (MARC) syndrome: A new variety of idiopathic central serous choroidopathy. *Doc. Ophthalmol.* 56:203–235, 1984.
   A variant of central serous chorioretinopathy characterized by patches of granular atrophy of the retinal pigment epithelium was present in 110 patients.
3. Gass, J.D.M. Pathogenesis of disciform detachment of the neuroepithelium. II. Idiopathic central serous choroidopathy. *Am. J. Ophthalmol.* 63:587–615, 1967.
   A classic description of the entity.
4. Gilbert, C.M., Owens, S.L., Smith, P.D., et al. Long-term follow-up of central serous chorioretinopathy. *Br. J. Ophthalmol.* 68:815–820, 1984.
   A follow-up of 73 patients with central serous chorioretinoptahy suggested no clinically significant effect of focal argon laser photocoagulation on final visual acuity or recurrence rate.
5. Klein, M.L., VanBuskirk, E.M., Friedman, F., et al. Experience with non-treatment of central serous choroidopathy. *Arch. Ophthalmol.* 91:247–250, 1974.
   Central serous chorioretinopathy is essentially a benign and self-limited disorder that seldom needs photocoagulation treatment.
6. Lewis, M.L. Idiopathic serous detachment of the retinal pigment epithelium. *Arch. Ophthalmol.* 96:620–624, 1978.
   This entity may be a variant of idiopathic central serous chorioretinopathy.
7. Spitznas, M. Pathogenesis of central serous retinopathy: A new working hypothesis. *Graefe's Arch. Clin. Exp. Ophthalmol.* 224:321–324, 1986.
   An editorial comment on the function of the choriocapillaris-Bruch's-retinal pigment epithelium complex and its role in the pathogenesis of central serous retinopathy.
8. Schatz, H., Yannuzzi, L.A., Gitter, K. Subretinal neovascularization following argon laser photocoagulation treatment for central serous chorioretinopathy. *Trans. Am. Acad. Ophthalmol. Otolaryngol.* 83:893–906, 1977.
   The development of subretinal neovascularization as a complication of argon laser photocoagulation in central serous chorioretinopathy is presented in six patients and 21 case reports.
9. Watzke, R.C., Burton, T.C., Leaverton, P.E. Ruby laser photocoagulation therapy of central serous retinopathy. *Trans. Am. Acad. Ophthalmol. Otolaryngol.* 78:205–211, 1974.
   Ruby laser photocoagulation was beneficial in shortening the duration of the serous detachment of the retina.
10. Watzke, R.C., Burton, T.C., Woolson, R.F. Direct and indirect laser photocoagulation of central serous choroidopathy. *Am. J. Ophthalmol.* 88:914–918, 1979.
    Direct photocoagulation of the leak in central serous choroidopathy is superior to indirect treatment away from the leak.

32. AGE-RELATED MACULAR DEGENERATION

Age-related macular degeneration (AMD) is the leading cause of blindness in adults over the age of 60 in the United States. AMD has a wide spectrum of clinical appearances that depend on the anatomic structures predominately affected. These ophthalmoscopic appearances include loss of the foveal reflex, fine granularity of the macular retinal pigment epithelium, drusen, geographic or areolar retinal pigment epithelial atrophy, serous or hemorrhagic retinal pigment epithelial or sensory retinal detachments, and disciform fibrovascular scars.

Pathogenesis
Normal aging produces histologic changes in the retinal pigment epithelium, Bruch's membrane, and the choriocapillaris. These include thickening, hyalinization, calcification, and patchy basophilia of Bruch's membrane and fine granular deposits (basal linear) beneath the retinal pigment epithelium. Such changes may be precursors of the degenerative changes in AMD: widespread basal linear deposits and thickening of Bruch's membrane, drusen, atrophy and proliferation of the retinal pigment epithelium, and the growth of choroidal capillaries through Bruch's membrane under the retinal pigment epithelium.

AMD can be conveniently divided into two clinical forms: an *atrophic* or *dry* type and an *exudative* type. More than 90 percent of eyes with severe visual loss have the exudative type. In the atrophic type, there are macular pigmentary changes but no neovascularization or exudation.

Drusen are the hallmark of AMD and are characteristically the earliest manifestation of atrophic macular degeneration. Pathologically, drusen are depositions of hyaline material between the retinal pigment epithelium and Bruch's membrane. This material may represent accumulated secretions of undigested material from the retinal pigment epithelium into the inner layer of Bruch's membrane. Isolated drusen may be present for many years asymptomatically and then lead to visual loss in the sixth or seventh decade of life. Such visual loss may occur when single drusen coalesce and involve the fovea, or when the overlying retinal pigment epithelium atrophies. The retinal pigment epithelium may also proliferate, which is clinically apparent as hyperpigmentation.

Diagnosis
Atrophic AMD manifests as a gradual loss of central vision; no medical or surgical treatment is available for these patients. Low-vision aids and supplemental lighting may improve visual function. These patients should also be monitored for the development of exudative changes, which may be detected early by distortion of Amsler grids. Copies of the Amsler grid should be given to the patient along with instructions for its use, and regular ophthalmoscopic examinations should be scheduled to detect subclinical changes.

Although most eyes with atrophic macular degeneration stabilize, a significant number progress to the exudative stage. Exudative macular degeneration is characterized by a serous detachment of the retinal pigment epithelium or a choroidal neovascular membrane, or both. Clinically, serous retinal pigment epithelial detachments appear as sharply demarcated, dome-shaped elevations that stain persistently in fluorescein angiography. A pure serous retinal pigment epithelial detachment is not accompanied by bleeding, lipid exudation, or a neovascular membrane. Photocoagulation has not been successful in stabilizing or improving serous retinal pigment epithelial detachments, and there is at present no satisfactory treatment. These patients should be followed, as a significant proportion eventually develop subretinal neovascularization.

Choroidal neovascular membranes may also develop in the absence of serous retinal pigment epithelial detachments. Such membranes may be dormant for a time and then cause a serous or hemorrhagic sensory retinal detachment in the macula. Initially, there may be only a small amount of subretinal fluid without hemorrhages or exudates. At this stage, patients may complain only of subtle distortion of central vision, which can be substantiated by Amsler grid testing. The macula should be examined carefully by stereoscopic slit lamp biomicroscopy for serous sensory retinal elevation. Angiography may demonstrate subtle leakage into the subretinal space. Most of these neovascular membranes eventually leak blood and serum under the retinal pigment epithelium and beneath the sensory retina, causing serous and hemorrhagic detachments. These cause subjective distortion and decrease in central vision. Left untreated, the end stage of the exudative process is organization of the blood products with development of a macular fibrovascular scar and severe visual loss.

Treatment

There is no convincing evidence that any medical therapy has value for patients with AMD. The randomized, controlled clinical study [7] of macular photocoagulation has demonstrated that argon laser photocoagulation applied to choroidal neovascular membranes lying outside the foveal avascular zone improves the visual prognosis. Photocoagulation effectively delayed visual loss in up to 60 percent of eyes with choroidal neovascular membranes. According to the criteria used in this study, this treatment was applicable to only a small percentage of patients with exudative AMD. Only the argon green light was used, and membranes inside the foveal avascular zone were not treated.

Other studies that are under way assess the effectiveness of different lasers (krypton red, krypton yellow, and argon green) and criteria. Until the results of these studies are available, a conservative approach to treatment of eyes that do not meet established treatment criteria is justified.

1. Bird, A.C., Chisholm, I.H., Grey, R.H.B., et al. Treatment of senile disciform macular degeneration: A single-blind randomized trial by argon laser photocoagulation. *Br. J. Ophthalmol.* 66:745–753, 1982.
   The results of this clinical trial show the beneficial effect of photocoagulation in the treatment of some patients with subretinal neovascularization secondary to aging.
2. Elman, M.J., Fine, S.L., Murphy, R.P., et al. The natural history of serous retinal pigment epithelium detachment in patients with age-related macular degeneration. *Ophthalmology* 93:224–230, 1986.
   In a retrospective study, one-third of eyes with serous detachment of the retinal pigment epithelium developed choroidal neovascular membranes.
3. Feeney-Burns, L., Ellersieck, M.R. Age-related changes in the ultrastructure of Bruch's membrane. *Am. J. Ophthalmol.* 100:686–697, 1985.
   A description of the ultrastructural changes occurring in Bruch's membrane of human eyes obtained from different decades of life.
4. Gass, J.D.M. Pathogenesis of disciform detachment of the neuroepithelium. IV. Fluorescein angiographic study of senile disciform macular degeneration. *Am. J. Ophthalmol.* 63:645–659, 1967.
   A classic paper on angiographic findings in senile disciform macular degeneration.
5. Gass, J.D.M. Drusen and disciform macular detachment and degeneration. *Arch. Ophthalmol.* 90:206–217, 1973.
   The natural course of drusen and disciform macular degeneration evaluated in 200 patients over a period of 4 years.
6. Gregor, Z., Bird, A.C., Chisholm, I.H. Senile disciform macular degeneration in the second eye. *Br. J. Ophthalmol.* 61:141–147, 1977.
   This study reports a risk of 12 to 15 percent per year for the development of senile macular degeneration in the other eye of patients who present with disciform degeneration in one eye.
7. Macular Photocoagulation Study Group. Argon laser photocoagulation for senile macular degeneration: Results of a randomized clinical trial. *Arch. Ophthalmol.* 100:912–918, 1982.
   This randomized, controlled clinical trial showed the beneficial results of treating certain subretinal neovascular membranes in patients with AMD.
8. Macular Photocoagulation Study Group. Argon laser photocoagulation for neovascular maculopathy: Three-year results from randomized clinical trials. *Arch. Ophthalmol.* 104:694–701, 1986.
   The beneficial results obtained during the initial phase of this study were maintained for 3 to 5 years.
9. Sarks, S.H. New vessel formation beneath the retinal pigment epithelium in senile eyes. *Br. J. Ophthalmol.* 57:951–965, 1973.
   Twenty percent of 150 senile eyes examined histologically showed evidence of new vessel proliferation through Bruch's membrane.
10. Sarks, S.H. Ageing and degeneration in the macular region: A clinico-pathological study. *Br. J. Ophthalmol.* 60:324–341, 1976.

An excellent article of the clinicopathologic relationship of changes occurring as a result of AMD in 378 eyes.

11. Smiddy, W.E., Fine, S.L. Prognosis of patients with bilateral macular drusen. *Ophthalmology* 91:271–277, 1984.

    Drusen confluence and associated focal hyperpigmentation were risk factors for the development of exudative maculopathy in patients with macular drusen.

12. Strahlman, E.R., Fine, S.L., Hillis, A. The second eye of patients with senile macular degeneration. *Arch. Ophthalmol.* 101:1191–1193, 1983.

    This study reports a risk of 3 to 7 percent per year for the development of disciform degeneration in patients who present with disciform macular degeneration in one eye and drusen in the other.

33. RHEGMATOGENOUS RETINAL DETACHMENT

Retinal detachment occurs when the sensory retina separates from the pigment epithelium. Three distinct types of retinal detachment occur: rhegmatogenous, tractional, and exudative.

Rhegmatogenous retinal detachments are secondary to retinal breaks. Fluid dissects through these breaks from the vitreous cavity into the potential subretinal space, separating the sensory retina from the retinal pigment epithelium. Rhegmatogenous retinal detachments that have no history of ocular trauma or disease are said to be *primary*. *Secondary* rhegmatogenous retinal detachments occur in eyes with trauma, uveitis, retinal vascular disease, or any antecedent disease that can cause a retinal hole or tear. The extent and location of the detachment determines whether it is *clinical* or *subclinical*. Subclinical denotes detachments that extend no more than one disk diameter from the break and no more than two disk diameters posterior to the equator. The incidence of primary rhegmatogenous retinal detachment in the general population is estimated to be under 1 per 10,000 (0.01% per year). Certain groups are particularly vulnerable to retinal detachment. Individuals with high myopia, surgical aphakia, trauma, and a history of detachment in the fellow eye are at higher risk for development of retinal detachment.

Pathogenesis

The fundamental mechanisms that lead to rhegmatogenous retinal detachment are not completely known. Of the pathologic changes that precede the detachment and are important in its genesis, *retinal breaks* and *vitreous traction* are the most important.

Retinal breaks in themselves do not produce retinal detachments. Asymptomatic retinal breaks are common, occurring in 5 to 10 percent of the general population. These breaks are usually small atrophic holes near the ora serrata, although some are horse shoe tears. The majority of retinas with these breaks have a low risk of subsequent detachment.

The most important vitreous change in the pathogenesis of rhegmatogenous retinal detachments is a *posterior vitreous detachment*. The vitreous, which in an entirely healthy state is a gel that is firmly apposed to the innermost retinal layers, may as a result of aging and degenerative changes liquefy, collapse, and separate from the retina. Factors other than aging that promote the liquefaction and collapse of the vitreous include myopia, aphakia, inflammation, trauma, and vitreous hemorrhage. The vitreous detachment starts posteriorly and spreads forward. If the separation continues, the vitreous will be adherent only to firm points of attachment (i.e., at the vitreous base and along retinal blood vessels). Thus, with posterior vitreous detachment, there will be vitreous traction at these points of attachment as well as at other abnormal vitreoretinal junctions (surrounding lattice degeneration), with the resultant formation of retinal breaks. In the presence of liquefied vitreous, posterior vitreous detachment, and a retinal break, fluid vitreous will pass through the break into the subretinal space. However, a retinal detachment will not occur until the forces that promote passage of fluid vitreous through the tear (ocular movement, gravity, vitreous traction at edge of break) overcome the forces that tend to promote continued attachment of the retina (negative pressure in the subretinal space created by the pigment epithelium acting as a pump, mucopolysaccharide "glue" between pigment epithelium and sensory retina, interdigitations of the retinal pigment epithelial cell processes with individual cells of the sensory retina).

Once a localized retinal detachment develops around a retinal break, it usually progresses to total retinal detachment. Rarely, a small retinal detachment will spontaneously reattach, or the detachment will stabilize and remain a subtotal detachment with surrounding demarcation lines.

If the detachment is not repaired, late secondary changes may occur, such as cataract, glaucoma or hypotony, uveitis, rubeosis, and phthisis. The retina itself may show evidence of massive proliferative vitreoretinopathy.

Diagnosis
The premonitory signs of rhegmatogenous retinal detachment are *flashes of light* caused by the vitreous traction on the retina and *sudden showers of floaters* due to vitreous hemorrhage resulting from retinal break formation. These symptoms are followed by the onset of a *field defect* caused by the detaching retina. The timing and presence of all three symptoms are variable; moreover, not all patients with rhegmatogenous retinal detachment have premonitory symptoms. Vitreous hemorrhage may be mild to severe and is usually a simple, single event. Occasionally, however, if a retinal vessel is avulsed from the surface of the retina, there may be multiple hemorrhages, which repeat over months or years. In some cases of rhegmatogenous retinal detachments, the symptoms of flashes, floaters, and field defects are absent, and the patient may be aware of only loss of his central vision. Inferior retinal detachments often have an insidious course with no symptoms until the detachment progresses to involve the macular area. Of course, *subclinical retinal detachments* that occur in the fundus periphery do not cause any symptoms and are usually found during routine examinations or during follow-up of patients with retinal detachments in the fellow eye.

The diagnosis of rhegmatogenous retinal detachment is confirmed by indirect ophthalmoscopy, during which every effort should be made to discover the retinal breaks. Since the majority of breaks involve the fundus periphery, scleral depression should be performed. Three-mirror contact lens slit lamp biomicroscopy is important to ascertain the presence of small holes and to assess the status of the vitreous gel and the presence or absence of preretinal membranes. With these techniques, a definite break can be found in 97 percent of rhegmatogenous retinal detachments. In the other 3 percent, even though a definite break cannot be found, it is presumed to be present because the retinal detachment has the other characteristics of rhegmatogenous retinal detachment. In such cases, other causes of retinal detachment should be considered (see Chap. 34).

Management
The treatment of rhegmatogenous retinal detachment is surgical. Management of an uncomplicated rhegmatogenous retinal detachment depends on identifying all the retinal breaks, closing them, and releasing any vitreoretinal traction. To that end, scleral buckling procedures combine in one surgical procedure the closure of retinal breaks and the release of vitreoretinal traction. The exact methodology varies from surgeon to surgeon. In general, the retinal breaks are closed through the production of a chorioretinal reaction around them by cryopexy, diathermy, or photocoagulation, while the vitreoretinal traction is released by a scleral buckle in which a variety of solid or expansile implants or explants of foreign material are used to indent the globe and release traction.

In eyes with severe proliferative vitreoretinopathy or detachments secondary to giant retinal tears (tears larger than 90 degrees), conventional scleral buckling procedures may not be adequate or successful in reattaching the retina. In these cases, sophisticated vitreoretinal surgical maneuvers such as vitrectomy, preretinal and subretinal membrane peeling, fluid-gas exchange, and endophotocoagulation may be necessary to obtain a reattachment.

The anatomic and visual results of surgical treatment of rhegmatogenous retinal detachment depend on many factors: the type and extent of the detachment, the status of the macula (on or off), the presence of vitreous blood, and the presence and extent of proliferative vitreoretinopathy. The prognosis is excellent in detachments that are localized, with the macula still attached and with minimal vitreous traction. The prognosis is poor when the detachment is total, with multiple tears, and with evidence of proliferative vitreoretinopathy. Even with excellent anatomic results, central vision may decrease secondary to macular edema or macular pucker.

Careful examination of the fellow eye should be done by indirect ophthalmoscopy and scleral depression to detect any retinal breaks or other abnormalities that predispose to retinal detachment. These should be managed accordingly.

1. Byer, N.E. The natural history of asymptomatic retinal breaks. *Ophthalmology* 89:1033–1039, 1982.
   Asymptomatic retinal breaks in phakic, nonfellow eyes have a benign natural history, and prophylactic treatment is not recommended.
2. Cousins, S., Boniuk, I., Okun, E., et al. Pseudophakic retinal detachments in the presence of various IOL types. *Ophthalmology* 93:1198–1208, 1986.
   The postsurgical anatomic and visual results of 600 pseudophakic retinal detachments were analyzed. In this series, pseudophakic detachment with anterior chamber intraocular lenses fared worse compared with those with posterior chamber and iris-fixed lenses.
3. Davis, M.D. Natural history of retinal breaks without detachment. *Arch. Ophthalmol.* 92:183–194, 1974.
   Symptomatic retinal breaks with evidence of vitreous traction may have a high rate of subsequent retinal detachment and may require prophylactic treatment.
4. Foulds, W.S. Aetiology of retinal detachment. *Trans. Ophthalmol. Soc. U.K.* 95:118–127, 1975.
   Different mechanisms involved in the production of retinal detachment are discussed.
5. Haimann, M.H., Burton, T.C., Brown, C.K. Epidemiology of retinal detachment. *Arch. Ophthalmol.* 100:289–292, 1982.
   The incidence of four types of retinal detachment in Iowa is calculated and discussed.
6. Machemer, R. The importance of fluid absorption, traction, intraocular currents, and chorioretinal scars in the therapy of rhegmatogenous retinal detachments. XLI Edward Jackson Memorial Lecture. *Am. J. Ophthalmol.* 98:681–693, 1984.
   The etiologic factors involved in rhegmatogenous retinal detachment and their proper manipulation to achieve reattachment.
7. McPherson, A., O'Malley, R., Beltangady, S.S. Management of the fellow eyes in patients with rhegmatogenous retinal detachment. *Ophthalmology* 88:922–934, 1981.
   The authors present their views of managing retinal breaks and lattice degeneration in the fellow eye of patients with rhegmatogenous retinal detachment.
8. Michels, R.G. Scleral buckling methods for rhegmatogenous retinal detachment. *Retina* 6:1–49, 1986.
   An excellent review of different methods of scleral buckling used in rhegmatogenous retinal detachment surgery.
9. The Retina Society Terminology Committee. The classification of retinal detachment with proliferative vitreoretinopathy. *Ophthalmology* 90:121–125, 1983.
   The most recent classification of proliferative vitreoretinopathy.
10. Schepens, C.L. *Retinal detachment and allied diseases*, Vols. 1 and 2. Philadelphia: Saunders, 1983.
11. Sigelman, J. Vitreous base classification of retinal tears: Clinical application. Review. *Surv. Ophthalmol.* 25:59–74, 1980.
    A survey of different retinal breaks and their significance in the etiology of rhegmatogenous retinal detachment.

34. NONRHEGMATOGENOUS RETiNAL DETACHMENT

Retinal detachments caused by a retinal break are called *rhegmatogenous* (see Chap. 33); those not caused by a retinal break are nonrhegmatogenous. Nonrhegmatogenous detachments may be subdivided into *traction* detachments, which result from vitreous traction on the retina, and *exudative* detachments, which are caused by the exudation of fluid into the subretinal space from the choroid or retina itself.

Pathogenesis

Traction Detachments
Traction retinal detachments have a characteristic clinical appearance: a smooth surface that is usually taut and immobile and concave toward the front of the eye. Traction retinal detachments are usually limited to the posterior fundus, only rarely extending to the ora serrata. Demarcation lines are common. Occasionally, vitreous traction also tears the retina, producing a combined traction and rhegmatogenous detachment. Total nonrhegmatogenous traction detachments are uncommon, and when they occur they are often accompanied by massive proliferative vitreoretinopathy.

In most cases the causative vitreous membrane is visible ophthalmoscopically, but it is best evaluated by contact lens slit lamp biomicroscopy. Any disease process that can induce the formation of vitreal membranes can produce traction detachments. These disease processes include the cicatricial stages of diabetic retinopathy, retinopathy of prematurity (see Chap. 38), sickle cell retinopathy, and traumatic retinopathy—especially when there is an intraocular foreign body and vitreous hemorrhage. Persistent hyperplastic primary vitreous, toxoplasmosis, toxocariasis, Eales' disease, and peripheral uveitis also occasionally lead to traction detachments.

Exudative Detachments
The retina in an *exudative detachment* is smooth and highly elevated, so high that it is sometimes visible just behind the lens. The detachment, however, does not usually reach the ora serrata. The subretinal fluid may be turbid, but biomicroscopy will usually reveal a clear vitreous, except in some inflammatory conditions in which there are cells and debris. The hallmark of the exudative detachment is the phenomenon of "shifting subretinal fluid," in which movements of the eye or head cause the subretinal fluid to shift easily to the dependent part of the eye.

The many causes of exudative retinal detachment are listed in Table 34-1. Benign or malignant tumors of the retina or choroid are an important cause of exudative detachments, and the detachment may be the initial manifestation of the tumor. In most instances, the tumor can be found by careful ophthalmoscopy. The extreme fundus periphery must be inspected carefully, since retinoblastomas and choroidal malignant melanomas may be harbored there. In difficult cases, transscleral illumination, ultrasonography, fluorescein angiography, and computed tomography may be required. Treatment of the tumor may lead to resolution of the exudative detachment.

Inflammatory disease is another important cause of exudative retinal detachments. Choroidal inflammation damages the retinal pigment epithelium, allowing fluid to leak into the subretinal space. Disease entities that combine inflammation and exudative detachment are Harada's syndrome, peripheral uveitis, and posterior scleritis.

Diagnosis

Harada's Syndrome
Harada's syndrome, one variant of the *Vogt-Koyanagi-Harada syndrome,* is a diffuse choroiditis of unknown etiology that typically develops in orientals, blacks, and darkly pigmented whites of either sex. Associated systemic manifestations include headaches, fever, anorexia, malaise, and vomiting. Neurologic findings include seizures, hemiparesis, coma, psychosis, and ataxia. Examination of the cerebrospinal fluid often reveals

Table 34-1. Exudative retinal detachments

Intraocular neoplasms
    Choroidal malignant melanoma
    Metastatic carcinoma
    Choroidal hemangioma
    Retinoblastoma

Inflammatory diseases
    Harada's syndrome
    Posterior scleritis
    Peripheral uveitis
    Infected scleral buckle

Idiopathic uveal effusion syndrome

Hydrostatic conditions
    Hypotony—wound leak
    Nanophthalmos

Retinal vascular diseases
    Coats's disease
    von Hippel-Lindau disease

Choroidal disorders
    Central serous chorioretinopathy
    Toxemia
    End-stage renal disease
    Dysproteinemia

pleocytosis and a high protein level. The presence of dysacousia from damage to the auditory nerve and the dermatologic manifestations of vitiligo, alopecia, and poliosis may aid in diagnosis.

The ophthalmic picture in Harada's syndrome is sudden bilateral visual loss caused by an exudative retinal detachment of the inferior fundus. The vitreous contains inflammatory cells, and an anterior uveitis may be present. The disks are hyperemic, and the choroid is thickened. Angiography demonstrates leakage from the choroid into the subretinal space. Initially, there are many irregular areas of fluorescein staining at the level of the retinal pigment epithelium. These areas gradually increase in size to form large areas of hyperfluoroescence. The disk leaks, and in the late stages of the angiogram, the subretinal fluid stains.

The exudative detachment of Harada's syndrome often resolves in 2 to 6 weeks, but may run a prolonged course and often recurs. High-dose systemic steroids shorten the duration. Even if the exudative detachment resolves, the retinal pigment epithelium may sustain extensive damage, with permanent visual loss.

Uveal Effusion Syndrome
The *uveal effusion syndrome* is a distinct clinical entity that affects otherwise healthy, middle-aged men almost exclusively. This syndrome is characterized by the spontaneous development of a serous retinal detachment accompanied by a serous detachment of the peripheral choroid and ciliary body. The disorder is bilateral, but both eyes may not be affected simultaneously. Minimal signs of anterior uveitis may be present, or there may be vitreous cells and flare. Other clinical findings include dilated episcleral vessels, blood in Schlemm's canal, choroidal thickening, retinal hemorrhages, disk edema, and retinal pigment epithelial changes, especially in chronic cases. There are usually no associated systemic findings.

Ultrasonography and fluorescein angiography are helpful in diagnosis. Ultrasonographically, the eye is of normal size, and there is a peripheral uveal tract detachment that is often difficult to appreciate by indirect ophthalmoscopy. The posterior choroid is also thickened. Angiographically, the background choroidal fluorescence is prolonged, with discrete or localized areas of leakage at the level of the retinal pigment epithelium. The optic disk capillaries also leak. Prominent retinal pigment epithelial changes are seen in chronic cases.

The etiology of the uveal effusion syndrome may relate to chronic venous obstruction. Medical treatment has been disappointing, but some success has been reported with surgical decompression of the vortex veins. In the differential diagnosis of exudative retinal detachment are other disorders that impair venous outflow. These include encircling scleral buckles, panretinal photocoagulation, nanophthalmos, aplasia or hypoplasia of vortex veins, diffuse primary and metastatic neoplasms involving the uvea, and inflammatory processes in the sclera and vortex veins, including rheumatoid scleritis, thyroid disease, and inflammatory pseudotumor of the orbit.

Coats's Disease
The most important of the primary retinal disorders that cause exudative detachments is *Coats's disease*, in which there is leakage from telangiectatic retinal vessels. In *von Hippel-Lindau disease*, retinal angiomas are the source of leakage. The retinal tumor often has dilated feeder vessels and is usually located in the periphery. Occasionally, the disk may be involved.

Treatment
In both Coats's and von Hippel-Lindau diseases, treatment of the vascular anomaly, usually by photocoagulation, leads to resolution of the detachment. The indications for treatment of traction retinal detachments are less clear. Localized detachments not involving the macula are probably best left alone. A progressive traction detachment that involves the macula may require vitrectomy to relieve the traction and return the retina to its normal anatomic location. Occasionally, a scleral buckling procedure or a lamellar scleral resection may also be indicated. If there is a combined traction and rhegmatogenous detachment, then scleral buckling will necessarily follow vitrectomy.

1. Aaberg, T.M., Pawlowski, G.J. Exudative retinal detachments following scleral buckling with cryotherapy. *Am. J. Ophthalmol.* 74:245–251, 1972.
   Exudative retinal detachments can occur subsequent to cryopexy utilized during scleral buckling procedures.
2. Brockhurst, R.J. Vortex vein decompression for nanophthalmic uveal effusion. *Arch. Ophthalmol.* 98:1987–1990, 1980.
   Successful attachments of exudative retinal detachments were obtained by surgical decompression of vortex veins in eyes with nanophthalmic uveal effusions.
3. Cohen, H.B., McMeel, J.W., Franks, E.P. Diabetic traction detachment. *Arch. Ophthalmol.* 97:1268–1272, 1979.
   The natural course of traction retinal detachment is presented in 124 patients followed for an average of 4.6 years.
4. Gass, J.D.M. Bullous retinal detachment: An unusual manifestation of idiopathic central serous choroidopathy. *Am. J. Ophthalmol.* 75:810–821, 1973.
   Large exudative retinal detachments may be a manifestation of central serous chorioretinopathy.
5. Gass, J.D.M., Jallow, S. Idiopathic serous detachment of the choroid, ciliary body, and retina (uveal effusion syndrome). *Ophthalmology* 89:1018–1032, 1982.
   Nine patients with the uveal effusion syndrome are presented. Obstruction of the venous outflow of the uveal tract may be an important etiologic factor.
6. Kanter, P.J., Goldberg, M.F. Bilateral uveitis with exudative retinal detachment. *Arch. Ophthalmol.* 91:13–19, 1974.
   Four cases of exudative retinal detachments are presented, and the various causes of the entity are discussed.

7. McMeel, J.W. Diabetic retinopathy: Fibrotic proliferation and retinal detachment. *Trans. Am. Ophthalmol. Soc.* 69:440–493, 1971.
   Proliferative diabetic retinopathy with its complications of traction and rhematogenous retinal detachments is discussed.

8. Schepens, C.L., Brockhurst, R.S. Uveal effusion. I. Clinical picture. *Arch. Ophthalmol.* 70:180–201, 1963.
   The clinical findings of the syndrome are presented.

9. Sears, M.L. Choroidal and retinal detachments associated with scleritis. *Am. J. Ophthalmol.* 58:764–766, 1964.
   Two patients with scleritis and choroidoretinal detachments are described.

10. Weiter, J.J., Brockhurst, R.S., Tolentino, F.I. Uveal effusion following panretinal photocoagulation. *Ann. Ophthalmol.* 11:1723–1727, 1979.
    Three patients developed exudative retinal detachments following panretinal photocoagulation.

35. RETINOSCHISIS

Retinoschisis is a condition characterized by splitting of the sensory retina into an inner and outer layer. Retinoschisis differs from retinal detachment in that, in the latter condition, the full thickness of the retina separates from the retinal pigment epithelium, whereas in retinoschisis, the outer retinal layer stays in apposition to the retinal pigment epithelium.

Retinoschisis can conveniently be classified into acquired and congenital forms. The acquired form is much more common and may result from a variety of causes. The most common cause of acquired retinoschisis is senescence, in which the retina gradually splits into two layers as a result of aging. This condition has been referred to as senile or degenerative retinoschisis, as well as by the terms giant cyst or macrocyst of the retina. Acquired retinoschisis can also be a consequence of any process that induces vitreal traction on the retina. Thus, diabetic retinopathy, retinopathy of prematurity, and vitreous traction secondary to trauma or inflammation all produce secondary tractional retinoschisis. A congenital and hereditary form of retinoschisis also occurs, characterized by both foveal and peripheral retinoschisis.

Pathogenesis

The most common form of retinoschisis, senile or degenerative retinoschisis, appears to be a pathologic extension of the process that causes peripheral cystoid degeneration. The microcystic spaces located at the ora serrata coalesce and eventually spread to become a system of spaces that split the retina in half. Histopathologic examinations confirm the splitting of the retina into inner and outer layers at the level of the outer plexiform layer. Thus, the inner layer usually consists of the ganglion cells, the nerve fiber layer, and the intraretinal vessels found in these layers. This layer is usually very thin and transparent and may harbor many tiny holes that may be very difficult to detect clinically. The outer layer of the retinoschisis remains attached to the retinal pigment epithelium. The schisis cavity is filled with a mucopolysaccharide material.

Histologically, two types of degenerative retinoschisis have been described: *flat* or *typical* and *bullous* or *reticular*. Flat retinoschisis is usually confined to the area anterior to the equator and does not harbor any holes in either the inner or outer layer. The bullous or reticular retinoschisis extends posterior to the equator and frequently harbors holes in the outer retinal layer. These histologic types usually cannot be distinguished by clinical examinations.

Degenerative or senile retinoschisis is a common condition that is present in approximately 3.5 percent of the general population. Rare in young people, it shows the highest prevalence in the group aged 50 to 69 years (7%). It occurs equally in males and females and is bilateral in about 85 percent of cases. Senile retinoschisis is more common in hyperopic eyes.

Diagnosis

Retinoschisis is usually found in asymptomatic patients during routine ophthalmic evaluation when dilated indirect ophthalmoscopy is performed. Some patients do complain of occasional photopsia and floaters. Central vision is rarely affected unless the retinoschisis involves the macular area. Few patients notice the peripheral visual field defects, regularly found on perimetry.

Retinoschisis is detected and diagnosed by indirect ophthalmoscopy and contact lens slit lamp biomicroscopy. On examination, either a shallow or a bullous elevation of the inner layer of the peripheral retina may be seen extending from the ora serrata to the equator. The areas of shallow retinoschisis resemble an exaggerated peripheral microcystic degeneration. In bullous retinoschisis, the inner layer of the retina is visible as a tense dome with no evidence of any shifting fluid phenomenon. The inner layer is very thin and transparent, and the blood vessels located in this area cast a shadow on the outer retinal layers. Occasionally, white dots are seen in this layer. Tiny atrophic holes are almost always present, but they are difficult to detect ophthalmoscopically. The outer layer of the retinoschisis has a rather mottled texture. On scleral indentation, the ophthalmoscopic sign of white with pressure may be observed. Holes in this area, if present, are large and may show raw edges. In assocation with these outer retinal holes, a schisis or detachment may be present. Here, a portion of the outer retinal layer becomes elevated above the retinal pigment epithelium, and the subretinal fluid communicates with the retinoschisis cavity through the hole in the outer layer. These schisis detachments are usually subclinical since they are asymptomatic and rarely progress.

Demarcation lines are not present unless there is a concomitant retinal detachment. In the presence of a concomitant retinal detachment, differentiation between the two conditions may be very difficult to make ophthalmoscopically. The retina outside the area of retinoschisis is normal ophthalmoscopically as well as histologically. The most common locations of acquired degenerative retinoschisis are the inferotemporal quadrant (72%) and the superotemporal quadrant (28%).

The clinical course of degenerative retinoschisis is usually benign. The vast majority of cases remain stationary with no enlargement of the schisis cavity. Infrequently, the cavity collapses spontaneously, resulting in a cure. In some patients, the schisis cavity extends into the posterior pole and in rare instances involve the macula causing visual loss. Early retinoschisis converts to a retinal detachment only rarely.

In the differential diagnosis, one should always consider ocular conditions that can produce traction with secondary retinoschisis, such as diabetic retinopathy and trauma and inflammation of the posterior pole. An old retinal detachment with a very thin retina and small atrophic holes may simulate retinoschisis.

Treatment

Since this entity has a benign clinical course and since the area of retinoschisis usually remains localized to the periphery of the retina, treatment is not indicated in the majority of patients. Some physicians advocate prophylactic photocoagulation or cryotherapy to prevent further extension of the retinoschisis to the posterior pole. This approach is controversial, but usually consists of placing a barrage of photocoagulation spots on the periphery of the schisis to produce chorioretinal scarring, which stops the extension of the schisis cavity. Cryopexy may also be utilized for the same purpose.

Surgery is indicated, however, when the retinoschisis progresses posteriorly beyond the equator and threatens the macula. This progression, which is extremely rare, must be documented with sequential fundus drawings and repeated visual field examinations. A controversial indication for surgery is the simultaneous presence of holes in both the inner and outer layers of the retinoschisis, since some believe that such cases may develop true retinal detachments. Here, the aim of the treatment is to close the holes in the outer layers of the retinoschisis before the retina detaches. Both cryopexy and photocoagulation may be used for treatment of such holes. In the presence of a true retinal detachment in association with the retinoschisis, a scleral buckling procedure will be necessary.

Hereditary Retinoschisis

Although not as common as degenerative retinoschisis, *hereditary retinoschisis*, also known as *X-linked juvenile retinoschisis*, congenital vascular veils, or congenital cystic detachment, is not a rare clinical entity. It is characterized by schisis of both the central and peripheral retina in association with vitreous degeneration. The disease is transmitted as a sex-linked recessive trait and thus is almost always encountered in males. Female carriers have no characteristic findings. The gene has a high degree of penetrance but a variable expressivity.

Pathologically, hereditary retinoschisis differs from degenerative retinoschisis in that the splitting of the retina in hereditary retinoschisis occurs in the nerve fiber layer, whereas in degenerative retinoschisis the split is at the level of the outer plexiform layer.

The most common clinical finding in hereditary retinoschisis is the foveal involvement that occurs in almost 100 percent of cases. *Foveal retinoschisis* may lead to decreased vision. Decreased vision may also occur secondary to vitreous hemorrhage. The foveal retinoschisis is the only retinal abnormality in 50 percent of the cases. In the other 50 percent of the patients, the peripheral retina also shows evidence of schisis. This peripheral schisis is commonly located in the temporal quadrants. Other ophthalmoscopic findings include vitreal veils or strands; sheathed vessels; grayish white arborescent and dendritiform structures; silver-gray, glistening spotty areas; disk pallor; and pseudopapillitis.

Ophthalmoscopically, the foveal retinoschisis consists of an optically empty zone delimited by two retinal layers, of which the most superficial one is very thin. This layer shows typical radial plications that are formed by small folds in the internal limiting membrane and that give a characteristic spoked or cartwheel appearance to the macula. Microcystic changes may also be present. Fluorescein angiography of the macula usually does not show any abnormalities.

The highly elevated inner layer of peripheral retinoschisis may be so thin as to be invisible unless retinal vessels are seen. The anterior border of the schisis rarely extends to the ora serrata, but the posterior edge may reach the macular area. Inner layer holes are more common and larger than outer layer holes. A true retinal detachment may occur, but is not common. In the differential diagnosis, one should consider other vitreoretinal dystrophies such as Wagner's vitreoretinal dystrophy, Goldmann-Favre's dystrophy, and retinal detachment and degenerative retinoschisis.

At this time, there is no treatment available to alter the foveal schisis. The treatment of peripheral retinoschisis is controversial, and prophylactic treatment by photocoagulation may be followed by retinal detachments. In those rare instances where a true rhegmatogenous retinal detachment develops, the treatment is the same as with rhegmatogenous detachments (see Chap. 33).

---

1. Byer, N.E. Clinical study of senile retinoschisis. *Arch. Ophthalmol.* 79:36–44, 1968.
   The author initiated a natural course study of senile retinoschisis, which was eventually carried out for 21 years (see refrences 2 and 3). This initial paper included 102 eyes of 56 patients.
2. Byer, N.E. The natural history of senile retinoschisis. *Trans. Am. Acad. Ophthalmol. Otolaryngol.* 81:458–471, 1976.
   Byer gives his observations on 193 eyes of 108 nonreferred patients who had senile retinoschisis. These eyes were followed without treatment for 2 to 11 years. Based on this author's as well as other reported series, the incidence of retinal detachment occurring in patients with retinoschisis was calculated to be 0.7 percent.
3. Byer, N.E. Long-term natural history study of senile retinoschisis with implications for management. *Ophthalmology* 93:1127–1137, 1986.
   An excellent long-term natural course study of senile retinoschisis, in which 218 eyes with senile retinoschisis were followed for 1 to 21 years. Controversial aspects of management of retinoschisis are discussed.
4. Deutman, A.F. Vitreoretinal dystrophies—X-linked juvenile retinoschisis. In E.

Krill, *Krill's Hereditary Retinal and Choroidal Diseases,* vol 2. Philadelphia: Harper & Row, 1977. Chap. 20, 1044–1062.
An excellent review of the subject.

5. Dobbie, J.G. Cryotherapy in the management of senile retinoschisis. *Trans. Am. Acad. Ophthalmol. Otolaryngol.* 73:1047–1059, 1969.
The author presents his indications for treating senile retinoschisis with cryotherapy, as the result of his successful treatment of 13 eyes in 11 patients.

6. Foos, R.Y. Senile retinoschisis: Relationship to cystoid degeneration. *Trans. Am. Acad. Ophthalmol. Otolaryngol.* 74:33–50, 1970.
The pathogenic relationship of typical and reticular cystoid degeneration to senile retinoschisis is presented in a study of 859 eyes obtained at autopsy.

7. Hagler, W.S., Woldoff, H.S. Retinal detachment in relation to senile retinoschisis. *Trans. Am. Acad. Ophthalmol. Otolaryngol.* 77:99–113, 1973.
Treatment of retinal detachment in association with senile retinoschisis with different modalities, including cryocoagulation, photocoagulation, and scleral buckling, is presented. The retinas were successfully attached in 97 percent of the eyes.

8. Lewis, R.A., Lee, G.B., Martonyi, C.L., et al. Familial foveal retinoschisis. *Arch. Ophthalmol.* 95:1190–1196, 1977.
Foveal retinoschisis, an X-linked recessive chromosomal disorder, is described in three females, daughters of ophthalmoscopically normal parents.

9. Straatsma, B.R., Foos, R.Y. Typical and reticular degenerative retinoschisis. XXVI Francis I. Proctor Memorial Lecture. *Am. J. Ophthalmol.* 75:551–575, 1973.
Clinical and histologic findings of the entity of degenerative retinoschisis, gathered from the study of 2319 eyes obtained at autopsy and 50 eyes examined clinically.

10. Sulonen, J.M., Wells, C.G., Barricks, M.E., et al. Degenerative retinoschisis with giant outer layer breaks and retinal detachment. *Am. J. Ophthalmol.* 99:114–121, 1985.
Five patients are presented who developed retinal detachments secondary to giant posterior breaks located in the outer layer of degenerative retinoschisis. Various surgical treatment modalities are described.

11. Yanoff, M., Rahn, E.K., Zimmermann, L.E. Histopathology of juvenile retinoschisis. *Arch. Ophthalmol.* 79:49–53, 1968.
The first histopathologic documentation of juvenile retinoschisis in which the retinal split was found to be at the level of the retinal nerve fiber layer.

12. Yassur, Y., Feldberg, R., Axer-Siegel, R., et al. Argon laser treatment of senile retinoschisis. *Br. J. Ophthalmol.* 67:381–384, 1983.
Successful treatment of senile retinoschisis by laser photocoagulation with a follow-up of 3 to 6 years.

36. RETINITIS PIGMENTOSA

Retinitis pigmentosa (RP) represents a set of progressive hereditary disorders that diffusely and primarily affect photoreceptor and retinal pigment epithelial function. RP is not an inflammatory disease, and the suffix "-itis," although entrenched in clinical usage, is inaccurate. Although there is no uniformly accepted classification, RP can be broadly divided into two categories: those disorders confined to the eye (Leber's congenital amaurosis), and those associated with systemic diseases (Usher's syndrome, abetalipoproteinemia, Bardet-Biedl syndrome, Refsum's syndrome, and mucopolysaccharidoses).

Approximately 1 of every 3,000 Americans has RP. There is no sex predilection, and several forms of inheritance exist. The most common is *autosomal recessive* inheritance (62%). *Autosomal dominant* inheritance (14%) is the mildest form of the disease, whereas the *X-linked recessive* form (6%) has the earliest age of onset and the worst visual prognosis. About 18 percent have *isolated* disease with no family history.

Pathogenesis

The exact pathogenesis in most cases is unknown. It is still uncertain whether this group of disorders is a primary photoreceptor disease or a combined photoreceptor-retinal pigment epithelial disease. Histopathologic studies show an absence of the photoreceptor layer involving both the rods and cones. In advanced cases, there is attenuation of all layers of the retina, which becomes thin and gliotic. The retinal pigment epithelium proliferates and migrates into the anterior retina. Melanin granules deposit in and around the walls of the retinal arterioles, and this deposition is responsible for the bone-spiculed pattern of pigmentation observed clinically. The retinal arterioles show moderate periarterial thickening and hyalinization of the wall.

Clinical

The diagnosis of RP is usually easily made on the basis of family history, subjective complaints, and ophthalmoscopic picture. Although RP is a hereditary disease, the visual signs and symptoms generally do not appear until early adult life. Symptoms of night blindness usually begin in the second decade of life, followed much later by decreased peripheral vision. About 50 percent of patients experience a decrease in central visual acuity attributable to macular pathology, i.e., cystoid macular edema, epiretinal membranes, and atrophy of the retinal pigment epithelium and choriocapillaris.

Ocular involvement is usually bilateral and symmetric. The clinical diagnosis is made by the ophthalmoscopic triad of pigmentary bone spicules, attenuated arterioles, and waxy, pale optic nerve head. The clumps and strands of pigment are usually scattered throughout the retina but are most prominent in the midperiphery or around blood vessels. Several variants of RP have been described, which include *sector RP* (focal fundus changes typical of RP), *unilateral RP* (only one eye shows the typical ophthalmoscopic and electrodiagnostic features of RP), and *inverse RP* (these probably represent cases of cone-rod dystrophy or more advanced atypical cases of fundus flavimaculatus). Other ocular findings that are frequently associated with RP include myopia, vitreous opacities, posterior subcapsular cataracts, keratoconus, optic nerve head drusen, and peripheral retinal vascular abnormalities.

Both subjective and objective tests are important in establishing the diagnosis. Of the subjective tests, visual fields and dark adaptation are the most important. Visual field examination usually reveals a ring scotoma that subsequently contracts from the periphery, leading to marked concentric constriction and eventual total blindness. Dark adaptometry shows elevation of the threshold of the dark adaptation curve of both rod and cone segments. Of the objective tests, the most definitive is the *electroretinogram* (ERG), which is a quite specific test for the evaluation of the outer retinal layers. Since in RP there is diffuse photoreceptor damage, the ERG is markedly reduced or, in most cases, extinguished. In some instances, the ERG is not extinguished, but the implicit time (the time period between the onset of flash and the peak of the response) is prolonged. The ERG is particularly important in making the diagnosis in atypical cases, in studying asymptomatic family members and carriers, and in evaluating infants and young children on whom subjective tests cannot be done.

In the differential diagnosis and especially in those individuals with unilateral RP, one should consider inflammatory, traumatic, and vascular etiologies that may present a clinical and ophthalmoscopic picture similar to that of RP.

Treatment

Specific treatment exists for only three systemic variants that have specific biochemical defects. Parenteral vitamin A is used in the Bassen-Kornzweig syndrome (abetalipoproteinemia); a diet low in phytanic acid is used in Refsum's syndrome (RP associated with peripheral neuropathy and cerebellar ataxia); and vitamin B_6 is used for gyrate atrophy. Unfortunately, for most people with RP, there is no effective therapy, and management consists of genetic counseling and low-vision aids. An important problem in genetic counseling is the accurate classification of the isolated (simplex) male. Characteristic retinal changes in X-linked carrier females may aid in differentiating the genetic variant. A certain number of female carriers have a scintillating golden reflex around the macular area or some peripheral pigment changes, or both. Grid laser photocoagulation has been advocated by some for treatment of macular edema associated with RP.

1. Berson, E.L. Retinitis pigmentosa and allied retinal diseases: Electrophysiologic findings. *Trans. Am. Acad. Ophthalmol. Otolaryngol.* 81:659–666, 1976.
   The ERG findings in early cases of RP are discussed and analyzed.
2. Carr, R.E. Retinitis pigmentosa: Recent advances. In Clinical, Structural, and Biomedical Advances in Hereditary Eye Disorders. In D.L. Daeth (ed.), *Progress in Clinical and Biological Research,* Vol. 82. New York: Alan R. Liss, 1982. Pp. 135–146.
   A concise summary of recent advances in the diagnosis and treatment of RP.
3. Carr, R.E., Noble, K. G. Retinitis pigmentosa. *Ophthalmology* 88:169–172, 1981.
   A résumé of the clinical and electrophysiologic findings in RP.
4. Fishman, G.A., Alexander, K.R., Anderson, R.J. Autosomal dominant retinitis pigmentosa. A method of classification. *Arch. Ophthalmol.* 103:366–374, 1985.
   An attempt to classify the heterogeneous group of patients with autosomal dominant RP.
5. Foxman, S.G., Heckenlively, J.R., Bateman, J.B., et al. Classification of congenital and early onset retinitis pigmentosa. *Arch. Ophthalmol.* 103:1502–1506, 1985.
   The authors propose a new classification of Leber's congenital amaurosis based on age of onset, severity of signs, and associated nonocular abnormalities.
6. Gartner, S., Henkind, P. Pathology of retinitis pigmentosa. *Ophthalmology* 89:1425–1432, 1982.
   Histopathologic study of 14 eyes with RP indicates that the initial pathology lies in the photoreceptors.
7. Jay, M. On the heredity of retinitis pigmentosa. *Br. J. Ophthalmol.* 66:405–416, 1982.
   The genetic makeup of the RP population seen at the Genetic Clinic at Moorfields Eye Hospital.
8. Jay, B., Bird, A. X-linked retinitis pigmentosa. *Trans. Am. Acad. Ophthalmol. Otolaryngol.* 77:641–651, 1973.
   In heterozygous female carriers, characteristic peripheral retinal changes were noted, including areas of retinal pigment epithelial atrophy with areas of pigment migration into the retina. It is important to recognize the heterozygous state for accurate genetic diagnosis and counseling.
9. Marmor, M.F., Aguirre, G., Arden, G., et al. Retinitis pigmentosa—a symposium on terminology and methods of examination. *Ophthalmology* 90:126–131, 1983.
   A preliminary report of opinions expressed by specialists in the field of RP regarding guidelines for unified terminology, classification, and methods of examination.
10. Merin, S., Auerbach, E. Retinitis pigmentosa. Review. *Surv. Ophthalmol.* 20:303–346, 1976.
    An extensive review of the subject with 480 references.

37. DIABETIC RETINOPATHY

Diabetes mellitus affects 1.5 percent of the population of the Western world. Diabetic retinopathy develops in almost half of all diabetics and is a major cause of blindness. The prevalence of diabetic retinopathy increases with the duration of the diabetes and the age of the patient. Diabetic retinopathy may be the first clinical sign of adult onset diabetes. Clinically, diabetic retinopathy can be classified into (1) *nonproliferative or background diabetic retinopathy* (BDR); (2) *preproliferative diabetic retinopathy;* and (3) *proliferative diabetic retinopathy* (PDR).

Pathogenesis
The cause and pathogenesis of diabetic microvascular disease are poorly understood. *Retinal capillary obliteration* and *increased retinal capillary permeability* are two major pathologic changes seen in the retinal vasculature that are thought to play a major role

in the pathogenesis of diabetic retinopathy. Retinal capillary obliteration leads to localized or widespread areas of retinal ischemia. With widespread retinal ischemia, retinal vascular endothelial proliferation occurs and eventually leads to neovascularization of the retina or optic disk or both. The neovascularization, which initially may be flat on the surface of the disk and retina, may extend into the vitreous cavity secondary to vitreous traction and cause major subhyaloid and vitreal hemorrhages. Fibrosis and organization of the vitreous may eventually lead to tractional or rhegmatogenous retinal detachments. The increased permeability of the retinal vasculature leads to localized or widespread areas of retinal edema. The retina shows evidence of thickening as a result of accumulation of edema fluid, and hard exudates may form surrounding areas of abnormally leaking capillaries and microaneurysms. In the macular area, the edema fluid may accumulate in cystic spaces, causing cystoid macular edema.

Diagnosis

The majority of patients with retinopathy (more than 90%) have BDR that is frequently mild and causes no visual loss. Clinically, BDR is characterized by the presence of retinal venous dilatation and beading, microaneurysms, cotton-wool infarcts, retinal exudates, superficial and deep retinal hemorrhages, macular edema, and intraretinal microvascular abnormalities (IRMA). Marked, irreversible central visual loss may occur in these patients secondary to chronic cystoid macular edema or to macular capillary occlusion and macular ischemia. Although ophthalmoscopy and slit lamp biomicroscopy permit visualization and study of most of these lesions, fluorescein angiography is essential in evaluating the ischemic and hyperpermeability changes. The angiography characterizes the extent and severity of these changes. Other causes of irreversible central visual loss secondary to BDR include subfoveal hemorrhages, macular cyst and hole formation, and preretinal fibrosis.

The *preproliferative* stage of the retinopathy is characterized by multiple, extensive areas of retinal ischemia (cotton-wool patches), IRMA, venous beading, and retinal hemorrhages. Fluorescein angiography, particularly of the preequatorial areas of the retina, shows extensive areas of capillary nonperfusion but no frank neovascularization. These patients are at high risk to develop PDR, which usually ensues within 12 months. In PDR, neovascular tufts become evident on the disk (NVD) or elsewhere in the retina (NVE). The neovascular fronds may be flat on the retina or elevated into the vitreous cavity and associated with subhyaloid or vitreous hemorrhages. Rhegmatogenous and tractional retinal detachments are major causes of visual morbidity. Late sequelae of PDR include anterior segment neovascularization with secondary glaucoma and subsequent total loss of vision.

Treatment

Treatment of diabetic retinopathy usually consists of medical control of the diabetes mellitus and photocoagulation therapy of the retina. Optimal medical control of the diabetes and associated systemic problems, such as hypertension and renal and cardiovascular disease, is essential. At this time, there is no conclusive evidence that tight metabolic control of diabetes with insulin infusion devices stabilizes or prevents the diabetic retinopathy.

The aim of photocoagulation therapy in BDR is to eliminate macular edema and areas of retinal ischemia. In the presence of clinically significant macular edema, laser treatment has been shown to be beneficial. Treatment involves focal coagulation of leaky microaneurysms and grid treatment of areas of diffuse leakage and of capillary nonperfusion greater than 500 μ from the center of the macula. Photocoagulation usually stabilizes the visual acuity, and in some instances visual acuity may improve. Patients with diffuse macular edema with moderate to severe visual loss usually do not fare well with photocoagulation, since the sources of leakage requiring treatment are difficult to identify and photocoagulate. At this time, the role of panretinal photocoagulation in treating diffuse macular edema in BDR has not been established. The results of the ongoing randomized clinical trial may clarify the role of this treatment. Lesions of the macula that are not amenable to photocoagulation treatment and yet may cause significant visual loss include macular cysts and holes, foveal hemorrhages, and macular preretinal membranes.

The efficacy of panretinal photocoagulation in the treatment of PDR has been established by the Diabetic Retinopathy Study. The aim of panretinal photocoagulation is to destroy large areas of ischemic retina that are thought to be the source of a stimulus (factor X) to neovascularization. The patients who show the greatest benefit are those who have high-risk characteristics of PDR. In these patients panretinal photocoagulation is definitely indicated. The high-risk characteristics include moderate to severe NVD, mild NVD associated with vitreous hemorrhages, and moderate to severe NVE associated with vitreous hemorrhages. Although panretinal photocoagulation has been beneficial in these patients, one should always remember the potential complications, which include decreased central visual acuity and reduced peripheral field. Treatment should be instituted only when indicated.

The role of panretinal photocoagulation in preproliferative diabetic retinopathy has not been established. It is not known whether treating severe preproliferative diabetic retinopathy with panretinal photocoagulation delays or prevents the development of PDR. The Early Treatment Diabetic Retinopathy Study is presently studying this question and whether prompt panretinal photocoagulation is indicated in preproliferative diabetic retinopathy. Vitreous and retinal surgery is indicated in patients who have complications of severe PDR, which include nonabsorbing vitreous hemorrhages, tractional retinal detachment involving the macula, and combined traction and rhegmatogenous retinal detachments.

1. Blankenship, G.W. Diabetic macular edema and argon laser photocoagulation: A prospective randomized study. *Ophthalmology* 86:69–75, 1979.
   Photocoagulation treatment of macular edema in patients with BDR was beneficial, with the treated eyes showing a tendency for visual improvement and a reduced rate of visual deterioration. This was a prospective study on 39 patients with symmetric BDR and macular edema in which one eye was treated while the other eye was followed without treatment.
2. Blankenship, G.W., Machemer, R. Long-term diabetic vitrectomy results. Report of 10-year follow-up. *Ophthalmology* 92:503–506, 1985.
   The long-term results of diabetic vitrectomy were quite satisfactory with 42 percent of patients maintaining 6/60 or better visual acuities for as long as 10 years.
3. Bresnick, G.H. Diabetic maculopathy: A critical review highlighting diffuse macular edema. *Ophthalmology* 90:1301–1317, 1983.
   The etiology of diabetic macular edema and ischemia is discussed, with the rationale for treatment.
4. The Diabetic Retinopathy Study Research Group. Four risk factors for severe visual loss in diabetic retinopathy. *Arch. Ophthalmol.* 97:654–655, 1979.
   Four risk factors were found in this study that increased the 2-year risk of developing severe visual loss. These factors include presence of vitreous or preretinal hemorrhages, presence of new vessels, location of new vessels on or near the optic disk, and severity of the new vessels.
5. The Diabetic Retinopathy Study Research Group. Photocoagulation treatment of proliferative diabetic retinopathy. *Ophthalmology* 88:583–600, 1981.
   The beneficial effects of photocoagulation in reducing the risk of severe visual loss are confirmed in the follow-up report of this study group.
6. The Diabetic Retinopathy Vitrectomy Study Research Group. Two-year course of visual acuity in severe proliferative diabetic retinopathy with conventional management. *Ophthalmology* 92:492–502, 1985.
   This report gives the results of the group N patients, recruited to study the visual acuity of patients with severe PDR who were managed by conventional methods.
7. The Diabetic Retinopathy Vitrectomy Study Research Group. *Early vitrectomy for severe vitreous hemorrhage in diabetic retinopathy. Arch. Ophthalmol.* 103:1644–1652, 1985.
   Early vitrectomy may be more beneficial in type I diabetic patients with severe vitreous hemorrhage, whereas such a benefit was not found in type II diabetic patients with severe vitreous hemorrhage.

8. Early Treatment Diabetic Retinopathy Study Research Group. Photocoagulation for diabetic macular edema. *Arch. Ophthalmol.* 103:1796–1806, 1985.
   Focal photocoagulation for "clinically significant" diabetic macular edema is indicated since it substantially reduces the risk of visual loss.
9. Michels, R.G. Proliferative diabetic retinopathy: Pathophysiology of extraretinal complications and principles of vitreous surgery. *Retina* 1:1–17, 1981.
   A comprehensive review of the subject with emphasis on surgical methodology.
10. Rice, T.A., Michels, R.G., Maguire, M.G., et al. The effect of lensectomy on the incidence of iris neovascularization and neovascular glaucoma after vitrectomy for diabetic retinopathy. *Am. J. Ophthalmol.* 95:1–11, 1983.
    Removal of the lens during vitrectomy contributed to a significant increase in postoperative iris neovascularization and neovascular glaucoma.
11. Rice, T.A., Michels, R.G., Rice, E.F. Vitrectomy for diabetic traction retinal detachment involving the macula. *Am. J. Ophthalmol.* 95:22–33, 1983.
    An analysis of 197 eyes that underwent vitrectomy for diabetic traction detachment of the macula is presented. A 66 percent success rate of retinal attachment was achieved.

38. RETINOPATHY OF PREMATURITY

Retinopathy of prematurity (ROP) is a proliferative retinopathy that affects the retinal vasculature of premature infants who are usually exposed to excessive oxygen and results in retinal neovascularization and its complications. It is a leading cause of childhood blindness in the United States and the rest of the industrialized world. Although this clinical entity is better known as *retrolental fibroplasia,* the term ROP more accurately characterizes the clinical and histologic features of this retinopathy.

Pathogenesis

The disease reached epidemic proportions in the late 1940s and early 1950s. This was linked to the administration of excessive amounts of oxygen to premature babies. The incidence of ROP dropped dramatically after rigid curtailment of oxygen use in nurseries. Recently, there has been a moderate increase in the incidence of ROP. This resurgence has been attributed to improve neonatology practices that have resulted in a marked reduction of mortality of very premature, low-birthweight infants, rather than as a result of excess oxygen use. As a matter of fact, many cases of ROP are now occurring despite meticulous control of oxygen administration and even when no supplemental oxygen has been administered. Those at greatest risk of developing ROP are premature infants with gestational ages of less than 37 weeks and birthweights of less than 1600 gm. Although use of oxygen and hyperoxia are additional major risk factors, other agents may also have a role in the etiology of this disease. Vitamin E deficiency, light toxicity, blood CO_2 tension and pH, and prostaglandins are additional factors that have been implicated and are being investigated. At the present time, the exact etiology of ROP remains unknown.

The retina is susceptible to oxygen damage only before its complete vascularization, that is, when it is immature. The main response of the immature retinal vessels to hyperoxia is severe vasoconstriction. This is most apparent in the temporal retinal periphery, where normal vascularization of the retina is not attained until after birth. With severe and sustained vasoconstriction, some degree of vascular closure eventually results. The anterior retina remains unvascularized. This stage is eventually followed (when the infant is returned to room air) by marked endothelial proliferation that arises from the residual vascular complexes immediately adjacent to retinal capillaries closed during hyperoxia. Retinal neovascularization eventually develops. This neovascularization starts on the surface of the retina but later extends into the vitreous cavity. The neovascularization, with its associated fibrous and glial tissue proliferation, eventually results in retinal and vitreal hemorrhages and tractional, rhegmatogenous, and exudative retinal detachments. Although the major pathology is in the retinal vasculature, recent studies have shown that hyperoxia can induce retinal neuronal necrosis, especially of ganglion cells. This may be responsible for subsequent poor vision.

Diagnosis

These active retinal changes, which initially occur in the fundus periphery, can be clinically detected and evaluated by binocular indirect ophthalmoscopy, fluorescein angiography, and fundus photography. These ophthalmoscopic findings have been incorporated into a classification system known as the *International Classification of ROP*, which specifies the location as well as the extent of the retinopathy. The severity of the active retinopathy is ranked in four stages, beginning with recognition of a definite demarcation line that separates avascular from vascular retina (stage 1) through progressive changes that may end with unequivocal detachment (stage 4).

Spontaneous regression is possible during any of the active stages of the retinopathy, especially in the early stages (80%). The rate of regression decreases with more advanced disease. Regardless of what stage of active disease regression occurs, some residual retinal damage may remain. These are referred to as the *cicatricial* stages of ROP. Although as yet there is no unified international classification for these changes of the retinopathy, cooperative efforts are now under way to reexamine the present classification, which divides the cicatricial stage into five grades. These cicatricial stage retinal changes range from minor areas of peripheral retinal pigmentation (grade 1) to temporally dragged retina and disk with retinal folds (grades 2 and 3) to the more advanced and late changes characterized by total retinal detachment with fibrovascular tissue and scarred and thickened retina that forms a retrolental mass (grades 4 and 5).

Children with the advanced cicatricial stages of ROP (grades 4 and 5) may present clinically with a white pupil (leukokoria). This must be differentiated from other important causes of leukokoria, such as retinoblastoma, persistent hyperplastic primary vitreous, congenital cataracts, nematode endophthalmitis, and rhegmatogenous retinal detachment.

Treatment

Treatment of this entity is controversial. The clinical management of *acute ROP* has been similar to the management of other proliferative retinopathies, i.e., either direct destruction of the neovascularization or destruction and elimination of the ischemic retina that is thought to be the stimulus for neovascularization. Photocoagulation (laser or xenon arc) and cryotherapy have been successfully used for these purposes. The therapeutic significance of these treatment modalities is not well known since a large number of patients with active ROP spontaneously regress. At this time, there is an ongoing clinical trial (the Multicenter Trial of Cryotherapy for Retinopathy of Prematurity) to evaluate the role of cryotherapy in treating patients with acute ROP.

Retinal detachments may occur during active disease. If these detachments are exudative in nature, then no treatment is indicated, since the majority will resolve spontaneously when the active disease regresses. Rhegmatogenous retinal detachments and occasional tractional retinal detachments, if present, can be treated with scleral buckling procedures. Patients with advanced cicatricial disease may need sophisticated vitreoretinal procedures, such as vitrectomy, membrane peeling, fluid-gas exchange, and scleral buckling, for repair of the detachment. Although good anatomic results have been obtained with these sophisticated vitreoretinal procedures, the visual results obtained have been disappointing.

Attempts at this time are directed toward measures to prevent ROP from occurring. The roles of vitamin E deficiency, phototoxicity, and prostaglandins are all being investigated in the prophylaxis of ROP.

---

1. Chong, L.P., Machemer, R., deJuan, E. Vitrectomy for advanced stages of retinopathy of prematurity. *Am. J. Ophthalmol.* 102:710–716, 1986.

Although the retinas were anatomically attached in 43 percent of patients with grades 4 and 5 cicatricial ROP, the visual results obtained were not encouraging.

2. The Committee for the Classification of Retinopathy of Prematurity. An international classification of retinopathy of prematurity. *Arch. Ophthalmol.* 102:1130–1134, 1984.
   This new classification of active ROP emphasizes the location and extent of the retinopathy.

3. Finer, N.N., Schindler, R.F., Peters, K.L., et al. Vitamin E and retrolental fibroplasia—improved visual outcome with early vitamin E. *Ophthalmology* 90:428–435, 1983.
   The authors produce clinical evidence that supports the use of vitamin E in decreasing the sequelae of ROP, especially in low-birthweight neonates who require oxygen therapy.

4. Flynn, J.T., O'Grady, G.E., Herrera, J., et al. Retrolental fibroplasia. I. Clinical observations. *Arch. Ophthalmol.* 95:217–223, 1977.
   The clinical findings in 97 premature infants with retrolental fibroplasia were studied by fundus photography and fluorescein angiography.

5. Glass, P., Avery, G.B., Siva Subramanian, K.N., et al. Effect of bright light in the hospital nursery on the incidence of retinopathy of prematurity. *N. Engl. J. Med.* 313:401–404, 1985.
   The authors present data incriminating light as a possible etiologic factor in the development of ROP.

6. Johnson, B.C., Ahdab-Barmada, M. Hyperoxemic retinal neuronal necrosis in the premature neonate. *Am. J. Ophthalmol.* 102:423–430, 1986.
   In an autopsy study of 30 premature neonates, retinal ganglion cell necrosis, especially in the macular area, was demonstrated, and this was speculated to be a result of oxygen toxicity.

7. Kushner, B.J., Essner, D., Cohen, I.J., et al. Retrolental fibroplasia. II. Pathologic correlation. *Arch. Ophthalmol.* 95:29–38, 1977.
   An excellent clinicopathologic correlation done on both eyes in each of six infants with retrolental fibroplasia.

8. Patz, A., Payne, J.W. Retinopathy of prematurity (retrolental fibroplasia). In T.D. Duane (ed.), *Clinical Ophthalmology,* vol 3. Philadelphia: Harper & Row, Chap. 20, 1–19.
   An excellent review of ROP.

9. Puklin, J.E., Simon, R.M., Ehrenkranz, R.A. Influence on retrolental fibroplasia of intramuscular vitamin E administration during respiratory distress syndrome. *Ophthalmology* 89:96–102, 1982.
   Prophylactic intramuscular vitamin E therapy was not beneficial in reducing or preventing the occurrence of ROP in neonates with the respiratory distress syndrome.

10. Tasman, W., Brown, G.C., Schaffer, D.B., et al. Cryotherapy for active retinopathy of prematurity. *Ophthalmology* 93:580–585, 1986.
    Cryotherapy was beneficial in treating patients with active ROP.

11. Trese, M.T. Visual results and prognostic factors for vision following surgery for stage V retinopathy of prematurity. *Ophthalmology* 93:574–579, 1986.
    Although good anatomic results are obtained by various vitreoretinal surgical procedures, the visual results obtained are not as satisfactory. Particularly poor visual results were obtained in patients who had subretinal exudates in the macular area.

39. SICKLE RETINOPATHY

The presence of one or more abnormal hemoglobins may cause the normally round to oval red blood cells to adopt a crescentic, elongated, sickle shape under conditions of hypoxia and acidosis. These sickled red blood cells are more rigid than normal red blood cells and consequently may impact in small blood vessels, causing hypoxia, ischemia, and necrosis of ocular or other tissues supplied by these vessels. These abnormal hemoglobins, which can occur either alone or in combination with each other and with normal hemoglobin, include hemoglobins S, C, D, E, and others. In patients with sickle cell thalassemia the rate of synthesis of hemoglobin is abnormal also.

Pathogenesis

Although sickling hemoglobinopathies may affect all the vascularized tissues of the eye, it is the retinal vascular involvement that is responsible for the major visual disturbances in these patients. Most of the ocular findings are attributable to the direct or indirect sequelae of vasoocclusions. Of the vascularized tissues of the eye, the conjunctiva shows highly characteristic isolated vascular segments that are comma or corkscrew in shape. These changes may aid in the diagnosis but in themselves do not cause any symptoms. The iris is occasionally involved, with circumscribed areas of ischemic atrophy and, rarely, with secondary iris neovascularization, which occurs in response to iris ischemia. The choroidal vasculature is seldom involved, although some chorioretinal scars seen in the fundus may be secondary to choroidal vasoocclusions.

The changes that damage vision the most are retinal and may be conveniently divided into nonproliferative and proliferative types. The *nonproliferative* retinal changes usually are asymptomatic lesions found on ophthalmoscopy and include retinal vascular tortuosity, iridescent spots with schisis cavities, salmon-patch retinal hemorrhages, pigmented lesions known as black sunbursts, angioid streaks, and areas of white without pressure and dark without pressure.

Some nonproliferative changes, however, do cause significant visual disturbances. This category includes central retinal artery occlusions, occlusions of the macular and perimacular capillaries, and, rarely, venous occlusions. Patients with central retinal artery, peripapillary, and macular arteriolar occlusions usually complain of sudden loss of vision or of sudden appearance of central and paracentral scotomas. Apart from major arteriolar occlusions, an appreciable number of patients (around 20–30%) sustain capillary occlusions in the macular and perimacular areas with subtle visual changes that may be detected only by meticulous perimetry. Fluorescein angiography best delineates these microvascular changes, which include microaneurysmlike dots, abnormal foveal avascular zones, and pathologic avascular zones. These changes in the macular area may be the etiology of reduced central vision in some patients. Venous occlusions (branch vein or central vein occlusions), although reported, are rare and probably fortuitous in occurrence.

The *proliferative* changes of sickle retinopathy (PSR) can be easily evaluated by indirect ophthalmoscopy and fluorescein angiography. These retinal changes have been classified by Goldberg [5] into five stages, which represent the chronology of events that take place in the retinal periphery of these patients. Goldberg's *stage I* is characterized by peripheral retinal arteriolar occlusions, which are usually the initiating event in PSR. The retina anterior to these occlusions remains avascular and probably is infarcted with loss of the inner retinal elements. From the site of arteriolar obstruction, runoff of blood into adjacent vessels occurs through dilated capillaries, developing a functional arteriovenular (AV) anastomosis (Goldberg's *stage II*).

Eventually, sprouts of neovascular tissue arise from these areas of AV anastomosis (Goldberg's *stage III*). These neovascular tufts are known as sea fans because of their characteristic configuration. They usually grow toward areas of retinal ischemia, which are usually located anterior to the AV anastomosis. These sea fans may be flat on the retina or elevated into the vitreous cavity secondary to vitreous syneresis and traction. Although sea fan neovascularization can occur in patients with sickle cell anemia and sickle cell trait, it is most frequently encountered in patients with sickle cell hemoglobin C (SC) disease and sickle cell B thalassemia (SB thal). Vitreous traction on the sea fans eventually causes localized or massive hemorrhages into the vitreous cavity (Goldberg's *stage IV*). Vitreoretinal traction adjacent or subjacent to fibrovascular tissue may produce retinal holes or tears with subsequent development of rhegmatogenous retinal detachment (Goldberg's *stage V*). The incidence of vitreal hemorrhages and retinal detachments roughly parallels that of the neovascular stage, that is, they occur primarily in patients with SC and SB thal disease. The hemorrhagic sequelae of the sea fans and the retinal detachments are the main reasons for these patients to consult the ophthalmologist, unless the early lesions of PSR were detected on routine or screening examinations.

Treatment

Since retinal neovascularization and its hemorrhagic and tractional complications are the major source of visual loss, treatment is aimed at eliminating these neovascular fronds to minimize their complications of vitreous hemorrhages and retinal detachment. The exact timing as well as the absolute indications for treatment are not well established, since some but not all patients with PSR will develop vitreous hemorrhages and retinal detachments, and 20 to 60 percent of these neovascular fronds will spontaneously regress (autoinfarct). At this time, the recommendation is to treat only one eye of any patient with bilateral PSR. In patients with unilateral disease with early neovascularizations, follow-up without treatment may be reasonable and acceptable if the patient is reliable.

Various approaches may be used to eradicate the neovascular fronds. Various small and flat sea fans may be directly treated by use of xenon arc or argon laser photocoagulation. Flat sea fans as well as elevated ones can also be treated by the feeder-vessel technique, in which the feeding arteriole and the draining venule are treated with xenon or argon photocoagulation. Although this method of treatment definitely reduces the incidence of vitreous hemorrhages in treated eyes, major complications may occur, including retinal tears and choroidal neovascularization. Another strategy is scatter photocoagulation, which is similar to methods used in treating proliferative diabetic retinopathy. Although patients have been treated successfully with scatter photocoagulation, its superiority to the feeder method has not been established. At this time, several randomized clinical trials are under way to study the effects of photocoagulation in PSR.

In patients in whom the vitreous hemorrhage is severe and persistent, vitrectomy may be employed. In eyes with vitreous hemorrhage where ultrasound examination reveals no retinal detachment, one should wait at least 6 months for spontaneous clearing of the hemorrhage. If clearing does not occur, vitrectomy may be considered, according to the needs of the individual patient. In patients with retinal detachment, conventional scleral buckling procedures are employed.

Patients undergoing vitrectomy, scleral buckling procedures, or combined procedures are at higher risk for the development of devastating ocular complications such as anterior segment necrosis and secondary glaucoma. Extreme care should be taken in evaluating these patients preoperatively, intraoperatively, and postoperatively and in designing measures that will maximize oxygenation and blood flow to the eye to protect it. These prophylactic regimens may include partial-exchange blood transfusions, erythropheresis, or use of a hyperbaric operating room. Medical and surgical maneuvers should be designed to keep the intraocular pressure as low as possible and the arterial perfusion pressure as high as possible. Even with all these precautions, the present success rate of combined scleral buckling and vitrectomy procedures is only approximately 50 percent.

1. Asdourian, G.K., Nagpal, K.C., Busse, B., et al. Macular and perimacular vascular remodelling in sickling haemoglobinopathies. *Br. J. Ophthalmol.* 60:431–453, 1976.
   Twenty-nine percent of patients with different sickling hemoglobins had macular and paramacular vascular abnormalities.
2. Asdourian, G.K., Nagpal, K.C., Goldbaum, M., et al. Evolution of the retinal black sunburst lesion in sickling haemoglobinopathies. *Br. J. Ophthalmol.* 59:710–716, 1975.
   The sequence of events leading to the formation of a black sunburst is described.
3. Condon, P.I., Hayes, R.J., Sergeant, G.R. Retinal and choroidal neovascularization in sickle cell disease. *Trans. Ophthalmol. Soc. U.K.* 100:434–439, 1980.
   The natural history of PSR and the factors related to its development are discussed.
4. Condon, P.I., Sergeant, G.R. Behavior of untreated proliferative sickle retinopathy. *Br. J. Ophthalmol.* 64:404–411, 1980.

There is a high incidence of spontaneous regression of neovascularization in patients who are followed without treatment for their PSR.

5. Goldberg, M.F. Classification and pathogenesis of proliferative sickle retinopathy. *Am. J. Ophthalmol.* 71:649–665, 1971.
   The events that led to the classification of PSR.
6. Goldberg, M.F. Natural history of untreated proliferative sickle retinopathy. *Arch. Ophthalmol.* 85:428–437, 1971.
   Definite progression documented in the severity of proliferative sickle retinopathy in 25 eyes with sickle-cell hemoglobin C disease.
7. Goldberg, M.F. Retinal vaso-occlusion in sickling hemoglobinopathies. *Birth Defects* 12:475–515, 1976.
   An excellent review of sickle retinopathy and the author's reasoning why retinal arteriolar vasoocclusions occur.
8. Goldberg, M.F., Jampol, L.M. Treatment of neovascularization, vitreous hemorrhage, and retinal detachment in sickle cell retinopathy. In *Symposium on Medical and Surgical Diseases of the Retina and Vitreous.* Transactions of the New Orleans Academy of Ophthalmology. St. Louis: Mosby, 1983. Pp. 53–81.
   An excellent review of PSR and the different modalities employed in treating PSR. Discusses results and complications.
9. Jampol, L.M., Green, J.L., Goldberg, M.F., et al. An update on vitrectomy surgery and retinal detachment repair in sickle cell disease. *Arch. Ophthalmol.* 100:591–593, 1982.
   The problems encountered and results obtained in treating patients with vitreous hemorrhage and retinal detachments with vitrectomy and scleral buckling procedures.
10. Lee, C.B. Woolf, M.B., Galinos, S.O., et al. Cryotherapy of proliferative sickle cell retinopathy. I. Single-freeze thaw cycle. *Ann. Ophthalmol.* 7:1299–1308, 1975.
    Patients with vitreous opacities and PSR can be treated with this modality with good results.
11. Nagpal, K.C., Asdourian, G.K., Goldbaum, M., et al. Angioid streaks and sickle haemoglobinopathies. *Br. J. Ophthalmol.* 60:31–34, 1976.
    Patients with sickling hemoglobinopathies are more prone to develop angioid streaks.
12. Nagpal, K.C., Goldberg, M.F., Rabb, M.F. Ocular manifestations of sickle hemoglobinopathies. *Surv. Ophthalmol.* 21:391–411, 1977.
    An excellent review of the subject.
13. Nagpal, K.C., Patrianakos, D., Asdourian, G.K., et al. Spontaneous regression (autoinfarction) of proliferative sickle retinopathy. *Am. J. Ophthalmol.* 80:885–892, 1975.
    Twenty percent of patients with PSR had evidence of spontaneous regression.
14. Romayanada, N., Goldberg, M.F., Green, W.R. Histopathology sickle cell retinopathy. *Trans. Am. Acad. Ophthalmol. Otolaryngol.* 77:652–676, 1973.
    A clinicopathologic correlation of changes seen in sickle retinopathy.

40. RETINOBLASTOMA

Retinoblastoma is a rare but highly malignant tumor of the retina. Despite its infrequent occurrence, it is the most common intraocular malignancy of childhood and is responsible for approximately 1 percent of all deaths from cancer in the age group under 15 years.

Retinoblastoma occurs in about 1 in every 17,000 to 34,000 live births. Recent studies have shown some apparent increase in its incidence (1/15,000 live births), but the cause for this is not known. The tumor occurs equally in both sexes, and there is no racial predilection. The tumor is probably present but not always detected at birth. About 90 percent of retinoblastomas become manifest by the age of 3 years, and it is extremely rare for the tumor to exhibit itself after the age of 6 years. Hereditary retinoblastomas are detected earlier (average, 12–14 months) as compared with sporadic retinoblastomas (average 24–30 months). This is probably the result of early screening and detection of children with a family history of retinoblastoma.

Pathogenesis

The tumor arises multicentrically in one or both retinas. Approximately 30 percent of retinoblastomas are bilateral. This is one consequence of the independent multicentric retinal origin of the tumor and not caused by extension from one eye to the other.

Retinoblastoma may be hereditary or nonhereditary. Six percent of patients with retinoblastoma have a family history of the disease and thus represent the hereditary form of the tumor. This is transmitted as an autosomal dominant trait with incomplete penetrance estimated to be between 60 and 95 percent. In the remaining 94 percent of patients with retinoblastoma, the tumor is sporadic, appearing without a family history of the disease. These sporadic cases occur as the result of a spontaneous mutation. Approximately 80 percent of these are thought to be somatic mutations, with the patient having no capacity to pass the gene to the offspring, whereas the remaining 20 percent are thought to represent germinal mutations, with the patient being capable of passing the gene to the offspring. Understanding the hereditary pattern of this disease is important for genetic counseling.

A small subset (5%) of patients with retinoblastoma harbor a host of other abnormalities, such as mental retardation, extra digits, imperforate anus, and failure to thrive. These patients usually have a partial deletion of the long arm of chromosome 13 that includes the q14 band. The 13q14 band is thought to be the genetic locus for retinoblastoma.

Clinical

The clinical presentation of retinoblastoma varies with the stage of the disease at the time of recognition. Most patients are initially seen with relatively advanced disease, which produces a white pupillary reflex (leukokoria). Tumors, even small ones, occupying the macular area may decrease vision with poor fixation and a secondary strabismus. An esotropia or an exotropia may be the first sign of the disease. Hence, it becomes imperative that every child presenting with a strabismus have a dilated ophthalmoscopic examination to rule out retinoblastoma. Other clinical signs at the time of presentation include dilated fixed pupil, heterochromia, hyphema, or noninfectious cellulitis and endophthalmitis. In patients with a family history of retinoblastoma, the tumor may be found on clinical examination when the patient does not have any signs or symptoms of the disease.

The findings on clinical examination depend also on the size of the tumor and the complications caused by the presence of the tumor in the eye. The early lesions of retinoblastoma are easily overlooked. The tumor appears to be flat and transparent or slightly white. Larger tumors are white, and their reflection causes the white pupillary reflex. The tumor may exhibit dilated and tortuous vessels, and there may be tumor particles in the vitreous. The retina may be attached or detached by exudation.

Two tumor growth patterns are recognized. *Endophytic tumors* grow from the retina inward toward the vitreous cavity. Vitreous seeds are common with this type of tumor, and if the tumor is advanced, the clinical picture mimics endophthalmitis. *Exophytic tumors* grow from the retina outward into the subretinal space. These tumors usually produce an exudative type of retinal detachment, with the detached retina being seen behind the lens with no apparent evidence of the tumor, making the diagnosis more difficult.

The tumor may seed into the vitreous cavity as well as into the anterior chamber, producing multiple iris nodules. Tumor infiltrating the iris may produce changes in the color of the iris, causing iris heterochromia. Rubeosis iridis as a consequence of posterior segment ischemia is seen especially in patients with retinal detachments (see Chap. 21).

With a delay in diagnosis, the tumor will eventually grow and show evidence of extraocular involvement, with invasion of the optic nerve, orbital extension, and distant metastasis. The tumor may spread directly through the optic nerve or subarachnoid space and extend intracranially. It may invade the skull bones, spinal cord, and regional lymph nodes. The tumor cells may enter the blood vessels and spread hematogenously to distant viscera.

The clinical features of various benign intraocular conditions may resemble those of retinoblastoma. These same benign conditions may cause leukokoria or strabismus or may present as an intraocular mass lesion. Some of the benign intraocular conditions that should be considered in the differential diagnosis include congenital cataracts, Coats's disease, Norrie's disease, retinal dysplasia, ocular toxocariasis, peripheral uveitis, metastatic endophthalmitis, retinopathy of prematurity, and retinal detachment.

A complete ophthalmologic examination, which includes dilated indirect ophthalmoscopy, may have to be done under general anesthesia. The clinician may use fluorescein angiography and radiologic examination of the globe including computed tomography scan and ultrasonography. Computed tomography is very sensitive to calcification, characteristic of retinoblastomas [7].

Retinoblastoma cells are thought to originate in the photoreceptor elements in the outer layers of the retina. Endophytic-type tumors are thought to originate in the internal nuclear layer, whereas exophytic-type tumors originate from the external nuclear layer. Histologically, the tumor is composed of uniform, small, round or polygonal cells with scant cytoplasm and a large, chromatin-rich nucleus. The cells grow luxuriantly around blood vessels but show evidence of ischemic coagulative necrosis some 90 to 110 μ away from the vessel. Calcification is seen mainly within these areas of necrosis. Most retinoblastomas are characterized by true rosette formation (the Flexner-Wintersteiner rosettes), in which large columnar cells are arranged radially around a central cavity to form spherical clusters. Almost all retinoblastomas have these characteristic areas of rosette formation associated with the less differentiated malignant cells. These rosettes represent areas of more differentiated cells, and the more numerous they are the better the prognosis. Certain areas of the tumor may show evidence of even higher maturation, with evidence of photoreceptor differentiation by individual tumor cells and small, bouquetlike clusters of benign-appearing tumor cells ("fleurettes"). Tumors composed only of such benign-appearing cells have been termed retinomas or retinocytomas.

Treatment

Treatment of retinoblastoma depends on the stage of the disease at the time treatment is undertaken. Unilateral retinoblastomas, especially when there is no hope of restoring any vision, are probably best treated by prompt enucleation after the fellow eye has been thoroughly studied and a search for metastasis has proved negative. In some instances, unilateral retinoblastomas may be treated conservatively with radiation or other treatment modalities rather than by enucleation.

In the rare bilateral cases, when both retinas are totally involved with the tumor, bilateral enucleation may be indicated. Generally, in bilateral cases the eye with the more advanced tumor is enucleated, while the remaining eye is treated.

Retinoblastoma may be treated with irradiation, chemotherapy, cryotherapy, diathermy, radioactive plaques, and light coagulation. Irradiation alone or combined with chemotherapy is employed as a primary form of treatment in almost all cases of retinoblastoma. Light coagulation, cryotherapy, and radioactive cobalt applications are other extremely valuable adjuncts in the management of this tumor.

Patients with bilateral retinoblastomas (heritable retinoblastomas) are at high risk of developing second nonocular tumors. The "retinoblastoma gene" is intimately related to proclivity to develop second tumors, which may occur in or away from the radiation field. Osteogenic sarcoma of the skull and the femur are the most common tumors. Patients with retinoblastoma should be followed for life for detection and management of these lethal nonocular malignancies.

1. Abramson, D.H. Retinoblastoma: Diagnosis and management. *Cancer* 32:130–140, 1982.
   A short review of the subject.

2. Abramson, D.H. Retinoblastoma, retinocytoma, and the retinoblastoma gene—editorial. *Arch. Ophthalmol.* 101:1517–1518, 1983.
   An editorial comment on the different names applied to different stages of retinoblastoma.
3. Abramson, D.H., Ellsworth, R.M., Kitchin, F.D., et al. Second nonocular tumors in retinoblastoma survivors. Are they radiation-induced? *Ophthalmology* 91:1351–1355, 1984.
   The incidence, time course, and pattern of second nonocular tumors in 711 retinoblastoma survivors were reviewed and analyzed. Sarcoma was the most common second tumor found.
4. Abramson, D.H., Ellsworth, R.M., Zimmerman, L.E. Nonocular cancer in retinoblastoma survivors. *Trans. Am. Acad. Ophthalmol. Otolaryngol.* 81:454–457, 1976.
   Patients with bilateral retinoblastoma are at high risk of developing a second nonocular malignancy, either in the field of radiation or distant from it.
5. Abramson, D.H., Fusco Marks, R., Ellsworth, R.M., et al. The management of unilateral retinoblastoma without primary enucleation. *Arch. Ophthalmol.* 100:1249–1252, 1982.
   In carefully selected patients (groups I–III of the Reese-Ellsworth classification) with monocular retinoblastoma, conservative treatment with radiation is a safe alternative to enucleation.
6. Bishop, J.O., Madson, E.C. Retinoblastoma. Review of the current status. *Surv. Ophthalmol.* 19:342–366, 1975.
   A general survey of the subject.
7. Char, D.H., Hedges, T.R. III, Norman, D. Retinoblastoma. CT diagnosis. *Ophthalmology* 91:1347–1350, 1984.
   Computed tomography is an excellent adjunct in the diagnosis and management of patients with retinoblastoma as well as in the evaluation of patients who present with leukokoria.
8. Ellsworth, R.M. The practical management of retinoblastoma. *Trans. Am. Ophthalmol. Soc.* 67:462–534, 1969.
   An extensive review of the subject.
9. Gallie, B.L., Phillips, R.A. Retinoblastoma: A model of oncogenesis. *Ophthalmology* 91:666–672, 1984.
   The possible genetic mechanisms involved in retinoblastoma are presented and discussed.
10. Margo, C., Hidayat, A., Kopelman, J., et al. Retinocytoma—a benign variant of retinoblastoma. *Arch. Ophthalmol.* 101:1519–1531, 1983.
    Pathologic findings in six cases of a "benign" variant of retinoblastoma.
11. Shields, J.A., Augsburger, J.J. Current approaches to the diagnosis and management of retinoblastoma. *Surv. Ophthalmol.* 25:347–372, 1981.
    A review of the subject with different modalities of treatment.

41. VIRAL RETINITIS

Viruses, both of the DNA group (herpes viruses) and of the RNA group (rubella and measles), have been documented as causing retinitis in humans; however, viral retinitis is still rare in healthy adults. These viruses, as obligatory intracellular parasites, proliferate, causing necrosis of cells and leading to irreversible damage to retinal structure and function. The cellular damage is usually accompanied by various degrees of inflammation and vasculitis secondary to the response of the immune system to the viral infection. These secondary inflammatory and vascular changes (vasoocclusion and retinal ischemia) add more insult to the original retinal damage, with disastrous effects on vision.

Diagnosis

Clinically, during the active phase of the infection, these patients may show evidence of mild to moderate anterior uveitis, episcleritis, or scleritis. In the posterior segment the uveitis manifests as solitary or confluent patches of whitening of the retina, which may be associated with cotton-wool spots, retinal hemorrhages, and exudates. In severe cases, the optic disk shows evidence of inflammation and swelling, and the vitreous is full of inflammatory cells. Exudative and rhegmatogenous retinal detachments may occur, with severe loss of vision. In the chronic and healed stages of the disease, the retina shows diffuse or localized pigmentary changes, while the optic disk becomes pale and atrophic. Clinically, different viral infections of the retina may thus have similar ophthalmoscopic appearances except for differences in severity of the retinitis and the associated inflammatory response. Thus, an exact etiologic diagnosis cannot be made solely on the ophthalmoscopic findings. The final etiologic diagnosis is usually made on the basis of the associated (nonophthalmic) clinical findings, viral cultures, and serology studies.

Rubella retinitis is one of the three most frequent abnormalities in a child with congenital rubella. The retinitis caused by the rubella virus during intrauterine infection usually consists of widespread fine, granular, symmetric mottling of the pigment epithelium that gives the fundus a "salt and pepper" appearance. The retinal vessels are normal, and the optic disk rarely shows evidence of atrophy. The retinitis causes minimal or no effect on retinal function. Cataract, glaucoma, and microphthalmia are major causes of poor vision in these patients. There is no treatment for the retinitis. It is hoped that by preventing maternal rubella infections (German measles) during pregnancy with vaccination, the retinopathy will be eradicated.

Retinitis also occurs during the course of *subacute sclerosing panencephalitis,* a devastating neurologic disease of childhood that is a complication of measles (rubeola). The ophthalmic manifestations include a bilateral necrotizing retinitis occurring in the macular or perimacular area with minimal evidence of inflammation. Retinitis may be associated with cotton-wool spots, retinal hemorrhages, and disk edema. In the late stages of the disease, only pigmentary changes with chorioretinal scars are seen associated with optic atrophy. Here also, medical treatment has been unsuccessful, and prevention of the measles infections remains the only sound thing to accomplish.

Herpes simplex, herpes zoster, and cytomegalovirus (CMV), members of the herpesvirus family, have all been implicated as etiologic agents in human retinitis.

Herpes simplex virus retinitis usually occurs in neonates with evidence of generalized herpetic infections and encephalitis; in children and adults with herpes encephalitis; and in patients with renal allografts who are on immunosuppressive therapy. The clinical picture is similar in all. White patches of active retinitis are seen associated with retinal hemorrhages, vascular sheathing, vitreous debris, and, in severe cases, exudative retinal detachment. Treatment involves both antiviral and anti-inflammatory medications and, in immunosuppressed patients, decreasing the immunosuppressive therapy.

Herpes zoster retinitis is rare. It appears weeks or months after the classic herpes zoster ophthalmicus. The posterior segment involvement is manifested by severe patchy vasculitis with secondary focal retinal necrosis. There is associated diffuse choroiditis. The pathologic changes in the posterior segment are due both to active viral destruction of retinal and vascular tissue as well as to severe acute inflammation secondary to type III hypersensitivity (immune complex deposition) within vessel walls that eventually leads to vasoocclusion and ischemia and necrosis of tissue supplied by the blood vessels. Treatment includes both antiviral and immunomodulating agents. Recently, acyclovir has shown promising results in treating this condition. Judicious use of anti-inflammatory medications may be necessary to control the severe secondary inflammation.

Recently, an unusual and visually devastating form of necrotizing retinitis has been described in otherwise healthy individuals. This condition, referred to as the *acute retinal necrosis syndrome* (ARN), is thought to be secondary to a viral infection of the retina. ARN typically presents with the insidious onset of diffuse anterior and posterior uveitis, followed by acute whitening of the peripheral retina, which occurs multifocally and in coalescent patches. There is associated vasculitis of both arteries and veins with secondary retinal hemorrhages. There is swelling of the optic disk and macular edema.

Initially, the vitreous shows evidence of mild inflammatory reaction, but eventually the vitreitis becomes severe, with eventual organization of the vitreous leading to traction and secondary retinal detachments. These detachments are difficult to repair surgically, and even in cases of successful therapy, vision is usually poor as a result of optic atrophy, macular edema, or pucker. In the healed stages of the disease, the involved retinal area evidences pigmentary changes.

ARN may occur at any age, either bilaterally or unilaterally (the majority of cases). There usually is no evidence of systemic disease or any evidence of immunologic compromise. There now exists histopathologic, electron microscopic, and tissue culture evidence that ARN is the result of infection by a herpes-type DNA virus (possibly herpes simplex or herpes zoster). Because of this evidence, systemic antiviral therapy has been recommended to treat the acute phase of the disease. However, at this time the role of antiviral therapy has yet to be proven.

Cytomegalovirus retinitis may occur as part of the clinical spectrum of congenital cytomegaloviral infections. It is seen as areas of focal necrotizing retinochoroiditis in both the central and peripheral retina. This congenital retinitis is often associated with optic atrophy. The disease is probably acquired transplacentally. Cytomegalovirus retinitis in healthy adults is rare. In recent years, the incidence of CMV retinitis has dramatically increased, and it occurs in specifically susceptible patients, including immunosuppressed individuals and persons who have received multiple blood transfusions. The immunosuppressed individuals include those who have neoplastic disorders of the hemopoietic and reticuloendothelial systems, those who are on chemotherapy for malignant diseases, and patients who are on immunosuppressive therapy following organ transplant. More recently, the recognition of CMV retinitis has become even more important because of its rising incidence in patients with the *acquired immune deficiency syndrome* (AIDS), a condition in which there is severe depression of cell-mediated immunity. In AIDS patients, CMV retinitis is a particularly devastating, relentless infection, especially in patients showing rapid clinical deterioration. Symptoms primarily relate to visual loss, which may occur dramatically over several days as the retinitis involves the macular region. Involvement is frequently bilateral and progressive.

Funduscopic examination characteristically reveals extensive areas of retinal necrosis and edema, with hemorrhages extending from the posterior pole along the major vascular arcades. Exudative retinal detachment accompanies CMV retinitis in approximately 60 percent of cases. Histologically, CMV retinitis typically involves all layers of the retina and the retinal pigment epithelium; the choroid is often involved in a patchy distribution not underlying areas of retinal involvement. There is neutrophilic infiltration of the retina with characteristic intranuclear and intracytoplasmic ("owl eye") viral inclusions.

Definite diagnosis of CMV retinitis may be made by direct viral cultures (e.g., of blood and urine), electron microscopy, and immunochemical techniques. However, these more sophisticated techniques are adjuncts to the diagnosis of CMV retinitis in an AIDS patient, as the funduscopic appearance is very characteristic.

Treatment

The development of CMV retinitis in a patient with AIDS is particularly ominous, with expected survival of less than 6 weeks from the time of diagnosis. No agent has been proved to be therapeutically beneficial in the treatment of CMV retinitis, including vidarabine, acyclovir, human leukocyte interferon, and alpha interferon. Recently, there was a report of relative success in suppressing aggressive CMV infection with continuous dihydroxypropoxymethyl guanine (DHPG), an acyclovir derivative [10]. However, on cessation of treatment the patient relapsed, and it is apparent that DHPG does not permanently eliminate the virus but acts as a suppressive agent and that long-term maintenance therapy may be needed.

1. Bachman, D.M., Rodrigues, M.M., Chu, F.C., et al. Culture proven cytomegalovirus retinitis in a homosexual man with the acquired immunodeficiency syndrome. *Ophthalmology* 89:797–804, 1982.

Retinal and vitreal cultures taken from a patient with AIDS and retinitis were positive for CMV but negative for herpes simplex and zoster.

2. Culbertson, W.W., Blumenkranz, M.S., Haines, H., et al. The acute retinal necrosis syndrome. Part 2: Histopathology and etiology. *Ophthalmology* 89:1317–1325, 1982.
   This article, together with the work cited below by Fisher, Lewis, Blumenkranz, et al. [5], reviews the clinical as well as the histopathologic findings in patients with the ARN syndrome, encompassing 11 cases seen in Bascom Palmer Eye Institute and 30 additional cases from the literature.

3. Culbertson, W.W., Blumenkranz, M.S., Pepose, J.S., et al. Varicella zoster virus is a cause of the acute retinal necrosis syndrome. *Ophthalmology* 93:559–569, 1986.
   Electron microscopy and immunocytopathologic studies done on two eyes with the ARN syndrome yield findings that incriminate the varicella-zoster virus as the infectious agent in these patients.

4. Fischer, D.H. Viral disease and the retina. In R.W. Darrell (ed.), *Viral Diseases of the Eye*. Philadelphia: Lea & Febiger, 1985. Pp. 487–497.
   A concise review of viruses that are implicated in human retinitis.

5. Fisher, J.P., Lewis, M.L., Blumenkranz, M., et al. The acute retinal necrosis syndrome. Part 1: Clinical manifestations. *Ophthalmology* 89:1309–1316, 1982. (See reference 2 above.)

6. Freeman, W.R., Thomas, E.L., Rao, N.A., et al. Demonstration of herpes group virus in acute retinal necrosis syndrome. *Am. J. Ophthalmol.* 102:701–709, 1986.
   Virus particles belonging to the herpes family were demonstrated in retinal tissues obtained from retinal biopsies during vitrectomy.

7. Friedman, A.H., Orellana, J., Freeman, W.R., et al. Cytomegalovirus retinitis: A manifestation of the acquired immune deficiency syndrome (AIDS). *Br. J. Ophthalmol.* 67:372–380, 1983.
   Cytomegalovirus was cultured from a vitreous biopsy taken from a patient with the typical findings of CMV retinitis.

8. Haltia, M., Tarkkanen, A., Vaheri, A., et al. Measles retinopathy during immunosuppression. *Br. J. Ophthalmol.* 62:356–360, 1978.
   Although measles retinitis is most commonly seen in patients with subacute sclerosing panencephalitis, this virus has the potential to infect the retina in immunosuppressed individuals. This is a case report of measles retinopathy following an attack of measles in a 14-year-old boy on chemotherapy for a testicular neoplasm.

9. Henry, K., Cantrill, H., Fletcher, C., et al. Use of intravitreal Ganciclovir (dihydroxy propoxymethyl guanine) for cytomegalovirus retinitis in patients with AIDS. *Am. J. Ophthalmol.* 103:17–23, 1987.
   This experimental antiviral medication was used via the intravitreal route since the patient had severe bone marrow suppression. Multiple intravitreal injections were necessary to control the retinitis.

10. Holland, G.N., Sakamoto, M.J., Hardy, D., et al. Treatment of cytomegalovirus retinopathy in patients with acquired immunodeficiency syndrome. Use of the experimental drug 9-[2-hydroxy-1-(hydroxymethyl)ethoxymethyl]guanine. *Arch. Ophthalmol.* 104:1794–1800, 1986.
    The results of treatment of 20 patients suffering from CMV retinopathy with this new antiviral medication are discussed. It seems the drug suppresses but does not eliminate the virus.

11. Krill, A.E. Retinopathy secondary to rubella. *Int. Ophthalmol. Clin.* 12(2):89–103, 1972.
    A general review of the subject with an additional four case reports.

12. Minckler, D.S., McLean, E.B., Shaw, C.M., et al. Herpesvirus hominis encephalitis and retinitis. *Arch. Ophthalmol.* 94:89–95, 1976.
    Herpesvirus retinitis is rare in healthy individuals but may occur in patients with simplex encephalitis. This case report proves such an association in a healthy 44-year-old individual.

13. Uninsky, E., Jampol, L.M., Kaufman, S., et al. Disseminated herpes simplex infection with retinitis in a renal allograft recipient. *Ophthalmology* 90:175–178, 1983.
    A case report of herpes retinitis in an immunosuppressed patient following renal transplant.

42. RETINAL ARTERIAL OCCLUSION

Retinal arterial occlusive disorders are among the most dramatic problems encountered in ophthalmology because of their rapid onset, their profound effects on vision, and their association with life-threatening systemic diseases. Occlusion may occur at any point from the ophthalmic artery to the main central retinal artery to the smallest precapillary arterioles. The signs and symptoms of arterial occlusions are thus dependent on the vessel obstructed. The mechanisms of retinal arterial occlusions may vary from disease to disease but usually are due either to *embolization* or *vasoobliterative processes* (for example, vasculitis) or to *pressure from outside.*

Pathogenesis
Precapillary arterial occlusions involve closure of precapillary arterioles in the posterior pole. Patients present with the clinical picture of cotton-wool spots, that represent a buildup of axoplasmic material in the inner retinal layers. Closure of the retinal precapillary arterioles may be related to embolization (talc retinopathy), vasculitis (lupus erythematosus), blockage by abnormal erythrocytes (sickle cell retinopathy), or abnormalities of the vascular endothelium (hypertension, diabetes mellitus, radiation retinopathy, and others) [8]. Clinically, the patients may be completely asymptomatic with normal visual acuities, color vision, and visual fields or they may complain of variable visual disturbances depending on the location and size of the involved retina. Closures involving the fovea produce the most profound loss of visual acuity. With sensitive perimetric testing, a scotoma may be elicited even in asymptomatic patients. With time, the cotton-wool patches fade away and the precapillary arterioles reperfuse. With careful ophthalmoscopy, especially with fluorescein angiography, some minute capillary abnormalities may be detected at the site of the occlusion and the surrounding capillary network. The resolved cotton-wool spot usually leaves behind a concave area of *retinal depression,* which is a result of loss of some of the inner retinal elements. This *depression sign* may be subtle and can be missed unless looked for specifically, but once detected it is a telltale sign of a previous vascular occlusion.

Branch Retinal Artery Occlusion (BRAO)
Most BRAOs affect the temporal branches of the central retinal arterial tree and are likely to involve part of the macular region. This results in symptomatic central or paracentral scotoma as well as a sectorial visual field defect. The obstruction, in rare instances, may involve the cilioretinal artery, which originates from either a short posterior ciliary artery or a choroidal vessel. Ophthalmoscopically, the involved retina appears white. The artery is narrow, and usually an embolus is seen at the site of the occlusion. With time the retinal edema gradually clears, but the inner retinal layers atrophy, with a permanent sectorial visual field defect. Recanalization of the obstructed arteriole may leave only subtle or absent ophthalmoscopic signs. BRAO usually occurs secondary to embolization or thrombosis. Embolic material from either the heart or the carotid arteries is usually responsible. Embolic material originating from the heart may be (1) *calcific,* emanating from diseased cardiac valves; (2) *vegetative,* secondary to subacute bacterial endocarditis; (3) *thromboembolic,* arising secondary to myocardial infarctions (mural thrombi) or mitral valve stenosis with atrial fibrillation; or (4) arising from a *rare atrial myxoma.* However, the most important cause of retinal embolization is atheroma at the origin of the internal carotid artery and the adjacent segment of the common carotid artery. Emboli from the carotids may be (1) *cholesterol emboli* (Hollenhorst plaques), (2) *fibroplatelet emboli,* or (3) *calcific emboli.*

Central Retinal Artery Obstruction (CRAO)
The central retinal artery supplies blood to the entire inner layers of the retina. Individuals with CRAO experience sudden, profound, painless loss of vision that usually ranges between counting fingers to light perception. In 10 to 25 percent of individuals, the fovea is spared with retention of central vision because of a patent cilioretinal artery. Although CRAO may occur in children and young adults, the entity is most often seen

in older adults, with a mean age in the early sixties. Upon examination, the retina appears white and edematous, especially in the posterior pole. However, the white area does not include the fovea, which is supplied by the intact choroidal circulation. This accounts for the "cherry-red spot" appearance. The retinal arterioles look narrowed and irregular in caliber, with evidence of sludging and segmentation of the blood column. With time, the retinal haze and "cherry-red spot" disappear, and the retina regains its normal translucent appearance. However, the retinal arterioles remain attenuated, and the optic disk becomes pale and atrophic.

Obstruction of the *ophthalmic artery* produces a clinical picture identical to that of CRAO. However, in this instance the choroidal circulation is also embarrassed, and vision may be diminished to no light perception. With time, the optic nerve shows marked atrophy, while the retina evolves diffuse pigmentary changes that are not seen when only the central retinal artery is occluded.

Similar to BRAO, CRAO occurs secondary to embolization, thrombosis, and vasculitis. However, CRAO may also occur secondary to local orbital or intraocular conditions, such as retrobulbar hemorrhage, retrobulbar anesthesia, trauma, and elevated intraocular pressure (for example, secondary to acute angle-closure glaucoma or intraoperative procedures such as vitrectomy). In young patients, CRAO may be caused by migraine, coagulation abnormalities, intravenous drug abuse, hemoglobinopathies, and oral contraceptives.

Treatment

Management of patients with retinal arterial occlusions also depends on the site of the occlusion. In patients with precapillary arterial occlusions, no specific treatment is possible except for identification of the underlying causative condition and its management. Similarly, in patients with BRAO, management is directed toward finding systemic etiologic factors. Acute CRAO is an ophthalmic emergency, and efforts should be directed toward restoring retinal circulation as soon as possible. Treatment should begin immediately after the diagnosis is made, even if the onset of visual loss was several hours earlier, since in most cases the period of complete cessation of flow to the retina cannot be determined. Therapeutic maneuvers include those that will increase retinal arterial perfusion. Carbon dioxide as a retinal arterial dilator can be given by allowing the patient to breathe a mixture of 5% carbon dioxide and 95% oxygen intermittently for several minutes out of every half hour. Other therapies include reduction in intraocular pressure by paracentesis and ocular massage. Still other methods that have been attempted include retrobulbar injection of vasodilators, ocular hypotensive agents (for example, acetazolamide), and systemic vasodilators. Although many clinicians believe these therapeutic maneuvers to be safe and occasionally beneficial, there is no clinically proven therapy available that will reliably reverse the effects of retinal arterial occlusions.

Retinal arterial occlusive disease is a manifestation of systemic disease. Thus, it is extremely important that the ophthalmologist makes the proper diagnosis.

1. Appen, R.E., Wray, S.H., Cogan, D.G. Central retinal artery occlusion. *Am. J. Ophthalmol.* 79:374–381, 1975.
   In a study of 54 patients with CRAO, follow-up examination revealed only two patients (5%) who had a stroke that was clearly related to the vessels involving the affected central retinal artery. However, multiple systemic diseases were found associated with this event.
2. Arruga, J., Sanders, M.D. Ophthalmologic findings in 70 patients with evidence of retinal embolism. *Ophthalmology* 89:1336–1347, 1982.
   The source of cholesterol and platelet fibrin emboli was found to be mainly the carotid arteries, whereas calcific emboli usually originated from the heart. Cholesterol emboli are the most common and are usually responsible for more transient visual complaints.
3. Brown, G.C., Magargal, L.E., Sergott, R. Acute obstruction of the retinal and choroidal circulations. *Ophthalmology* 93:1373–1382, 1986.

Eight patients who probably had ophthalmic artery occlusions are presented. The difficulties inherent in making this diagnosis versus combined central retinal artery and choroidal occlusions are discussed.

4. Brown, G.C., Magargal, L.E., Shields, J.A., et al. Retinal arterial obstruction in children and young adults. *Ophthalmology* 88:18–25, 1981.
   Systemic diseases causing CRAO in young adults may be different from those causing the occlusion in older patients. In contrast to the situation in adults, atheromatous disease was not a cause of CRAO in young individuals.

5. Brown, G.C., Shields, J.A. Cilioretinal arteries and retinal arterial occlusions. *Arch. Ophthalmol.* 97:84–92, 1979.
   Patients with CRAOs that spare the cilioretinal artery do much better visually than patients without cilioretinal sparing. Of 107 cases of CRAO, 26 percent showed some degree of macular sparing attributable to a patent cilioretinal artery.

6. Gold, D. Retinal arterial occlusion. *Trans. Am. Acad. Ophthalmol. Otolaryngol.* 83:OP392–468, 1977.
   An excellent review of the subject.

7. Hayreh, S.S., Kolder, H.E., Weingeist, T.A. Central retinal artery occlusion and retinal tolerance time. *Ophthalmology* 87:75–78, 1980.
   The ophthalmoscopic, angiographic, electrophysiologic, and morphologic results of experimental CRAOs in rhesus monkeys are given. The retina of the rhesus monkey can tolerate acute ischemia up to 97 to 98 minutes with full recovery with rare exceptions.

8. Jampol, L.M. Arteriolar occlusive diseases of the macula. *Ophthalmology* 90:534–539, 1983.
   The clinical manifestation and the various systemic diseases that present with retinal arteriolar occlusions are presented in this excellent short review.

9. Karjalainen, K. Occlusion of the central retinal artery and retinal branch arterioles. *Acta Ophthalmol.* 109(Suppl.):5–96, 1971.
   An extensive review of 175 patients with retinal arterial occlusions.

10. Klein, M.L., Jampol, L.M., Condon, P.I., et al. Central retinal artery occlusion without retrobulbar hemorrhage after retrobulbar anesthesia. *Am. J. Ophthalmol.* 93:573–577, 1982.
    Retrobulbar injection may cause CRAO even in the absence of retrobulbar hemorrhage, presumably either by direct trauma to the central retinal artery behind the globe or by the pharmacologic and compressive effects of the injected solution. Four case reports are discussed.

43. RETINAL VEIN OCCLUSION

Retinal vein occlusions are common retinal vascular disorders that are clinically classified as branch, hemispheric, and central vein occlusions.

Pathogenesis of Branch Retinal Vein Occlusion

Branch retinal vein occlusion involves one of the branch retinal veins. The vast majority of symptomatic branch vein occlusions involve either the superior or inferior temporal arcades, and occur almost invariably at an arteriovenous crossing where the vein is compressed by a sclerotic artery. An occlusion limited to one of the small venous tributaries draining a sector of the macula located between the superior and inferior temporal arcades may also occur *(macular vein occlusion)*, with profound effect on vision. Branch vein occlusion may also occur in the nasal quadrant. However, these occlusions are usually asymptomatic and are found on routine examinations. A *hemispheric vein occlusion* occurs if the occlusion involves the venous drainage of either the superior or inferior retina. Similar to branch vein occlusions elsewhere, these occur at arteriovenous crossings but close to the optic disk. These occlusions should be distinguished from hemi-central vein occlusions, which are variants of central vein occlusion.

Branch vein occlusions affect male and female patients equally, occurring most frequently in individuals in the age group of 60 to 70 years. There is controversy regarding the pathogenesis of branch vein occlusions. It is not known whether primary venous disease per se with thrombosis or arterial disease with secondary venous disease is the primary factor that eventually leads to branch vein occlusion. Irrespective of the primary pathogenic processes underlying branch vein occlusions, it is clear that disease of the arterial wall and the presence of a common adventitia between artery and vein at arteriovenous crossings play a role in the pathogenesis. Branch vein occlusion is a complex disorder. The factors associated with it include both local ocular problems (phlebitis, arteritis) and systemic disorders (most importantly systemic hypertension and diabetes mellitus).

Diagnosis of Branch Retinal Vein Occlusion

The most common symptoms of branch vein occlusion are blurring and distortion of vision. Some patients complain of central and paracentral scotomas. The ophthalmoscopic picture is characteristic. During the early acute stage, multiple superficial and deep retinal hemorrhages are seen in a pie configuration in the distribution of the affected vein, with the apex of the obstructed tributory vein almost always lying at an arteriovenous crossing. The veins in the occluded segment are usually dilated and tortuous. Nerve fiber layer infarcts (cotton-wool spots) and macular edema are often present. Dilated collateral channels may be evident in the vicinity of the occlusion.

Fluorescein angiography at this stage is helpful in delineating the hemodynamic changes occurring in the retinal vasculature. The angiography usually shows that the vein is not completely occluded but that the venous return is slow. Multiple dilated capillaries and collateral channels are seen, with delineation of areas of capillary closure with retinal ischemia. Most of the affected vessels show evidence of leakage with secondary macular edema. At this acute hemorrhagic stage, no ocular treatment is beneficial, and none is recommended. However, an evaluation for risk factors (e.g., hypertension, diabetes) should be undertaken.

The structural and functional recovery following acute branch occlusion depends on many factors, including the order of the affected vein, the status of the arterial perfusion, and the adequacy of the collateral channels. Ophthalmoscopy during the healing and chronic stages of branch vein occlusion reveals the presence of collaterals and shunt vessels, microaneurysms, sheathed vessels, macular exudates, and edema.

Approximately 50 percent of patients recover good visual acuity following the branch vein occlusion. However, two complications of branch vein occlusion may lead to reduced visual acuity. *Macular edema* develops in more than 50 percent of patients with temporal branch vein occlusion. This edema reduces vision. Other macular changes that cause decreased vision include surface-wrinkling retinopathy, macular holes, intraretinal hemorrhages of the fovea, foveal capillary nonperfusion, foveal cysts, and macular retinal pigment epithelial changes. The second major complication of branch vein occlusion is *retinal neovascularization,* both of the disk and of the retina, with the risk of vitreous hemorrhage. The retinal neovascularization is thought to be secondary to retinal ischemia. Its development is correlated with the presence of large areas of capillary nonperfusion as seen on fluorescein angiography. Because of the limited retinal area involved, neovascularization does not follow macular vein occlusions. Other less common but visually debilitating complications that may occur secondary to branch vein occlusions include exudative and rhegmatogenous retinal detachments.

Treatment of Branch Retinal Vein Occlusion

Management of both of the major complications of branch vein occlusion (macular edema and retinal neovascularization) involves laser photocoagulation. The macular edema may be treated with grid pattern photocoagulation. The Collaborative Branch Vein Occlusion Study, a multicenter, randomized control clinical trial, showed the beneficial effect of such treatment in improving visual acuity for certain eyes with macular edema. Foveal hemorrhages and foveal capillary nonperfusion, other major causes of decreased vision in these patients, are not amenable to laser photocoagulation. The same study also showed the beneficial effect of photocoagulation in treating disk and retinal neovascularizations secondary to branch vein occlusions. The recommended treatment is to ablate the peripheral ischemic retina with scatter photocoagulation. Such treatment can prevent the development of both neovascularization and vitreous hemorrhage.

If vitreous hemorrhage does not resolve, then vitrectomy may be utilized to clear the vitreous. Patients with exudative retinal detachments have been successfully treated with laser photocoagulation; however, those with rhegmatogenous retinal detachments will need surgical correction of their detachment. Every effort should also be made to detect associated systemic conditions and treat them accordingly.

Pathogenesis of Central Retinal Vein Occlusion

Central retinal vein occlusion (CRVO) involves occlusion of the main central vein, which usually occurs at the level of the lamina cribrosa. This occlusion will interfere with the drainage of the whole retina. In approximately 20 percent of the population, the central retinal vein has a dual trunk, each trunk draining either the superior or inferior retina. Occlusion of either trunk will result in *hemicentral retinal vein occlusion*. The pathogenesis, classification, clinical features, and management of both hemicentral and central retinal vein occlusions are similar.

The mechanisms producing the clinical picture of CRVO is not known. It is not clear whether complete or partial thrombosis of the central retinal vein is sufficient to produce the characteristic clinical picture of CRVO or whether concomitant arterial disease with arterial insufficiency is essential in the pathogenesis of the disease. Although the exact pathogenesis of CRVO remains unclear, several *local* and *systemic* factors are known to predispose eyes to CRVO. The most important local factor is *chronic open-angle glaucoma*, which is present in over 20 percent of patients with CRVO. Other, less common, local predisposing factors include papilledema, subdural hemorrhage, optic nerve hemorrhage, and drusen of the optic nerve head. Frequent systemic associations include cardiovascular disease, hypertension, diabetes, and hyperviscosity syndromes. CRVO is primarily a disease of the elderly, but its occurrence in younger persons is well documented.

There is still confusion in the ophthalmic community as to the clinical classification and nomenclature of CRVO. However, on the basis of the clinical presentation, clinical findings, fluorescein angiography, and natural course findings, CRVO has been clinically divided into two distinct types. However, some cases still occur that cannot be classified in either category on initial presentation.

Diagnosis of CRVO

Nonischemic CRVO (partial CRVO, venous stasis retinopathy, hyperpermeable CRVO) is the more common form of the disease. It is milder and more variable than ischemic CRVO. Visual complaints vary from none (discovered on routine examination), to mild or moderate blurring of vision, which may be transient. Visual fields are usually normal except for occasional central scotomas. Ophthalmoscopic features include moderate dilatation and tortuosity of all of the retinal branch veins, with multiple punctate hemorrhages in the peripheral retina and a few scattered retinal hemorrhages in the posterior pole. There is mild hyperemia and swelling of the optic nerve head. Macular edema may or may not be present. This form of CRVO can be easily confused with a similar retinopathy that in the literature has the etiologically imprecise designation of venous stasis retinopathy, a condition secondary to severe occlusive disease of the carotid artery. The two entities can be separated by measuring the central retinal arterial pressure, which will always have a low value in patients with carotid disease. Fluorescein angiography is very helpful and shows no capillary obliteration in the vast majority of patients (except for occasional patchy capillary obliteration where cotton-wool spots are present). The retinal veins and the disk show mild staining and leakage, whereas the macula shows evidence of edema, which is the main cause of decreased vision in these patients. The course is relatively benign. Most of the hemorrhagic activity resolves over several months. Some patients may be left with some permanent visual loss from the nonresolving cystoid macular edema, macular cystic degeneration, macular retinal pigment epithelial changes and preretinal fibrosis. Retinal or anterior segment neovascular complications are very rare. There is no known effective treatment for this condition.

Ischemic CRVO (complete CRVO, hemorrhagic retinopathy, combined occlusion of retinal vessels) occurs in older individuals who have a higher incidence of systemic vascular disease, preexisting glaucoma, and ocular hypertension. These patients usually present with sudden painless loss of vision. Vision is usually markedly decreased, usually less than 6/60. The majority of these patients will have a vision of counting fingers or hand motion. Peripheral visual fields are almost always normal, with a dense central or centrocecal scotoma. The ophthalmoscopic features include marked tortuosity and dilatation of all of the retinal branch veins, diffuse retinal hemorrhages extending from the optic disk to the periphery of the fundus, and multiple cotton-wool patches. There is marked hyperemia and swelling of the optic disk. The macula shows marked edema with large cystic spaces that may contain hemorrhages. On fluorescein angiography, the capillary obliteration is universal, and it may vary from mild to almost complete obliteration of the retinal capillary bed.

The prognosis is very poor. Central vision is seldom recovered due to ischemic maculopathy or cystic macular degeneration, macular holes and cysts, and macular epithelial fibrosis. The retinal pigment epithelium under the macula may show moderate to marked changes. However, the more serious complication of ischemic CRVO is neovascularization, with iris neovascularization being the most frequent type. The iris neovascularization will eventually lead to neovascular glaucoma. The more extensive the retinal ischemic process, the more likely anterior segment neovascularization will occur. The average time for the development of neovascular glaucoma is 3 to 5 months after the occlusion.

Treatment of CRVO

There is no known effective treatment for ischemic CRVO. Many modalities of treatments have been tried, including steroids, anticoagulants, fibrinolytic agents, and photocoagulation. However, none has been shown to be effective in restoring vision. However, photocoagulation (panretinal photocoagulation) causes regression of iris neovascularization or even prevents its development. Thus, a major complication (neovascular glaucoma) can possibly be prevented by panretinal photocoagulation of the retina. Although there is no treatment per se for the CRVO, the physician should look for associated medical conditions and treat them accordingly.

---

1. Branch Vein Occlusion Study Group. Argon laser photocoagulation for macular edema in branch vein occlusion. *Am. J. Ophthalmol.* 98:271–282, 1984.
   Laser photocoagulation is beneficial in treating macular edema secondary to branch vein occlusion. The criteria of treatment and the results of this multicenter, randomized controlled clinical trial are given.
2. Branch Vein Occlusion Study Group. Argon laser scatter photocoagulation for prevention of neovascularization and vitreous hemorrhage in branch vein occlusion. *Arch. Ophthalmol.* 104:34–41, 1986.
   The results of this randomized, controlled clinical trial are given. Laser photocoagulation was beneficial in controlling vitreous hemorrhage and retinal neovascularization that occurred secondary to branch retinal vein occlusion.
3. Finkelstein, D. Argon laser photocoagulation for macular edema in branch vein occlusion. *Ophthalmology* 93:975–977, 1986.
   Argon laser photocoagulation was beneficial in certain forms of macular edema secondary to branch retinal vein occlusion. During an average follow-up of 3.1 years, vision improved in 65 percent of treated eyes compared with 37 percent of control eyes.
4. Green, W.R., Chan, C.C., Hutchins, G.M., et al. Central retinal vein occlusion: A prospective histopathologic study of 29 eyes in 28 cases. *Trans. Am. Ophthalmol. Soc.* 79:371–422, 1981.
   A clinicohistopathologic study of 29 eyes with CRVO demonstrates the presence of a fresh or a recanalized thrombus in each case.

5. Gutman, F.A., Zegarra, H. The natural course of temporal retinal branch vein occlusion. *Trans. Am. Acad. Ophthalmol. Otolaryngol.* 78:OP178–192, 1974.
   The natural course of temporal retinal vein occlusion in 40 patients was observed. Macular edema and retinal neovascularization were the two most serious complications of this condition.
6. Hayreh, S.S. Classification of central retinal vein occlusion. *Ophthalmology* 90:458–474, 1983.
   The author's reasoning and data for classifying CRVO into ischemic and nonischemic types is given and discussed.
7. Hayreh, S.S., Hayreh, M.S. Hemi-central retinal vein occlusion. Pathogenesis, clinical features, and natural history. *Arch. Ophthalmol.* 98:1600–1609, 1980.
   Hemicentral vein occlusion occurs in patients who have a congenital variant of central vein, that is, a two-trunked central retinal vein instead of a vein with one trunk. Occlusion of either trunk results in hemicentral vein occlusion, in which clinical features and natural history are similar to those of CRVO.
8. Joffe, L., Goldberg, R.E., Magargal, L.E., et al. Macular branch vein occlusion. *Ophthalmology* 87:91–97, 1980.
   A subset of temporal branch vein occlusion, this condition is difficult and more subtle to recognize. It may adversely affect central vision. Its variable clinical presentation is discussed.
9. Kohner, E.M., Laatikainen, L., Oughton, J. The management of central retinal vein occlusion. *Ophthalmology* 90:484–487, 1983.
   After discussing several treatment modalities, the authors conclude that at present no treatment is available to prevent vision loss or improve vision in patients with CRVO.
10. Orth, D.H., Patz, A. Retinal branch vein occlusion. *Surv. Ophthalmol.* 22:357–376, 1978.
    An excellent review of the subject.
11. Priluck, I.A., Robertson, D.M., Hollenhorst, R.W. Long-term follow-up of occlusion of the central retinal vein in young adults. *Am. J. Ophthalmol.* 90:190–202, 1980.
    CRVO was studied retrospectively in 42 patients aged 40 years and younger. A 12 percent early mortality rate was discovered in this group of patients. Photocoagulation remains the only modality helpful in preventing and improving rubeosis and thrombotic glaucoma.

44. ANGIOID STREAKS

Aging and a constellation of systemic conditions have been associated with breaks of Bruch's membrane and associated retinal pigment epithelial changes. These breaks, known as *angioid streaks*, have a characteristic clinical appearance. Ophthalmoscopically, they are seen as irregular, linear, jagged lines radiating from the region of the optic disk in all directions, sometimes reaching the equator of the eye. Originally, these streaks were thought to represent choroidal vessels seen through the retinal pigment epithelium (hence the name angioid). In reality, the streaks represent linear, cracklike dehiscences in a calcified and thickened Bruch's membrane.

Angioid streaks are almost always bilateral. The streaks are most prominent in the posterior pole of the eye, and they taper as they reach the periphery of the fundus. Near the disk they are often interconnected by circumferential breaks in Bruch's membrane. The color of the streak ranges from reddish orange to dark red or brown. The color of the streaks is dependent on the fundus pigmentation as well as on the secondary changes of the retinal pigment epithelium and choriocapillaries that are associated with the streaks.

The general significance of angioid streaks is their association with a host of systemic disorders, including pseudoxanthoma elasticum, sickle cell disease, and Paget's disease.

A long list of other conditions has been compiled in which the association may be only coincidental. In approximately 50 percent of patients, however, no definite systemic condition is found. In such patients the streaks are thought to be the result of calcification and breaks in Bruch's membrane secondary to aging processes.

Pseudoxanthoma elasticum is the most common systemic disease associated with angioid streaks. An estimated 80 to 90 percent of patients with pseudoxanthoma elasticum have evidence of angioid streaks. This systemic disease, which is characterized by a primary degeneration of the elastic fibers of the body with their secondary calcification, affects the skin, the eye, the cardiovascular system, and other organs. The angioid streaks are thought to be one manifestation of these generalized elastic tissue degenerations. The skin findings are confluent, yellowish papules along body folds at the side of the neck and in the flexor surfaces of the extremities, axillae, and creases of the groin. There are premature calcification of the peripheral arteries and symptoms of arterial insufficiency. In the eye, apart from the angioid streaks, the fundus shows evidence of diffuse mottling of the retinal pigment epithelium, an appearance described as peau d'orange. There may be associated peripheral subretinal yellowish spots (salmon spots), which represent isolated dehiscences of Bruch's membrane. These peripheral changes resemble the histo spots seen in the periphery of the fundus in patients with presumed ocular histoplasmosis syndrome (see Ch. 46).

Sickle cell disease, a hereditary hemoglobinopathy, may also be associated with angioid streaks. The reported incidence of angioid streaks in sickle cell disease is between 1 and 2 percent. These patients, however, do not have any evidence of associated elastic tissue disease. The exact etiology of angioid streaks in sickle cell disease is not known, although it is speculated that it may be due to either vasoocclusive disease of the choriocapillaries or deposition of iron in Bruch's membrane.

Paget's disease is a hereditofamilial disease of the bone characterized by gradual development of deformities of the skull, spine, pelvis, and femora. In severe cases, there is an increase in the size of the head and a gorillalike deformity of the skeleton. It is estimated that around 8 percent of patients with Paget's disease develop angioid streaks.

Angioid streaks in themselves do not cause any visual morbidity except where the streaks excite secondary ingrowth of fibrovascular tissue from the choriocapillaries. These choroidal neovascular membranes may cause a secondary serous or hemorrhagic detachment of the overlying retina. This complication usually occurs in the macular area, presenting as metamorphopsia and a central scotoma.

Fluorescein angiography has helped greatly in understanding the structural changes that occur in the posterior segment of eyes with angioid streaks. Fluorescein angiography usually reveals areas of hyperfluorescence and hypofluorescence that reflect the secondary changes in the retinal pigment epithelium and the choriocapillaries. In the initial phases of the angiogram, the streaks may appear as hyperfluorescent areas. The late phases will show staining of the streaks. In pigmented individuals, however, the initial appearance of the streaks may be as areas of hypofluorescence. Although fluorescein angiography is not necessary to make a diagnosis in a patient with characteristic angioid streaks, angiography is helpful in diagnosing early cases and in detecting the occasional streaks that are not obvious on ophthalmoscopy. However, the most important role of angiography is visualization of subretinal choroidal neovascular membranes. Since this complication is the most important cause of decreased vision in these patients, its early detection and treatment are very important. The angiography reveals tufts of neovascular tissue growing from the choriocapillaries through the streaks into the subretinal/subretinal pigment epithelial space. There may be associated subretinal, subretinal pigment epithelial, or intraretinal hemorrhages.

These fibrovascular tufts when left untreated will eventually evolve into a disciform scar of the macula, with secondary decrease of central vision. If the neovascular membrane is detected and found to be outside the foveal avascular zone, then efforts directed at obliterating the membrane with photocoagulation may be successful. Laser photocoagulation has been used with good long-term results. As these neovascular membranes can recur even after treatment, long-term follow-up is indicated in these patients.

Since Bruch's membrane is very brittle in patients with angioid streaks, these patients should also be warned regarding ocular trauma and the need for protective devices if they are involved in any kind of sports. Minimal trauma to the eye may cause loss of central vision secondary to choroidal ruptures and submacular hemorrhages.

1. Clarkson, J.G., Altman, R.D. Angioid streaks. *Surv. Ophthalmol.* 26:235–246, 1982.
   An excellent review of the subject.
2. Clarkson, J.G., Gass, J.D. Angioid streaks and disciform macular detachment in Paget's disease (osteitis deformans). *Am. J. Ophthalmol.* 75:576–586, 1973.
   The funduscopic, angiographic, and histologic findings in an eye with angioid streaks and macular degeneration are presented. The patient had Paget's disease.
3. Federman, J.L., Shields, J.A., Tomer, T.L. Angioid streaks. Fluorescein angiographic features. *Arch. Ophthalmol.* 93:951–962, 1975.
   Different angiographic patterns of 31 patients with angioid streaks are presented.
4. Hamilton, A.M., Pope, F.M., Condon, P.I., et al. Angioid streaks in Jamaican patients with homozygous sickle cell disease. *Br. J. Ophthalmol.* 65:341–347, 1981.
   Twenty-one of 242 patients with homozygous sickle cell disease had angioid streaks.
5. Hull, D.S., Aaberg, T.M. Fluorescein study of a family with angioid streaks and pseudoxanthoma elasticum. *Br. J. Ophthalmol.* 58:738–745, 1974.
   Discussion of the ophthalmoscopic and angiographic findings of angioid streaks in members of two consecutive generations in a family with pseudoxanthoma elasticum.
6. Nagpal, K.C., Asdourian, G., Goldbaum, M., et al. Angioid streaks and sickle haemoglobinopathies. *Br. J. Ophthalmol.* 60:31–34, 1976.
   Five of 356 patients with different sickle hemoglobinopathies had angioid streaks. None of these five patients had an elastic tissue disorder.
7. The Relation of Angioid Streaks to Systemic Disease. In D. Paton, *Thomas American Lecture Series.* Springfield, Ohio: Charles C Thomas, 1972.
   The book discusses the different systemic diseases associated with angioid streaks.
8. Peabody, R.R., Warren, H. Angioid streaks in macular disease. In F.A.J. Esperance (ed.), *Current Diagnosis and Management of Chorioretinal Diseases.* St. Louis: Mosby, 1977. Pp. 527–539.
   The author's results of photocoagulation treatment of six patients with angioid streaks complicated with subretinal neovascular membranes.
9. Shields, J.A., Federman, J.L., Tomer, T.L., et al. Angioid streaks—ophthalmoscopic variations and diagnostic problems. *Br. J. Ophthalmol.* 59:257–266, 1975.
   Fifty-six patients with angioid streaks were evaluated photographically, and the varied ophthalmoscopic findings in these patients are presented.
10. Singerman, L.J., Hatem, G. Laser treatment of choroidal neovascular membranes in angioid streaks. *Retina* 1(2):75–83, 1981.
    Laser treatment was beneficial in treating patients with angioid streaks complicated with choroidal neovascular membranes.

45. TOXIC RETINOPATHY

Numerous ocular side effects of drugs used in treating systemic diseases have been documented. Most agents that are toxic to the retina usually do not affect the retina as a whole, but primarily affect various substructures within the retina. There are numerous known retinotoxic agents, of which chloroquine and the phenothiazine derivatives are the most widely used and studied. Other retinal toxins include methyl alcohol, heavy metals, quinine, and digitalis.

Chloroquine and *hydroxychloroquine* have been effective in the treatment of various connective tissue disorders, including rheumatoid and juvenile arthritis, systemic lupus erythematosus, and mixed connective tissue disease. Their prolonged use has been associated with a toxic maculopathy which, if not detected early, may progress to severe visual loss.

The *phenothiazine derivatives* are used in the management of depressive, involutional, or organic psychosis and various forms of schizophrenia. The most widely used phenothiazine derivatives are chlorpromazine and thioridazine, and it is with the chronic use of these medications that significant side effects appear. Chronic use of chlorpromazine causes pigmentary deposits in or on the eye, and, rarely, a retinopathy develops when the recommended dosages are exceeded. Pigmentary retinopathy with thioridazine is similarly dose-related and occurs only after long-term use.

Pathogenesis

Experimental studies have shown that chloroquine given systemically concentrates in the eye and binds to melanin-containing tissues (iris, retinal pigment epithelium, choroid). The tissue concentration is cumulative over time. Although the drug is highly concentrated in these tissues, the exact mechanism of damage to the ocular structures in general, and to the retina, retinal pigment epithelium, and choroid in particular, is not known. It is not known whether the insult is primarily in the retinal pigment epithelium, with the retinal degenerative changes occurring secondarily, or whether the deleterious effects of chloroquine directly involve specific retinal elements, such as the ganglion cells. Histopathologically, there are considerable changes in the retinal pigment epithelium, with migration of melanin granules into the sensory retina and destruction of rods and cones. Membranous inclusions have also been noted in the ganglion cell layer.

The phenothiazines, similar to chloroquine, concentrate in uveal tissue and retinal pigment epithelium by absorption to melanin granules. They may remain in these tissues. Here also, the exact mechansim of damage is not known. However, it is speculated that phenothiazine retinal toxicity is the result of a primary injury to the ellipsoids of rods that is the result of a loss of ATPase activity in rod mitochondria. This causes a secondary degeneration of the outer segment of the rods, which are then phagocytized by pigment epithelial cells.

Diagnosis

The ocular toxic effects of chloroquine are related to the duration of treatment, total dose, and patient age. Ocular toxicity rarely occurs with a total dose of less than 300 gm. Hydroxychloroquine causes fewer toxic reactions and is more commonly used. Toxic reactions are more likely when the daily dose exceeds 750 mg. Subjective evaluation reveals, depending on the stage of the retinopathy, decreased visual acuity with central, paracentral, and peripheral visual field defects. The early ophthalmoscopic findings of chloroquine retinopathy include mild retinal pigment epithelial changes (loss of the foveal reflex and increased pigmentation of the macula) with mild macular edema. With time, the pigmentary changes become more extreme, leading to the characteristic "bull's eye" lesion. The peripheral retina is normal except for occasional pigment clumps. The retinal blood vessels and the optic nerve generally are not affected. The macular pigmentary lesions are usually bilateral and symmetrical. Color vision may be abnormal. The electroretinogram (ERG) and the electrooculogram (EOG) may show some abnormalities. Dark adaptation is usually normal. Other ophthalmologic manifestations of chloroquine toxicity include corneal deposits, diplopia, and defects of accommodation and convergence.

The pigmentary chorioretinopathy secondary to thioridazine is different from that of chloroquine. The initial fundus changes include pigmentary mottling or stapling, followed by rather uniform clumps of pigment at the level of the retinal pigment epithelium. This may be followed by a stage characterized by discrete nummular areas of atrophy of the retinal pigment epithelium and choriocapillaries. In advanced stages, a diffuse and extensive atrophy of both the retinal pigment epithelium and the choriocapillaries is seen. Patients complain of night vision defects and blurred vision associated with central scotomas. The ERG, EOG, and dark adaptation may be normal in the early stages of the retinopathy; however, in advanced stages of the retinopathy, all of these tests become abnormal.

Treatment

The only treatment consists of discontinuing the medication at the earliest sign of retinal toxicity. Early detection of chloroquine toxicity is not easy, and careful and total ophthalmoscopic evaluation with visual acuity, visual fields (static, kinetic, and Amsler grid), color testing, and fundus photography may be needed since measurable loss of visual function may precede subjective visual symptoms. Patients should be followed up every 6 months and seen as soon as symptoms occur. Even after cessation of the medication, follow-up examinations are important because the toxic effects can progress despite stopping the drug.

The same principles of surveillance apply to phenothiazine retinal toxicity. Again, the medication should be discontinued at the earliest sign of retinal toxicity.

1. Bernstein, H.N. Chloroquine ocular toxicity. *Surv. Ophthalmol.* 12:415–447, 1967.
   A comprehensive review of the subject.
2. Davidorf, F.A. Thioridazine pigmentary retinopathy. *Arch. Ophthalmol.* 90:251–255, 1973.
   Progressive, irreversible changes of the retinal pigment epithelium are documented in a patient with thioridazine retinopathy even after cessation of the medication. The author speculates that the initial insult occurs at the level of the choriocapillaris.
3. Easterbrook, M. The use of Amsler grids in early chloroquine retinopathy. *Ophthalmology* 91:1368–1372, 1984.
   The Amsler grid is a simple and inexpensive way of detecting scotomas in early chloroquine retinopathy.
4. Henkind, P., Carr, R.E., Siegel, I.M. Early chloroquine retinopathy: Clinical and functional findings. *Arch. Ophthalmol.* 71:157–165, 1964.
   Reduction of EOG and ERG was noted in patients with early chloroquine retinopathy; ERG and EOG examinations are recommended for patients receiving chloroquine.
5. Maksymowych, W., Russell, A.S. Antimalarials in rheumatology: Efficacy and safety. *Seminars Arthr. Rheumat.* 16:206–221, 1987.
   A review of the efficacy and complications of antimalarial agents (chloroquine and hydroxychloroquine) in rheumatology.
6. Meredith, T.A., Aaberg, T.M., Willerson, W.D. Progressive chorioretinopathy after receiving thioridazine. *Arch. Ophthalmol.* 96:1172–1176, 1978.
   A distinctive nummular chorioretinopathy described in three patients who were on high doses of orally administered thioridazine. The retinopathy was progressive even after discontinuation of the drug.
7. Miller, F.S. III, Bunt-Milam, A.H., Kalina, R.E. Clinical-ultrastructural study of thioridazine retinopathy. *Ophthalmology* 89:1478–1488, 1982.
   A clinicohistopathologic presentation of a patient with advanced thioridazine retinopathy. On the basis of the ultrastructural change, the author postulates an initial photoreceptor damage followed by pigmentary degeneration.
8. Nozik, R.A., Weinstock, F.J., Vignos, P.J. Jr. Ocular complications of chloroquine. *Am. J. Ophthalmol.* 58:774–778, 1964.
   Color testing may be important in detecting early chloroquine retinopathy.
9. Tobin, D.R., Krohel, G.B., Rynes, R.I. Hydroxychloroquine—seven-year experience. *Arch. Ophthalmol.* 100:81–83, 1982.
   With patients maintained on no more than 400 mg of hydroxychloroquine daily, the incidence of toxicity was very low.
10. Wetterholm, D.H., Winter, F.C. Histopathology of chloroquine retinal toxicity. *Arch. Ophthalmol.* 71:82–87, 1964.
    In a histopathologic study of chloroquine retinopathy, selective destruction of the photoreceptors was noted.

VIII. UVEA

George K. Asdourian

The presumed ocular histoplasmosis syndrome (POHS) is a distinct clinical entity characterized by the ophthalmoscopic triad of: (1) *peripapillary chorioretinal scarring,* the result of presumed circumpapillary choroiditis; (2) *scattered peripheral atrophic chorioretinal scars* (referred to as *histo spots*), the result of presumed disseminated choroiditis; and (3) *histoplasmic maculopathy,* which in the inactive stage may appear as a histo spot. In the active stage histoplasmic maculopathy is characterized by a pigment ring, with or without associated serous or hemorrhagic detachment of the sensory retina.

Pathogenesis

The peripheral histo spots are usually asymptomatic, but aid in diagnosis. The peripapillary scarring, although asymptomatic in the majority of patients, may lead to a serous or hemorrhagic detachment of the peripapillary retina with extension into the macular area, causing visual dysfunction. It is the maculopathy, however, that will bring the majority of patients with POHS to the ophthalmologist's attention with symptoms of metamorphopsia or central scotoma, or both.

Ophthalmic examination will reveal the characteristic ophthalmoscopic traid. Inflammatory signs are absent in both the anterior and posterior segments. The vitreous is clear with no inflammatory cells. A history of systemic histoplasmosis cannot be elicited from the majority of patients although most of them come from areas endemic for histoplasmosis, the largest areas in the United States being the Ohio River and Mississippi River valleys.

In a minority of patients, the maculopathy at initial presentation may resemble that of central serous chorioretinopathy, i.e., a serous detachment of the sensory retina (see Chap. 31). However, in the majority of symptomatic patients, the macular involvement is *hemorrhagic.* The macular hemorrhages are the result of bleeding from tufts of capillaries that grow from the choriocapillaris and through Bruch's membrane under the retinal pigment epithelium or the sensory retina or both. These new capillary tufts grow through dehiscences of Bruch's membrane that are thought to result from the original attack of choroiditis. For unknown reasons, such choroidal neovascular membranes occur mostly in the macular area. Thus, patients with inactive histo spots in the disk to macular area are at risk of developing symptomatic active hemorrhagic maculopathy. Rarely, maculopathy develops even in the absence of any apparent histo spots in the macular area. The peripheral histo spots rarely neovascularize; even if they do, they do not produce any significant ocular morbidity.

Bleeding from the neovascular tufts under the retinal pigment epithelium produces a characteristic pigment ring. With more exudation and hemorrhages, the sensory retina in the macular area detaches. The process eventually ends with disciform scarring of the macula and marked reduction of central vision.

Diagnosis

Fluorescein angiography is an excellent clinical tool for evaluating patients with POHS maculopathy. Some atrophic histo spots not detected ophthalmoscopically are visible angiographically. Where there are nonhemorrhagic lesions, areas of retinal edema appear as hyperfluorescence. The most important role of angiography, however, is in the detection and characterization of subretinal neovascular tufts. These tufts are seen in the configuration of a sea fan or a bicycle wheel. In these configurations, the capillaries typically radiate outward from their points of entry through Bruch's membrane into the subpigment epithelial or subretinal space. Such capillaries typically leak fluorescein that stains the subretinal space. Angiography not only detects the neovascularization but also delineates its extent and location in relation to the foveal avascular zone. The location of the border of the neovascular membrane in relation to the foveal avascular zone determines the advisability and feasibility of photocoagulation as a means of treatment.

Although the ophthalmoscopic triad is characteristic of POHS, other entities should also be considered in the differential diagnosis. Among inflammatory diseases, toxoplasmosis, syphilis, sarcoidosis, and toxocariasis may produce similar ophthalmic pictures. Myopic chorioretinal degeneration, drusen of the optic disk, angioid streaks, and the idiopathic subretinal neovascular syndrome are noninfectious entities that should also be considered.

Although *Histoplasma capsulatum* has been demonstrated histologically in some patients with the clinical picture of POHS, most evidence for an association between POHS and histoplasmosis has been derived from epidemiologic studies. Similar ocular findings have been reported from countries where histoplasmosis is either not endemic or not known to occur. Thus, other unknown causative agents may be producing an ophthalmologic picture similar to the one we associate with histoplasmosis.

Treatment

The prognosis for retaining good visual acuity is guarded if the maculopathy is not treated. The final visual outcome depends on the location and severity of the maculopathy. Inactive lesions do not require any treatment. Patients with macular histo spots should be warned to seek immediate ophthalmic care in the event of any central visual disturbances. Steroids and photocoagulation have been the two main modalities of treatment for symptomatic histoplasmic maculopathy. The results of steroid use (topical and systemic) have been equivocal, and no randomized prospective controlled clinical trials have been performed to show the efficacy of steroids. Laser photocoagulation is beneficial in certain circumstances. If the choroidal neovascular membrane is situated 200 to 2500 μ from the center of the foveal avascular zone, then photocoagulation with an argon blue green laser may prevent visual acuity loss. Although neovascular membranes closer than 200 μ to the center of the foveal avascular zone may be treated with photocoagulation, the efficacy of such treatment has not been demonstrated.

1. Braunstein, R.A., Rosen, D.A., Bird, A.C. Ocular histoplasmosis syndrome in the United Kingdom. *Br. J. Ophthalmol.* 55:893–898, 1974.
   Fifteen patients from the United Kingdom with the ophthalmologic criteria of POHS are reported. They did not find any evidence of infection with H. capsulatum.
2. Krill, A.E., Chrishti, M.I., Klien, B.A., et al. Multifocal inner choroiditis. *Trans. Am. Acad. Ophthalmol. Otolaryngol.* 73:222–245, 1969.
   Classic paper describing the entity referred to as POHS.
3. Macular Photocoagulation Study Group. Argon laser photocoagulation for ocular histoplasmosis. *Arch. Ophthalmol.* 101:1347–1357, 1983.
   Reports the beneficial results of photocoagulation in preventing severe visual loss in eyes with choroidal neovascular membranes as a result of POHS.
4. Macular Photocoagulation Study Group. Argon laser photocoagulation for neovascular maculopathy. Three-year results from randomized clinical trials. *Arch. Ophthalmol.* 104:694–701, 1986.
   The beneficial long-term results (3 years) of treating neovascular membranes in POHS are reported.
5. Roth, A.M. Histoplasma capsulatum in the presumed ocular histoplasmosis syndrome. *Am. J. Ophthalmol.* 84:293–298, 1977.
   Histologic demonstration of the fungus in a case of POHS.
6. Schlaegel, T.F. Jr. (ed.). Ocular histoplasmosis. *Int. Ophthalmol. Clin.* 15(3), 1975.
   This entire issue of this publication series reports the proceedings of a 2-day symposium on ocular histoplasmosis held in Indianapolis. All aspects of ocular histoplasmosis are addressed.
7. Schlaegel, T.F. Jr. *Ocular Histoplasmosis.* Orlando: Grune & Stratton, 1977.
   This entire 301-page monograph is devoted to ocular histoplasmosis.
8. Schlaegel, T.F. Jr., O'Connor, G.R. Fungal uveitis. *Int. Ophthalmol. Clin.* 17(3):121–141, 1977.
   An excellent short review of POHS.
9. Scholz, R., Green, W.R., Kutys, R., et al. Histoplasma capsulatum in the eye. *Ophthalmology* 91:1100–1104, 1984.

The ocular pathologic findings as described in an immunosuppressed patient who died of disseminated histoplasmosis.
10. Watzke, R.C., Claussen, R.W. The long-term course of multifocal choroiditis (presumed ocular histoplasmosis). *Am. J. Ophthalmol.* 91:750–760, 1981.
Forty patients with POHS were followed using stereoscopic color fundus photography and fluorescein angiography.

47. TOXOPLASMOSIS

Toxoplasmosis is one of the most common causes of posterior uveitis in humans. It accounts for approximately 30 to 50 percent of all posterior uveitis.

Pathogenesis
The etiologic agent for toxoplasmosis is an obligate intracellular protozoan parasite called *Toxoplasma gondii*. This organism is an intestinal parasite of the cat (the definitive host), in whose intestinal tract it reproduces sexually. The parasite is shed in cat feces and insect vectors transmit the parasite and contaminate food, as well as infect other herbivorous animals. Humans acquire the parasite by eating contaminated food, mainly raw meat.

Once the parasite is acquired by humans, it enters human cells, where it replicates asexually and forms cysts to protect the progeny protozoa. These cysts may remain dormant for many years but occasionally rupture, releasing protozoa that then infect nearby cells. This stimulates the host immune response, and the end result is an inflammation at or near the site of infection.

Clinical
Infection by *T. gondii* manifests in a variety of ways. It may cause a *primary systemic infection,* which is subclinical in most cases. The normal human immune system is adequate to contain the infection. The commonest clinical manifestation of acquired toxoplasmosis is a lymphadenopathy, often associated with fever, skin rash, and hepatosplenomegaly. Toxoplasmic myocarditis, pneumonitis, and encephalitis may occur, but are rare.

Although the human immune system can sequester the parasite, it cannot totally eliminate it. Thus, recovery from the primary acute infection is followed by a chronic form of the disease that may persist throughout the host's lifetime. Humans infected with the parasites will produce antibodies for a long time, and it is estimated that approximately 50 percent of the adult population in the United States test positive for these antibodies.

Ocular lesions occurring with acquired toxoplasmosis are rare, but have been reported. Ocular involvement is most common with toxoplasmic encephalitis. Posterior uveitis, papillitis, and optic atrophy have been reported to occur with approximately 3.1 percent of acquired systemic toxoplasmosis.

If toxoplasmosis is acquired by a pregnant woman, the parasite may be transmitted to the fetus, resulting in *congenital toxoplasmosis.* Transmission to the fetus occurs through either maternal parasitemia during pregnancy or implantation of the placenta into a portion of the uterus that contains latent cysts of the organism. Clinical evidence suggests that congenital toxoplasmosis results from acute infection of the mother during pregnancy, and only rarely from chronic infection. Consequently, mothers who have given birth to toxoplasmic infants are unlikely to infect subsequent offspring, presumably because of protection by maternal immunity. However, a few cases of toxoplasmic retinochoroiditis occurring in siblings have been reported. Acute infection during the first trimester may cause severe fetal infection with death of the newborn. The clinical features of congenital toxoplasmosis in a neonate may include convulsions, intracranial calcifications, mental retardation, and chorioretinal lesions.

Infection occurring late in pregnancy may be mild or subclinical. A purely ocular form of congenital toxoplasmosis is the most common variety. The ocular findings in these children are chorioretinal scars, which usually remain asymptomatic unless there is a flare-up of the infection later in life. These children may also develop esotropia or fail vision-screening tests secondary to macular scarring.

In recent years, opportunistic systemic infections with toxoplasmosis and toxoplasmic retinochoroiditis have been implicated in patients suffering from various acquired immunodeficiency states caused by viruses, malignancies, or intensive corticosteroid and cytotoxic chemotherapy regimens. These are all considered flare-ups of congenitally acquired infections secondary to breakdown of the host immune system. These infections may be severe and difficult to control.

In the eye, *T. gondii* has a predilection for the nerve fiber layer of the retina. Here, cysts containing the protozoa may remain dormant and inactive for many years, until for unknown reasons (perhaps stress or immunologic imbalance), the cysts rupture and release the protozoa. The protozoa then incite a severe inflammatory reaction in the inner retina, which is seen clinically as a focal area of necrotizing retinitis. Thus, *ocular toxoplasmosis* is thought to be a reactivation of congenital toxoplasmosis. Patients seen by the ophthalmologist usually have a chief complaint of blurry vision or floaters. The floaters are usually due to vitreous inflammatory cells, whereas the decreased vision is mainly secondary to cystoid macular edema, papillitis, or severe vitreous reaction in front of the macula.

Diagnosis

Examination of the anterior segment often reveals few signs of inflammation. The eye may be white and quiet, with the anterior chamber showing only occasional cells and mild flare. Occasionally moderate to severe granulomatous and nongranulomatous iridocyclitis may be associated with the posterior retinochoroiditis. This anterior segment reaction is thought to be a hypersensitivity reaction and not direct infection. The vitreous shows multiple opacities and inflammatory cells. A posterior vitreous detachment is often present, with multiple punctate precipitates on the back surface. These precipitates may resemble keratitic precipitates. A characteristic whitish-yellowish, slightly elevated lesion represents the actual site of the retinochoroiditis and is usually located in the posterior pole, in the macula or close to it, and in the juxtapapillary retina. This lesion has fuzzy borders and is usually located adjacent to an old chorioretinal scar. In a minority of patients, the focus of inflammation may be at the immediate edge or within the superficial optic nerve head, simulating the clinical picture of severe papillitis. The inflammatory reaction in the vitreous may occasionally be so intense that even with indirect ophthalmoscopy the exact location of the lesion cannot be definitely identified. Segmental periarteritis and diffuse sheathing of the venules may accompany toxoplasmic retinitis. These phenomena are also thought to represent sites of local antigen-antibody reaction.

Although the only way of making a definitive diagnosis of toxoplasmosis is by demonstrating the *T. gondii* organisms in diseased tissue, a clinical diagnosis is usually reached by observing the characteristic exudative focal retinochoroiditis, by serologic testing for antitoxoplasma antibodies, and by excluding other causes of exudative retinochoroiditis. Several serologic tests are used to detect the antitoxoplasma antibodies. These include the toxoplasma dye test of Sabin and Feldman, the hemagglutination test, the indirect fluorescent-antibody test, and the enzyme-linked immunosorbent assay for toxoplasmosis. The serum titers determined by any of these tests may be extremely low in patients with ocular toxoplasmosis. *Any* titer of serum antibodies should be significant, especially in patients with characteristic fundus lesions. In doubtful cases, the aqueous may be used to confirm the presence of antibodies. If the titer of antibodies in the aqueous is higher than that in the serum, then this finding becomes very significant.

Since the most common presentation of ocular toxoplasmosis is a focal necrotizing retinitis, other conditions that present with a similar clinical picture should be considered in the differential diagnosis. Lesions of tuberculosis, syphilis, sarcoidosis, cytomegalovirus, herpes simplex, candida, and acute retinal necrosis may mimic those of toxoplasmosis and should be considered in the differential diagnosis, even with a positive antitoxoplasma antibody level.

Treatment
The retinochoroiditis of toxoplasmosis is thought to be the result of actively multiplying parasites and the associated inflammatory reaction. Thus, treatment is aimed at destroying the parasite with antimicrobial medications and minimizing the inflammatory tissue damage, especially to sensitive areas of the retina such as the macula and the optic nerve, with anti-inflammatory medications. The antimicrobial agents used to treat toxoplasmosis include pyrimethamine, sulfonamides, and clindamycin. Corticosteroids are used in association with the antimicrobial agents to minimize the inflammatory reaction. Light photocoagulation and cryotherapy have also been used to destroy the organisms at the site of infection as well as to eliminate dormant cysts. At this time, there is no effective treatment of the encysted form of the parasite, and treatment is principally aimed at controlling an acute recurrent infection.

1. Asabell, P.A., Vermund, S.H., Hofeldt, A.J. Presumed toxoplasmic retinochoroiditis in four siblings. *Am. J. Ophthalmol.* 94:656–663, 1982.
   Four siblings with presumed toxoplasmic retinochoroiditis are presented.
2. Dobbie, J.G. Cryotherapy in the management of toxoplasma retinochoroiditis. *Trans. Am. Acad. Ophthalmol. Otolaryngol.* 72:364–373, 1968.
   Six patients were treated with cryotherapy to control severe toxoplasmic retinochoroiditis.
3. Folk, J.C., Lobes, L.A. Presumed toxoplasmic papillitis. *Ophthalmology* 91:64–67, 1984.
   Six patients with ocular toxoplasmosis presenting with unilateral disk inflammation and swelling.
4. Haller Yeo, J., Jakobiec, F.A., Iwamoto, T., et al. Opportunistic toxoplasmic retinochoroiditis following chemotherapy for systemic lymphoma. *Ophthalmology* 90:885–898, 1983.
   Microscopic documentation of toxoplasmosis in an immunocompromised patient.
5. Perkins, E.S. Ocular toxoplasmosis. *Br. J. Ophthalmol.* 57:1–17, 1973.
   An excellent review of the literature on ocular toxoplasmosis with emphasis on ocular complications in acquired and congenital toxoplasmosis.
6. Scott, E. New concepts in toxoplasmosis. *Surv. Ophthalmol.* 18:255–274, 1974.
   A general review of the subject.
7. Tabbara, K.F., Dy-Liacco, J., Nozik, R.A., et al. Clindamycin in chronic toxoplasmosis. *Arch. Ophthalmol.* 97:542–544, 1979.
   Results of subtenon injections of clindamycin to control chronic toxoplasmosis in experimental animals show promise.
8. Tabarra, K.F., O'Connor, G.R. Treatment of ocular toxoplasmosis with clindamycin and sulfadiazine. *Ophthalmology* 87:129–134, 1980.
   This study shows the efficacy of combining two antimicrobial agents that operate on unrelated metabolic pathways of toxoplasma in treating recurrent active toxoplasmic retinochoroiditis in humans.
9. Tessler, H.H. Diagnosis and treatment of ocular toxoplasmosis. In *Clinical Modules for Ophthalmology—American Academy of Ophthalmology.* Focal points, Vol 3, module 2. San Francisco: American Academy of Ophthalmology, 1985.
   Review of ocular toxoplasmosis and different treatment modalities.

48. TOXOCARIASIS

Toxocariasis is a common ocular and systemic infection of children that is found worldwide. It frequently causes visual impairment of children in the United States. The etiologic agent of the infection is the common dog roundworm *Toxocara canis,* which is capable of infecting humans and producing serious systemic and ocular disease.

Pathogenesis
Demographic surveys indicate that between one-third and one-half of all households in the United States have one or more dogs, most of which are infected with *T. canis* as puppies. The adult form of the worm lives in the dog's proximal small intestine. The female worm produces 200,000 eggs per day, so infected animals contaminate the environment with millions of eggs. The eggs can survive for long periods of time under adverse conditions. Ten to 32 percent of the soil samples collected from parks, playgrounds, and other public places in North America are contaminated with toxocara eggs. Thus, dogs, contaminated household environments, and playgrounds are potential sources of infection to children, especially those with earth-eating habits.

The ova, once swallowed by children, hatch into larvae in the stomach and the small intestines. After hatching, the larvae penetrate the bowel wall and enter the systemic circulation, by which they are disseminated to distant organs, especially the liver, lungs, heart, and eyes. The larvae do not develop into adult worms in humans, which explains why stool cultures of *T. canis* are negative in infected children. The sequelae of this generalized systemic infestation by the parasite is a clinical syndrome known as *visceral larva migrans* (VLM), which is characterized by fever, cough, malaise, hepatosplenomegaly, leukocytosis, eosinophilia, and hypergammaglobulinemia.

Ocular toxocariasis is thought to be a late sequela of systemic infection, although it is usually impossible to elicit a clear-cut history of VLM from patients (usually children) or their parents. Ocular toxocariasis is rarely seen in association with systemic disease and is almost never seen concurrently with VLM. Children with ocular toxocariasis are usually older, 7.5 years of age compared with 2 years of age with VLM. A history of pica is less common than in children with VLM. The exact incidence of ocular toxocariasis is not known. Ten percent of all cases of uveitis in Britian are presumed to be caused by this infection. There is no sex or racial predilection.

Diagnosis
Once the parasite gains access to the eye, it initiates a granulomatous reaction. Clinically, ocular toxocariasis may manifest itself in a variety of ways. The most common clinical presentation is a solitary *submacular granuloma* in a quiet eye with no evidence of associated inflammation. There may be associated preretinal gliosis with evidence of retinal traction lines radiating from the lesion. These lesions are usually discovered as a result of school vision-screening tests or in a child with strabismus. The next most common clinical presentation is a *peripheral retinal granuloma,* which occasionally may involve the pars plana and simulate pars planitis. The granuloma frequently appears as a white, uninflamed, hemispheric mass that is usually solitary and unilateral. The granuloma may show prominent traction bands and retinal folds, which may extend back to the macula and disk, causing macular traction and detachment. The traction bands may produce retinal holes and dialyses, eventually resulting in localized or total retinal detachments.

A third common clinical manifestation of ocular involvement is a *chronic intraocular inflammation* that on occasion is so intense that it resembles endophthalmitis. This severe intraocular inflammation results in a red eye with a white pupillary reflex and poor vision. There may be a cataract and secondary retinal detachment. This clinical picture is very difficult or impossible to differentiate from that of retinoblastoma, and these eyes may be enucleated for suspected retinoblastomas. Diseases other than retinoblastoma that should be considered in the differential diagnosis include primary persistent hyperplastic vitreous, retinopathy of prematurity, familial exudative vitreoretinopathy, toxoplasmosis, and cataract.

The diagnosis of ocular toxocariasis is usually presumptive, based on the clinical findings with a history of pica and a household pet at home or in the neighborhood, but it can be confirmed by immunologic tests. The most sensitive and specific of these tests is the enzyme-linked immunosorbent assay (ELISA). In patients with ocular toxocariasis, the ELISA is 90 percent sensitive and 90 percent specific at a serum titer of 1 : 8. The 10 percent false-positive rate in ocular serodiagnosis is attributed to the 10 percent prevalence of serum titers of 1 : 8 or higher among healthy children. Antibody titers have also been tested in vitreous samples in patients undergoing vitrectomy for the complications of ocular toxocariasis. These vitreous titers have been found to be equal or greater than the serum titers, suggesting the possibility of local antibody production or concentration in the vitreous.

Treatment

There is no effective treatment for ocular toxocariasis. Various anthelmintic compounds (thiabendazole, diethylcarbamazine) have been used with disappointing results. Steroids have also been used in association with the above anthelmintic medications to control the intraocular inflammation. Although the parasite cannot be directly eliminated, the rhegmatogenous or traction retinal detachments secondary to the vitreous bands that form as a result of intraocular inflammation can be treated successfully by various surgical methods, mainly vitrectomy and scleral buckling procedures [4].

The most important aspect of treatment of ocular and systemic toxocariasis is prevention. The public health hazards posed by toxocariasis and other helminth infections of pet dogs should be explained to the public and to pet owners. Veterinarians should also warn pet owners of the potential zoonotic risks and provide the necessary advice and chemotherapeutic intervention to minimize them.

1. Ashton, N. Larval granulomatosis of the retina due to Toxocara. *Br. J. Ophthalmol.* 44:129–148, 1960.
   The original article describing four cases of ocular toxocariasis presenting as posterior pole granulomas.
2. Biglan, A.W., Glickman, L.T., Lobes, L.A. Jr. Serum and vitreous Toxocara antibody in nematode endophthalmitis. *Am. J. Ophthalmol.* 88:898–901, 1979.
   Vitreous titers of antibody to toxocara are equal or greater than serum titers in five patients undergoing vitrectomy.
3. Glickman, L.T., Schantz, P.M. Epidemiology and pathogenesis of zoonotic toxocariasis. *Epidemiol. Rev.* 3:230–250, 1981.
   A review of the epidemiology and pathogenesis of toxocariasis.
4. Hagler, W.S., Pollard, Z.F., Jarrett, W.H., et al. Results of surgery for ocular Toxocara canis. *Ophthalmology* 88:1081–1086, 1981.
   Results of vitreoretinal surgery on 17 patients with complications secondary to T. canis *are presented and discussed.*
5. Molk, R. Ocular toxocariasis: A review of the literature. *Ann. Ophthalmol.* 15:216–231, 1983.
   Excellent review of ocular toxocariasis.
6. Pollard, Z.F., Jarrett, W.H., Hagler, W.S., et al. ELISA for diagnosis of ocular toxocariasis. *Ophthalmology* 86:743–749, 1979.
   The authors stress the importance, sensitivity, and specificity of the ELISA in the diagnosis of ocular toxocariasis.
7. Shields, J.A. Ocular toxocariasis: A review. *Surv. Ophthalmol.* 28:361–381, 1984.
   Another good review of ocular and systemic toxocariasis with 200 references.
8. Wilder, H.C. Nematode endophthalmitis. *Trans. Am. Acad. Ophthalmol. Otolaryngol.* 55:99–109, 1950.
   The author demonstrates that many cases of enucleated eyes with the diagnosis of pseudolipoma were cases of nematode endophthalmitis and establishes ocular toxocariasis as a clinical entity.
9. Wilkinson, C.P., Welch, R.B. Intraocular toxocara. *Am. J. Ophthalmol.* 71:921–930, 1971.
   Different clinical presentations of 40 patients with presumed or proven intraocular toxocara are presented.

49. CANDIDIASIS

Candida albicans, a yeastlike fungus, is not usually highly infectious. It is a frequent commensal organism of the human gastrointestinal tract, mouth, and vagina. Although *Candida* may cause occasional bouts of candidemia in normal individuals by invading the blood stream, infection is usually controlled by the immunologic defenses of the host. However, if these host defense mechanisms are interfered with either by disease processes or iatrogenically, such individuals may lose resistance to this yeast and candidemia may be followed by hematogenous candida endophthalmitis.

Pathogenesis
The clinical setting for the development of endogenous *C. albicans* endophthalmitis includes the following: (1) a history of gastrointestinal or biliary tract surgery followed by prolonged systemic administration of antibiotics through indwelling catheters; (2) prolonged use of indwelling cathethers for hyperalimentation; (3) immunosuppressive therapy for organ transplant patients; (4) chronic steroid therapy for patients with chronic, progressive collagen diseases; (5) chronic disease states in which cell-mediated defenses are definitely compromised, such as diabetes, sarcoidosis, chronic liver disease, and malignant diseases; and (6) drug addiction in people who administer heroin and other narcotic agents to themselves by the intravenous route. Drug addicts with ocular candidiasis may present a more difficult diagnostic problem than the other predisposed patients since the majority appear generally well and healthy and without other evidence of disseminated candidemia [1]. In these cases, ocular involvement probably follows an intravenous infection rather than resorption of fungus from the gut.

Infection in the eye appears to arise in the choroid as a focal granulomatous inflammation. In some cases, the retina may be the site of this granulomatous reaction, without choroidal involvement. Bruch's membrane usually offers no barrier to the infection. Lesions progress anteriorly from the choroid into the retina and overlying vitreous, thus producing a picture of generalized endophthalmitis. Histopathologic examination of eyes with candida endophthalmitis has revealed a combination of suppurative and granulomatous inflammation in the inner choroid with evidence of subretinal abscess. In some eyes, the inflammation was confined to the retina alone and appeared to originate from the deep capillary plexus of the retina. Organisms were found in most of these lesions.

Diagnosis
Clinical infection of the eye initially is characterized by the painless onset of blurred vision and floaters in one or both eyes. The eyes are usually white, and photophobia is rare. As the infection progresses, the eye may become red and painful. Slit lamp examination reveals occasional mild anterior uveitis. Ophthalmoscopy shows multiple, white, cottonlike, circumscribed exudates with filamentous borders located in the chorioretina and extending into the vitreous with an accompanying overlying vitreous haze. Occasional retinal hemorrhages with white centers (Roth's spots) are seen. The vitreous may contain multiple small white puff balls. The chorioretinitis clinically resembles the lesions of acute toxoplasmic retinochoroiditis. However, the fundi of patients with candidiasis do not have any stigmata of old, healed toxoplasma-chorioretinal scars. Other entities that should be considered in the differential diagnosis include herpetic retinitis, cytomegalovirus inclusion disease, reticulum cell sarcoma, and other fungi. The clinical picture of chorioretinitis associated with vitreous haze in a patient with any of the predisposing factors mentioned previously should alert the clinician to the possibility of candida endophthalmitis.

The clinical diagnosis may be substantiated by positive blood cultures or by positive cultures from the tip of an intravenous catheter. Blood cultures, however, are positive in only approximately 50 percent of patients with candida endophthalmitis. Skin tests and serum levels of precipitins and agglutinins for *Candida* are not very helpful diagnostic tools. If a definite diagnosis cannot be reached clinically and with cultures, a vitreous tap may be justified to establish the etiology of the endophthalmitis. This aggressive diagnostic modality has been supported on the grounds that treatment of candidiasis involves highly toxic drugs and that unless a definite diagnosis is established, such treatment should not be given. Recovery of the yeast from the vitreous gel is difficult, because the yeast appears to be localized by necrotic inflammatory cells. Thus, it is essential to remove a focal vitreous lesion in which organisms are present in large numbers and can usually be seen on a direct smear. Cultures of the vitreous aspirate on blood agar or Sabouraud's agar should confirm the presence of fungi in 24 hours.

Treatment

This disease has an extremely poor prognosis unless the etiology can be established quickly and early treatment is initiated with antifungal agents. The ideal antifungal therapy for candida endophthalmitis has yet to be defined. The mainstay of therapy has been intravenous amphotericin B, which is often used in conjunction with oral 5-fluorocytosine. Intravenous amphotericin has poor ocular penetration and severe side effects. Treatment is often accompanied by fever, chills, and nausea. The drug is also highly toxic to the kidney and liver, and the functions of these organs should be carefully monitored. Amphotericin is most effective if started before the vitreous is involved. Oral 5-fluorocytosine may be used in conjunction with amphotericin B if no clinical improvement occurs after amphotericin B treatment alone or when severe toxic effects occur. This combined treatment has a synergistic effect, presumably because of the different mechanisms of action of each drug on *Candida*. 5-Fluorocytosine has its own limitations as an antifungal drug. Fifty percent of all *Candida* isolates show primary resistance to it, and 30 percent emerge resistant to it after brief therapy. The drug also has significant liver toxicity, and hepatic function should be tested frequently. Despite its shortcomings, amphotericin B is still the drug of choice and is frequently successful in treating candida endophthalmitis.

Other, more aggressive treatment modalities have been proposed for ocular candidiasis. These include injection of amphotericin B under Tenon's capsule or directly into the vitreous. Sub-Tenon's injection may be accompanied by a great deal of local irritation and superficial tissue necrosis, and vitreous injection may produce retinal toxicity. Several case reports, however, have shown that intraocular amphotericin B injection has the potential to treat ocular candidiasis without retinal toxicity [6, 8].

Other antifungal medications that are being investigated either alone or in combination with existing drugs include the imidazole derivatives (including miconazole and ketoconazole). Experience with these drugs is limited, and only future research will establish their role in treating candida endophthalmitis.

Once the vitreous is massively involved with infection, then systemic and local treatment may not be adequate and curative. Untreated massive vitreous gliosis with secondary retinal detachment and eventual phthisis will occur. In these cases, a more radical treatment has been proposed that involves vitrectomy for removal of the entire vitreous gel to rid the eye of the bulk of organisms and the mass of inflammatory cells. Vitrectomy is accompanied by intravitreal injection of amphotericin B. These radical treatment modalities are presently used in desperate clinical situations with fulminating infection.

Since early diagnosis and treatment is the best way to control infection and preserve vision, physicians should question any patient with candidemia specifically about visual disturbances. Even in the absence of symtoms, frequent dilated funduscopic examinations should be performed in all patients with proven candidemia.

1. Aguilar, G.L., Blumenkrantz, M.S., Egbert, P.R., et al. Candida endophthalmitis after intravenous drug abuse. *Arch. Ophthalmol.* 97:96–100, 1979.
   Three cases of candida endophthalmitis occurring in intravenous drug addicts. The patients did not have evidence of systemic candidemia.
2. Edwards, J.E. Jr., Foos, R.Y., Montgomerie, J.Z., et al. Ocular manifestations of Candida septicemia: Review of seventy-six cases of hematogenous Candida endophthalmitis. *Medicine* 53:47–75, 1974.
   A fine review of the ocular manifestations of candida endophthalmitis.

3. Elliott, J.H., O'Day, D.M., Gutow, G.S., et al. Mycotic endophthalmitis in drug abusers. *Am. J. Ophthalmol.* 88:66–72, 1979.
   Candida endophthalmitis occurred in a husband and wife who were both intravenous drug addicts.
4. Griffin, J.R., Pettit, T.H., Fishman, L.S., et al. Blood borne Candida endophthalmitis. A clinical and pathologic study of 21 cases. *Arch. Ophthalmol.* 89:450–456, 1973.
   An excellent article about the clinical and pathologic findings in candida endophthalmitis.
5. Michelson, P.E., Stark, W., Reeser, F., et al. Endogenous Candida endophthalmitis— Report of 13 cases and 16 from the literature. *Int. Ophthalmol. Clin.* 11:125–147, 1971.
   Clinical and pathologic findings in 29 cases of endogenous candida endophthalmitis.
6. Perraut, L.E. Jr., Perraut, L.E., Bleiman, B., et al. Successful treatment of Candida albicans endophthalmitis with intravitreal amphotericin B. *Arch. Ophthalmol.* 99:1565–1567, 1981.
   An excellent visual recovery after treatment of candida endophthalmitis with intravitreal and systemic amphotericin B.
7. Salmon, J.F., Partridge, B.M., Spalton, D.J. Candida endophthalmitis in a heroin addict: A case report. *Br. J. Ophthalmol.* 67:306–309, 1983.
   Unilateral panuveitis was the presenting sign of candida endophthalmitis, which was confirmed by vitrectomy. Treatment with new antifungal medications controlled the infection.
8. Stern, G.A., Fetkenhour, C.L., O'Grady, R.B. Intravitreal amphotericin B treatment of candida endophthalmitis. *Arch. Ophthalmol.* 95:89–93, 1977.
   A patient was successfully treated for candida endophthalmitis with intravitreal amphotericin B. The eye, obtained after the accidental death of the patient, did not show any evidence of retinal toxicity from the intravitreal amphotericin B.
9. Stone, R.D., Irvine, A.R., O'Connor, G.R. Candida endophthalmitis: Report of an unusual case with isolation of the etiologic agent by vitreous biopsy. *Ann. Ophthalmol.* 7:757–762, 1975.
   A case of candida endophthalmitis was diagnosed by vitreous needle biopsy.

50. UVEAL MALIGNANT MELANOMA

Melanocytic neoplasms are the most common primary tumors of the uvea. These rather pigmented neoplasms may be benign *(nevi* and *melanocytomas)* or malignant *(melanomas)* and are thought to arise from mature melanocytes within the stroma of the iris, ciliary body, and choroid. Light-skinned white persons are predisposed to melanocytic neoplasms, which are rare in blacks.

Iris Melanomas
Malignant melanomas of the iris represent 3 to 10 percent of all malignant melanomas of the uvea. Clinically, they often resemble iris nevi and present as a solitary mass that may be pigmented or nonpigmented. A diffuse type, involving the iris stroma circumferentially, is another unusual form of iris melanoma that may produce heterochromia and is difficult to diagnose. Iris melanomas also may involve the angle and infiltrate the trabecular meshwork and ciliary body, producing glaucoma, uveitis, and iris neovascularization as their presenting signs. The diagnosis may be delayed or made difficult if there is corneal clouding secondary to the glaucoma and uveitis. The clinician confronted with a suspicious iris lesion should have a high index of suspicion as well as an awareness of the many other clinical lesions that can simulate an iris melanoma. The differential diagnoses include epithelial tumors, metastatic tumors, foreign bodies in the iris, and iris cysts.

The treatment of localized iris melanomas is either observation or surgical excision.

An iris melanoma may be observed with periodic photography until definite growth has been documented. The surgical treatment is simple iridectomy for localized lesions. Iridotrabeculectomy (trabecular meshwork involvement), iridocyclectomy (ciliary body involvement), or iridocyclochorioretinectomy (ciliary body and anterior pars plana involvement) may be necessary if the tumor has extended beyond the boundaries of the iris proper. Enucleation is indicated on rare occasions for extensive melanomas of the iris. The prognosis for both vision and survival is excellent. Vision is usually preserved unless secondary complications occur, and death from metastases is rare.

Posterior Uveal Melanomas

Posterior uveal melanomas (melanomas of the choroid and ciliary body), like iris melanomas, are thought to arise from uveal melanocytes. The basis for the malignant transformation is not known. Environmental factors as well as areas of increased choroidal pigmentation and existing nevi are thought to be predisposing factors. Three specific conditions appear to be associated with the higher incidence of melanomas: ocular melanocytosis, oculodermal melanocytosis, and neurofibromatosis. Posterior uveal melanomas differ from iris melanomas in that they are composed of more malignant cell types, carry a worse prognosis, and produce more profound visual disturbances. Posterior uveal melanomas occur in older white individuals of both sexes (average age, 50 years), are extremely rare in blacks, and are usually unilateral.

The symptomatology of posterior uveal melanomas depends on the location and size of the tumor. Anteriorly located tumors, especially those arising from the ciliary body or anterior choroid, may be asymptomatic and found on routine examinations. Eventually, the growth of these tumors produces shallowing of the anterior chamber, dislocation of the lens, and cataract formation. Pigmented episcleral nodules and dilated episcleral vessels may be the initial manifestation of the tumor. More posteriorly located lesions may produce increasing hyperopia and metamorphopsia secondary to associated serous detachment of the retina. Other symptoms include scotomas, floaters, photopsias, and ocular pain.

Indirect ophthalmoscopy is the most important diagnostic test for choroidal melanomas. Ophthalmoscopy of a typical tumor reveals an elevated globular mass protruding into the vitreous cavity. Occasionally, the tumor may be flat and diffuse, and such tumors carry a poorer prognosis. There may be an associated serous detachment of the retina or the retina may show cystic changes overlying the tumor. If the tumor has broken through Bruch's membrane, then it may have a characteristic "mushroom" or "collar-button" shape. The color of the tumor is not of great prognostic importance; however, the presence of pigment in the tumor aids in the diagnosis. Many, however, are amelanotic. The retinal pigment epithelium overlying the tumor may be degenerated or totally absent. An orange to golden brown pigment may be seen overlying the tumor. This orange coloration is due to the presence of macrophages that are filled with lipofuscin and melanin granules released from damaged pigment epithelial cells. Retinal pigment epithelial changes can be better evaluated by fluorescein angiography. Angiography is also helpful in demonstrating the presence or absence of large blood vessels within the tumor. This finding is important in that blood vessels are more frequently seen in malignant melanomas than in nevi.

A number of ocular lesions clinically simulate malignant melanomas of the posterior uvea, including suspicious choroidal nevi, hemorrhagic disciform degenerations, choroidal hemangiomas, melanocytomas of the optic nerve, metastatic carcinomas, and choroidal osteomas.

Once the diagnosis of melanoma is made, then the size and thickness of the tumor should be accurately determined by both ophthalmoscopy and ultrasonography, since these two parameters are very important prognostic indicators. Lesions less then 5 mm in diameter and 2 mm thick are most likely benign. Tumors with diameters of 5 to 10 mm and thicknesses of 2 to 3 mm are considered small tumors, those with diameters of 10 to 15 mm and thicknesses of 3 to 5 mm are considered medium-sized tumors, and those with diameters larger than 15 mm and thicknesses above 5 mm are considered large tumors. Another important prognostic sign that cannot be determined clinically is the histologic type of the tumor. Tumors are histologically classified as spindle A, spindle B, epithelioid, mixed, and necrotic. The spindle A and B types carry a better prognosis than the mixed or necrotic types; the epithelial cell tumors carry the worst prognosis.

Advanced tumors frequently cause opaque media as a result of corneal edema, hyphema, cataract, and vitreous hemorrhage. Any patient with unexplained unilateral opaque media should be suspected of having a uveal melanoma until proven otherwise. Here, ultrasonography is of paramount importance in making the diagnosis.

Metastatic disease from posterior malignant melanomas may occur with extrascleral extension into the orbit, whereas distant metastases occur hematogenously. The liver and the lung are the most common sites of distant metastases from posterior malignant melanomas.

Once the diagnosis of malignant melanoma is made and its dimensions are determined and documented photographically, then a decision must be made as to the best way of managing the tumor. Management of malignant melanomas of the posterior uvea remains a very controversial subject, with different authorities advocating different treatment modalities.

The historic and traditional treatment of malignant melanoma of the posterior uvea has been enucleation of the tumor-containing eye. In 1979, this modality of treatment was challenged by Zimmerman and McLean [11], who hypothesized that enucleating an eye with choroidal malignant melanoma may produce metastatic disease. At present, alternative methods of management are being used more often. These include periodic observations with photography (usually of small lesions), photocoagulation, radiotherapy, and local resection, especially in eyes with useful and salvageable vision. Enucleation is still the treatment of choice for large tumors and for eyes in which there is no hope for useful vision. When there is definite evidence of extraocular extension into the orbit, exenteration is the accepted treatment.

1. Char, D.H., Castro, J.R. Helium ion therapy for choroidal melanoma. *Arch. Ophthalmol.* 100:935–938, 1982.
   Forty patients were treated with helium ion therapy.
2. Ferry, A.P. Lesions mistaken for malignant melanoma of the iris. *Arch. Ophthalmol.* 74:9–18, 1965.
   Ferry investigates the incidence of incorrect clinical diagnosis of malignant melanoma of the iris in eyes submitted to the Armed Forces Institute of Pathology.
3. Gass, J.D.M. Comparison of prognosis after enucleation vs cobalt 60 irradiation of melanomas. *Arch. Ophthalmol.* 103:916–923, 1985.
   The probability of dying of metastatic melanoma within 5 years after cobalt 60 therapy was 50 percent, compared with 16 percent after enucleation. This study was not randomized and had a small number of patients.
4. Gass, J.D. Comparison of uveal melanoma growth rates with miotic index and mortality. *Arch. Ophthalmol.* 103:924–931, 1985.
   Widely varied growth rates were documented in different melanomas, which argues against the theory that melanomas have a relatively uniform slow growth rate before enucleation.
5. Gonder, J.R., Shields, J.A., Albert, D.A., et al. Uveal malignant melanoma associated with ocular and oculodermal melanocytosis. *Ophthalmology* 89:953–960, 1982.
   This study shows that white persons with ocular or oculodermal melanocytosis have a higher incidence of uveal malignant melanoma than white persons without these conditions.
6. Gragoudas, E.S., Seddon, J., Goitein, M., et al. Current results of proton beam irradiation of uveal melanomas. *Ophthalmology* 92:284–291, 1985.
   241 uveal melanomas have been treated with proton beam irradiation.
7. Manschot, W.A., van Peperzeel, H.A. Choroidal melanoma—enucleation or observation? A new approach. *Arch. Ophthalmol.* 98:71–77, 1980.
   The authors are proponents of early enucleation of all choroidal melanomas, and they argue against those who prefer to observe small melanomas.
8. Peyman, G.A., Raichand, M. Full thickness eye wall resection of choroidal neoplasms. *Ophthalmology* 86:1024–1036, 1979.

The technique of full-thickness eye wall resection and the results of treatment of 19 eyes with choroidal neoplasms are described.

9. Shields, J.A., Augsburger, J.A., Brown, G.C., et al. The differential diagnosis of posterior uveal melanomas. *Ophthalmology* 87:518–522, 1980.

This article summarizes the findings in 400 patients who were referred to the oncology center at Wills Eye Hospital with the initial diagnosis of malignant melanoma but who were found to have lesions simulating malignant melanoma.

10. Shields, J.A., Augsberger, J.J., Grady, L.W., et al. Cobalt plaque therapy of posterior uveal melanomas. *Ophthalmology* 89:1201–1207, 1982.

Cobalt plaque therapy was used on 100 patients with choroidal melanomas, and a 1- to 5-year follow-up on these patients is given. Tumor regression was noted in 96 percent of patients.

11. Zimmerman, L.E., McLean, I.W. An evaluation of enucleation in the management of uveal melanomas. *Am. J. Ophthalmol.* 87:741–760, 1979.

The authors hypothesize that enucleation for uveal melanomas may promote metastatic disease.

IX. OPTIC NERVE

John W. Gittinger, Jr.

51. PSEUDOTUMOR CEREBRI

Increased intracranial pressure in the absence of a mass lesion or mechanical obstruction of cerebrospinal fluid flow is called *pseudotumor cerebri*. The alternative descriptions *idiopathic intracranial hypertension* and *benign intracranial hypertension* are inappropriate because an etiology can sometimes be defined and because pseudotumor cerebri does in some cases lead to blindness. In older literature, the form of pseudotumor cerebri caused by thrombosis of the lateral sinus following middle ear infection with mastoiditis was called *otitic hydrocephalus*. Of course, pseudotumor cerebri has no relationship to inflammatory pseudotumor of the orbit (see Chap. 8).

Pathogenesis
The majority of cases of pseudotumor cerebri are indeed idiopathic, although in all series there is a preponderance of young, obese women. This has led to the implication of abnormalities of endocrine function, especially elevation of estrones, in pathogenesis. Detailed evaluations with available testing techniques have so far failed to identify a consistent endocrine abnormality [19]. The relationship of menarche and pregnancy to pseudotumor cerebri has also been called into question, since the prevalence of pregnancy in young women is so high [8]. There are, however, instances in which pseudotumor had its onset with pregnancy and resolved with miscarriage, and in fact the major risk of pseudotumor cerebri in pregnancy may be to the fetus [1].

The major definable cause of pseudotumor cerebri is reduction in venous outflow from the head. In many people, the right-sided venous outflow predominates, and only a unilateral or partial obstruction is necessary to raise the intracranial pressure. In addition to mastoiditis, surgery (e.g., radical neck dissection), small tumors impinging on the sinuses [15], and various conditions causing thrombosis of the sinuses or jugular vein [5, 9] may cause a pseudotumor syndrome.

A variety of other associations have been proposed. Using relatively strict criteria, Ahlskog and O'Neill [1] identified corticosteroid therapy and its withdrawal, hypoparathyroidism, hyper- and hypovitaminosis A, anemia, nitrofurantoin and tetracycline administration, and kepone poisoning as associated with pseudotumor cerebri. When one considers the wide usage of corticosteroids and tetracycline, pseudotumor cerebri must be a rare complication of these therapies.

In some malnourished children, pseudotumor cerebri develops upon refeeding [7]. Additionally, the central venous line used in total parenteral nutrition may serve as a focus for thrombophlebitis and venous outflow obstruction.

Diagnosis
The clinical diagnosis of pseudotumor cerebri is based on the presence of papilledema (although increased intracranial pressure has been confirmed by continuous monitoring even in the absence of papilledema), neuroradiologic studies that exclude intracranial mass lesions or hydrocephalus, a normal neurologic examination except for the manifestations of increased intracranial pressure, and normal cerebrospinal fluid except for elevated pressure. The presentations of pseudotumor cerebri are headache, diplopia, and blurred vision. A few cases are discovered incidentally by ophthalmoscopy.

Computed tomography has become the neuroradiologic study most often used to diagnose pseudotumor cerebri. The lateral and third ventricles are either normal or small ("slit" or difficult to visualize). Optic nerve enlargement is probably just a manifestation of the increased intracranial pressure, and a prominent cisterna magna and empty sella are encountered [22]. Angiography may be necessary to identify those cases in which there is venous sinus or jugular obstruction. Digital subtraction venous angiography, which can be performed as an outpatient study, is particularly suitable [9].

The major neurologic complication of pseudotumor cerebri is blindness as the result of secondary optic nerve atrophy. A few instances of acute vascular occlusions causing visual loss have also been reported [3], and chronic papilledema occasionally stimulates juxtapapillary subretinal neovascularization [6]. Manual visual field tests performed on the Goldmann perimeter probably remain the best way of following visual status [21], although other techniques such as contrast sensitivity may have a place [20]. Increased intracranial pressure also produces sixth nerve palsies with resulting horizontal diplopia. Instances of vertical deviations with diplopia are also encountered [2], but the mechanism of this is unclear.

The differential diagnosis of increased intracranial pressure with a normal computed tomogram and normal cerebrospinal fluid includes so-called gliomatosis cerebri, in which a neoplastic process is so diffuse that identification is difficult, and atypical or early encephalitides in which the spinal fluid is normal [16]. Small tumors compressing the dural sinuses are not easy to visualize on computed tomography.

Treatment

Pseudotumor cerebri has been considered a self-limited process. In those patients in whom visual loss does not ensue and in whom headaches are not disabling, observation alone may be appropriate, assuming the diagnosis is firmly established. There is increasing evidence, however, that many cases of pseudotumor cerebri are chronic and that the proportion of patients who eventually lose vision is significant [14, 17].

One time-honored therapy is repeated lumbar punctures. Studies of cerebrospinal fluid dynamics indicate that the pressure-lowering effect of a lumbar puncture is transient, perhaps lasting only a few hours. On the other hand, as many as one-quarter of patients have spontaneous remissions of their pseudotumor cerebri after an initial lumbar puncture. Thus, it seems reasonable to consider repeating the diagnostic lumbar puncture after 48 hours or more to be sure that the elevation in pressure persists before contemplating more vigorous therapy, especially since the ophthalmoscopic findings of papilledema persist for long periods even after intracranial pressure is normalized.

The next level of treatment is medical: diuretics and systemic steroids. Dramatic responses to short courses of oral corticosteroids have been reported; however, prolonged administration is contraindicated. If there are any precipitating factors identified, these should be removed if possible. Simple weight loss may ameliorate pseudotumor cerebri, but this may be surprisingly difficult to accomplish.

If progressive visual loss is recognized, surgical intervention must be considered. The most common surgical procedure now used is a lumboperitoneal shunt, since the small ventricles make ventriculoperitoneal shunting technically difficult. Optic nerve decompressions have also been performed in a few cases [11]; the protection of vision is probably the result of scarring of the optic nerve sheath. Subtemporal decompressions have fallen out of favor because of serious complications such as seizures, and surgical procedures to produce weight loss have not been widely performed [13].

1. Ahlskog, J.E., O'Neill, B.P. Pseudotumor cerebri. A review. *Ann. Intern. Med.* 97:249–256, 1982.
   A careful review with 83 references.
2. Baker, R.S., Buncic, J.R. Vertical ocular motility disturbance in pseudotumor cerebri. *J. Clin. Neuro-ophthalmol.* 5:41–44, 1985.
   Three patients with both sixth nerve palsies and vertical deviations are described. See also Smith's editorial in the same issue (pp. 55–56).
3. Baker, R.S., Buncic, J.R. Sudden visual loss in pseudotumor cerebri due to central retinal artery occlusion. *Arch. Neurol.* 41:1274–1276, 1984.
   Pseudotumor cerebri caused by sinus thrombosis in a 16-year-old boy was complicated by deep vein thrombosis in the legs, a retinal vascular occlusion, and neovascularization.
4. Baker, R.S., Carter, D., Hendrick, E.B., et al. Visual loss in pseudotumor cerebri of childhood: A follow-up study. *Arch. Ophthalmol.* 103:1681–1686, 1985.
   Contrary to previous reports, children are at risk for visual loss from the chronic papilledema of pseudotumor cerebri.
5. Byrne, J.V., Lawton, C.A. Meningeal sarcoidosis causing intracranial hypertension secondary to dural sinus thrombosis. *Br. J. Radiol.* 56:755–757, 1983.
   Neurosarcoidosis as the cause of a pseudotumor syndrome.

6. Copetto, J.R., Monteiro, M.L.R. Juxtapapillary subretinal hemorrhages in pseudotumor cerebri. *J. Clin. Neuro-ophthalmol.* 5:45–53, 1985.
   Two more cases of subretinal neovascularization from chronic papilledema.
7. Couch, R., Camfield, P.R., Tibbles, J.A.R. The changing picture of pseudotumor cerebri in children. *Can. J. Neurol. Sci.* 12:48–50, 1985.
   The commonest cause of childhood pseudotumor cerebri in this Canadian series was refeeding following nutritional deprivation early in life.
8. Digre, K.B., Varner, M.W., Corbett, J.J. Pseudotumor cerebri and pregnancy. *Neurology* 34:721–729, 1984.
   A study with age-matched controls indicates that pseudotumor occurs no more frequently in pregnancy than would be expected by chance and offers a number of recommendations concerning management.
9. Harper, C.M., O'Neill, B.P., O'Duffy, J.D., et al. Intracranial hypertension in Behçet's disease: Demonstration of sinus occlusion with use of digital subtraction angiography. *Mayo Clin. Proc.* 60:419–422, 1985.
   Intracranial hypertension in Behçet's disease is caused by thrombosis of the intracranial dural venous sinuses. Venous digital subtraction angiography is the procedure of choice to demonstrate this.
10. Hoffmann, H.J. How is pseudotumor cerebri diagnosed? *Arch. Neurol.* 43:167–168, 1986.
    The first of three editorials in the same issue that offer different perspectives.
11. Knight, R.S.G., Fielder, A.R., Firth, J.L. Benign intracranial hypertension: Visual loss and optic nerve sheath fenestration. *J. Neurol. Neurosurg. Psychiatry* 49:243–250, 1986.
    Five cases in which optic nerve fenestration protected vision in patients with pseudotumor cerebri.
12. Lessell, S., Rosman, N.P. Permanent visual impairment in childhood pseudotumor cerebri. *Arch. Neurol.* 43:801–804, 1986.
    Further evidence that the visual system of children is not spared the ravages of chronic papilledema.
13. Noggle, J.D., Rodning, C.B. Rapidly advancing pseudotumor cerebri associated with morbid obesity: An indication for gastric exclusion. *So. Med. J.* 79:761–763, 1986.
    A surgical partitioning of the stomach produced weight loss and resolution of papilledema. When the gastric staple line gave way 3 years later, the patient gained weight and papilledema recurred.
14. Orcutt, J.C., Page, N.G.R., Sanders, M.D. Factors affecting visual loss in benign intracranial hypertension. *Ophthalmology* 91:1303–1312, 1984.
    In this series, 49 percent of patients had some visual loss; in 6 percent it was severe. Various factors are considered: the patient at highest risk is over 40 years old, highly myopic, and has atrophic or high-grade papilledema.
15. Powers, J.M., Schnur, J.A., Baldree, M.E. Pseudotumor cerebri due to partial obstruction of the sigmoid sinus by a cholesteatoma. *Arch. Neurol.* 43:519–521, 1986.
    A small tumor compressing the left sigmoid sinus was not initially detected by computed tomography.
16. Raucher, H.S., Kaufman, D.M., Goldfarb, J., et al. Pseudotumor cerebri and Lyme disease: A new association. *J. Pediatr.* 107:931–933, 1985.
    Two children who fulfilled the diagnostic criteria for pseudotumor cerebri may have had a cerebrospinal fluid-negative encephalitis.
17. Repka, M.X., Miller, N.R., Savino, P.J. Pseudotumor cerebri. *Am. J. Ophthalmol.* 98:741–746, 1984.
    Two women in whom lumboperitoneal shunts were removed years after they were placed and in whom pseudotumor recurred, supporting the proposition that this is not necessarily a self-limited disease.
18. Rush, J.A. Pseudotumor cerebri: Clinical profile and visual outcome in 63 patients. *Mayo Clin. Proc.* 55:541–546, 1980.
    Rush offers his characteristically thorough and even-handed analysis of the Mayo Clinic experience between 1961 and 1978.
19. Sørensen, P.S., Gjerris, F., Svenstrup, B. Endocrine studies in patients with pseu-

dotumor cerebri: Estrogen levels in blood and cerebrospinal fluid. *Arch. Neurol.* 43:902–906, 1986.
      No distinctive endocrinologic abnormality was identified.
20. Wall, M. Contrast sensitivity in pseudotumor cerebri. *Ophthalmology* 93:4–7, 1986.
      In this series, contrast sensitivity testing with Arden gratings was useful in following visual status.
21. Wall, M., George, D. Visual loss in pseudotumor cerebri: Incidence and defects related to visual field strategy. *Arch. Neurol.* 44:170–175, 1987.
      Manual perimetry on a Goldmann perimeter with an Armaly-Drance strategy is recommended over automated perimetry in the follow-up of patients with pseudotumor cerebri.
22. Weisberg, L.A. Computed tomography in benign intracranial hypertension. *Neurology* 35:1075–1078, 1985.
      Acceptable abnormalities include small ventricles, a prominent cisterna magna, an empty sella, and enlarged optic nerves.

52. ISCHEMIC OPTIC NEUROPATHY

The relationship between the two types of optic nerve infarction, *anterior ischemic optic neuropathy* and *posterior ischemic optic neuropathy,* is analogous to that between papillitis and retrobulbar optic neuritis. Unilateral disk swelling with visual loss in a young person usually represents papillitis, the anterior form of optic neuritis. A similar picture in an older individual is recognized as anterior ischemic optic neuropathy. Visual loss without disk swelling is characteristic of both retrobulbar optic neuritis and posterior ischemic optic neuropathy.

The differential diagnosis between retrobulbar optic neuritis and posterior ischemic optic neuropathy is at once more difficult to define and less often a clinical problem. Although hundreds of cases of anterior ischemic optic neuropathy have been collected and reported, posterior ischemic optic neuropathy is seldom recognized.

The distinction between an inflammatory and an ischemic process has clinical importance, as both the prognosis and the underlying disorder differ. The vision in an eye with papillitis or retrobulbar optic neuritis usually improves; that in an eye with ischemic optic neuropathy usually does not. While the majority of cases of both ischemic optic neuropathy and optic neuritis are idiopathic, ischemic optic neuropathy has a significant association in the elderly with a generalized arteritis (so-called giant-cell or temporal arteritis), and optic neuritis is a frequent manifestation of multiple sclerosis.

Pathogenesis

Even with nonarteritic anterior ischemic optic neuropathy, the fellow eye is at increased risk for the subsequent development of anterior ischemic optic neuropathy [13]. Several studies point to disk structural features as predispositions to anterior ischemic optic neuropathy [1, 4, 5]. The cup-disk ratio in the fellow eye of patients with anterior ischemic optic neuropathy is reduced in comparison to the ratio in normal eyes, suggesting that the disks that develop anterior ischemic optic neuropathy are anomalous. Also, optic disk drusen—which are known to be a feature of anomalous disks—and anterior ischemic optic neuropathy may affect the same eye [6].

The vascular supply of the anterior optic nerve is complex, and despite considerable attention to the problem, the actual vessel whose occlusion produces anterior ischemic optic neuropathy remains unknown. The leading candidates for this role are the posterior ciliary arteries, but the vascular territory supplied by these vessels is segmented vertically, whereas disk infarction tends to segment horizontally.

Diagnosis

The first task of the physician confronted with a patient who has unilateral disk swelling and visual loss is to diagnose and treat any associated disease. The most important association of anterior ischemic optic neuropathy is with giant-cell arteritis, an autoimmune vasculitis of the elderly with inflammation centered in the elastica of middle-sized arteries. Other signs of ocular ischemia may be present: retinal infarction, choroidal infarction, and ischemic myopathy with ophthalmoplegia. Most patients also have systemic symptoms: malaise, headache, weight loss, and the virtually pathognomonic complaint of pain on chewing, called *jaw claudication*. Marked elevation of the erythrocyte sedimentation rate is characteristic, and the diagnosis is confirmed pathologically by temporal artery biopsy.

Rarely, ischemic optic neuropathy is encountered in the course of other vasculitides such as polyarteritis nodosa. There is a loose association between nonarteritic ischemic optic neuropathy and diabetes and hypertension. When the diagnosis of anterior ischemic optic neuropathy is made in young persons on the basis of disk swelling followed by a permanent, characteristic field defect, a history of migraine is often elicited [11, 12]. Ischemic optic neuropathy has also been reported after cataract extraction [16], nonocular surgery [10], blood loss (see Chap. 20), and trauma. Eyes subjected to therapeutic radiation may develop both a retinopathy and an ischemic optic neuropathy [3].

The relationship between anterior ischemic optic neuropathy and carotid disease is uncertain. Anterior ischemic optic neuropathy is one possible feature of the ischemic eye sometimes produced by carotid occlusion [2]. Carotid embolic disease only rarely precipitates ischemic optic neuropathy [17], and there is no demonstrated increase in the incidence of carotid disease in persons with ischemic optic neuropathy. On the other hand, the combination of hypertension and ischemic optic neuropathy increases the risk of stroke and myocardial infarction [7]. This observation has led to the suggestion that these patients should be evaluated for preventable causes of stroke, including carotid artery disease. There is, however, no clear evidence that the strokes that these hypertensive patients have are carotid in origin, and the question of effective surgical prophylaxis for carotid strokes remains open even if this relationship is accepted.

Treatment

When giant-cell arteritis is suspected, immediate administration of systemic corticosteroids is warranted, pending obtaining and interpreting a temporal artery biopsy. Even in arteritic anterior ischemic optic neuropathy, the administration of corticosteroids does not ordinarily result in recovery of vision, but may protect the fellow eye and other organs from infarction. Steroid administration in nonarteritic ischemic optic neuropathy is controversial. Hayreh [8] believes that early treatment with systemic corticosteroids improves visual prognosis, but this has not been confirmed by controlled studies. Most physicians have had little success with steroid treatment of nonarteritic ischemic optic neuropathy.

In the majority of patients with nonarteritic anterior ischemic optic neuropathy, in whom no treatable element has been identified, an extensive evaluation is probably not warranted. Fortunately, many eyes with ischemic optic neuropathy retain useful vision, and recurrent anterior ischemic optic neuropathy in the same eye is uncommon. The patient, however, has lost some vision in one eye and is at risk to lose vision in the other. This is an unsatisfactory situation for both patient and doctor and demands considerable skill on the part of the physician in explaining the problem and providing support for the patient.

1. Beck, R.W., Savino, P.J., Repka, M.X., et al. Optic disc structure in anterior ischemic optic neuropathy. *Ophthalmology* 91:1334–1337, 1984.
   The physiologic cup was lacking in a high percentage of eyes of patients with anterior ischemic optic neuropathy.
2. Brown, G.C. Anterior ischemic optic neuropathy occurring in association with carotid artery obstruction. *J. Clin. Neuro-ophthalmol.* 6:39–42, 1986.

This case report suggests the premise that evaluation of the carotid circulation in a patient with anterior ischemic optic neuropathy is warranted when there are other ischemic signs.

3. Brown, G.C., Shields, J.A., Sanborn, G., et al. Radiation optic neuropathy. *Ophthalmology* 89:1489–1493, 1982.
   The development of 14 cases of ischemic optic neuropathy after radiation is documented. Diabetics developed the optic neuropathy with smaller doses, probably because their vessels are more sensitive to radiation-induced damage.

4. Doro, S., Lessell, S. Cup-disc ratio and ischemic optic neuropathy. *Arch. Ophthalmol.* 102:1143–1144, 1985.
   The fellow eyes of patients with optic neuritis and with ischemic optic neuropathy were compared. The cup–disk ratio was smaller in the patients with ischemic optic neuropathy.

5. Feit, R.H., Tomsak, R.L., Ellenberger, C. Jr. Structural factors in the pathogenesis of ischemic optic neuropathy. *Am. J. Ophthalmol.* 98:105–108, 1984.
   The cup–disk ratio in the unaffected eye of patients with anterior ischemic optic neuropathy is significantly smaller than that in age-matched controls.

6. Gittinger, J.W. Jr., Lessell, S., Bondar, R.A. Ischemic optic neuropathy associated with optic disc drusen. *J. Clin. Neuro-ophthalmol.* 4:79–84, 1984.
   Four patients with optic disk drusen developed anterior ischemic optic neuropathy.

7. Guyer, D.R., Miller, N.R., Auer, C.L., et al. The risk of cerebrovascular and cardiovascular disease in patients with anterior ischemic optic neuropathy. *Arch. Ophthalmol.* 103:1136–1142, 1985.
   Review of the records of 217 patients revealed a significantly increased risk of strokes and myocardial infarcts in hypertensives with ischemic optic neuropathy over a control group. Subsequent correspondence challenged the interpretation of these observations (Arch. Ophthalmol. 103:1633–1634, 1985).

8. Hayreh, S.S. Ischemic optic neuropathy. *Int. Ophthalmol.* 1:9–18, 1978.
   Hayreh presents a brief summary of his understanding of this entity.

9. Hayreh, S.S. Anterior ischemic optic neuropathy. V. Optic disc edema an early sign. *Arch. Ophthalmol.* 99:1030–1040, 1981.
   One of a long series of contributions, identifying eyes in which the disk swelling preceded the visual loss.

10. Jaben, S.L., Glaser, J.S., Daily, M. Ischemic optic neuropathy following general surgical procedures. *J. Clin. Neuro-ophthalmol.* 3:239–244, 1983.
    Three cases of atypical anterior ischemic optic neuropathy followed uncomplicated general surgery. One patient had improvement of vision following transfusion.

11. Katz, B., Bamford, C.R. Migrainous ischemic optic neuropathy. *Neurology* 35:112–114, 1985.
    Ischemic optic neuropathy developed in a 38-year-old woman with migraine.

12. O'Hara, M., O'Connor, P.S. Migrainous optic neuropathy. *J. Clin. Neuro-ophthalmol.* 4:85–90, 1984.
    Two more instances of ischemic optic neuropathy in migraineurs, with a tabulation of previously reported cases.

13. Repka, M.X., Savino, P.J., Schatz, N.J., et al. Clinical profile and long-term implications of anterior ischemic optic neuropathy. *Am. J. Ophthalmol.* 96:478–483, 1983.
    Twenty of 83 patients with nonarteritic anterior ischemic optic neuropathy developed contralateral ocular involvement during follow-up. Diabetes and hypertension were significantly increased only in patients between 45 and 64 years of age.

14. Shimo-oku, M., Miyazaki, S. Acute anterior and posterior ischemic optic neuropathy. *Jpn. J. Ophthalmol.* 28:159–170, 1984.
    These Japanese clinicians report an experience quite different from that of American workers.

15. Shults, W.T. Ischemic optic neuropathy: Still the ophthalmologist's dilemma. *Ophthalmology* 91:1338–1341, 1984.
    A series of questions are addressed by a panel of experts.

16. Spedick, M.J., Tomsak, R.L. Ischemic optic neuropathy following secondary intraocular lens implantation. *J. Clin. Neuro-ophthalmol.* 4:255–257, 1984.
    A case report occasions a review of this association.

17. Tomsak, R.L. Ischemic optic neuropathy associated with retinal embolism. *Am. J. Ophthalmol.* 99:590–592, 1985.

Three cases of ischemic optic neuropathy developed in patients who also had evidence of retinal emboli following coronary artery bypass surgery or cardiac catheterization, suggesting that embolic occlusion of small disk vessels is causative in some instances.

18. Toshniwal, P. Anterior ischaemic optic neuropathy secondary to cluster headache. *Acta Neurol. Scand.* 73:213–218, 1986.

Ischemic optic neuropathy and a cluster had their onset on the same day in a 42-year-old man.

53. LEBER'S OPTIC ATROPHY

Leber's optic atrophy, also called *Leber's optic neuropathy, Leber's hereditary optic neuroretinopathy,* or simply *Leber's disease,* must be distinguished from the several other ocular syndromes named after Theodor Leber. The most frequent nosologic confusion is with *Leber's congenital amaurosis,* a congenital retinal pigmentary degeneration that presents as visual loss in infancy. Leber's optic atrophy must also be separated from various other types of hereditofamilial and degenerative optic atrophy.

Pathogenesis

The inheritance of Leber's optic atrophy may be through the genes encoded in mitochondrial DNA [2]. There is no well-documented instance of transmission from a male to his offspring. Females, on the other hand, have an almost 100 percent carrier rate; about half the sons of carriers develop the disease [6]. (As with sex-linked recessive disorders, the most important relatives to inquire about are the maternal uncles.) This non-Mendelian matrilineal inheritance suggests transmission via a cytoplasmic factor, since cytoplasm is present in ova but not spermatozoa, and mitochondrial DNA is the leading candidate.

Thiosulfate sulfur transferase—a mitochondrial enzyme also known as rhodanese—was decreased in the livers of patients with Leber's optic atrophy [1]. In another study its activity in red cells was normal [14]. The role of zinc deficiency is uncertain [14]. Other neurologic disorders are occasionally associated with Leber's optic atrophy, and in at least one of them—a familial dystonia, perhaps a variant of infantile bilateral striatal necrosis—a mitochondrial disorder is postulated [11].

Leber's optic atrophy—like tobacco amblyopia, with which it shares some clinical similarities—has also sometimes been considered a disorder of cyanide metabolism [14]. The package insert for the conventional form of vitamin B_{12}, cyanocobalamin, actually mentions Leber's optic atrophy as a possible contraindication since cyanocobalamin contains the cyanide radical. Conversely, hydroxocobalamin, a vitamin B_{12} cogener that lacks a cyanide radical, is thought to bind free cyanide. There is, however, no biochemical evidence linking elevated plasma cyanide levels to the onset of Leber's optic atrophy.

Diagnosis

The clinical syndrome called Leber's optic atrophy is usually distinct, with occasional variants that are difficult to classify. Acute or subacute visual loss develops simultaneously or sequentially, usually with the second eye involved within a few months of the first. Central acuity is reduced, with development of a centrocecal scotoma to visual field testing. Males around the age of 20 years are the largest group affected in most series. Women make up only about 20 percent of cases and tend to develop the disease between the ages of 30 and 50 years.

Clinically, the early stages of Leber's optic atrophy are unique. Unaffected family members sometimes have circumpapillary telangiectasia and tortuosity of larger retinal vessels [5]. Increased arteriovenous shunting at the capillary level just before the onset of visual loss has been demonstrated by fluorescein angiography in a few cases in which this study has been performed [9]. During the period of acute visual loss, the disk hyperemia and the swelling and glistening opacification of peripapillary nerve fibers produce an appearance characterized as "pseudoedema," since angiographically, there is no leakage of dye. Retinal hemorrhages are occasionally seen at this stage.

Subsequently, the pseudoedema resolves with evolution of optic atrophy. The large-vessel tortuosity persists, but the microangiopathy is no longer apparent. Visual acuity at this point is often 20/400 or worse, but varies over a wide range. After a year or two, in a small minority of patients, visual acuity returns spontaneously to near normal levels [3]. The pathophysiologic basis for this remarkable improvement is not known.

Treatment

There is no compelling evidence that any treatment improves the prognosis for vision in Leber's optic atrophy. Systemic steroids have no demonstrated long-term effect. Because of the question of a relationship with cyanide metabolism, high doses of parenteral hydroxocobalamin have been administered. Cystine, a sulfur-containing amino acid, has also been given orally to encourage conjugation of exogenous cyanide with sulfur, forming nontoxic thiocyanate [14]. There are no controlled series demonstrating favorable responses to these regimens. In still another unproven therapy, Japanese surgeons performed craniotomies to lyse arachnoidal adhesions, with subsequent visual improvement.

A major problem in evaluating any treatment of Leber's optic atrophy is those patients in whom vision recovers without any intervention. Unless new evidence is produced, the clinician would be well advised to let the disease run its natural course.

1. Cagianut, B., Rhyner, K., Furrer, W., et al. Thiosulfate-sulphur tranferase (Rhodanase) deficiency in Leber's hereditary optic atrophy. *Lancet* 2:981–982, 1981.
   The activity of the liver enzyme thiosulfate sulfur transferase was reduced in two patients with Leber's optic neuropathy, supporting the suggestion of a defect in cyanide detoxification.
2. Egger, J., Wilson, J. Mitochondrial inheritance in a mitochondrially mediated disease. *N. Engl. J. Med.* 309:142–146, 1983.
   Reviews the evidence for mitochondrial inheritance.
3. Lessell, S., Gise, R.L., Krohel, G.G. Bilateral optic neuropathy in young men: Variation on a theme by Leber? *Arch. Neurol.* 40:2–6, 1983.
   Five young men with optic neuropathy had delayed spontaneous improvement. The authors suggest that the absence of the typical vascular findings is related to the capacity to recover.
4. Lopez, P.F., Smith, J.L. Leber's optic neuropathy: New observations. *J. Clin. Neuro-ophthalmol.* 6:144–152, 1986.
   The probands did not have telangiectatic microangiopathy, but another family member did. These families are thought to manifest "atypical Leber's disease."
5. McCluskey, D.J., O'Connor, P.S., Sheehy, J.T. Leber's optic neuropathy and Charcot-Marie-Tooth disease: Report of a case. *J. Clin. Neuro-ophthalmol.* 6:76–81, 1986.
   A profusely illustrated case report of this association.
6. Nikoskelainen, E. The clinical findings in Leber's hereditary optic neuroretinopathy: Leber's disease. *Trans. Ophthalmol. Soc. U.K.* 104:845–852, 1985.
   An updated clinical overview.
7. Nikoskelainen, E.K., Savontaus, M-L., Wanne, O.P., et al. Leber's hereditary optic neuroretinopathy, a maternally inherited disease: A genealogic study in four pedigrees. *Arch. Ophthalmol.* 105:665–671, 1987.
   Some family members with peripapillary microangiopathy remain asymptomatic. A cardiac preexcitation syndrome appears to be linked with Leber's.
8. Nikoskelainen, E., Hoyt, W.F., Nummelin, K. Ophthalmoscopic findings in Leber's hereditary optic neuropathy. I. Fundus findings in asymptomatic family members. *Arch. Ophthalmol.* 100:1597–1602, 1982.
9. Nikoskelainen, E., Hoyt, W.F., Nummelin, K. Ophthalmoscopic findings in Leber's

hereditary optic neuropathy. II. The fundus findings in the affected family members. *Arch. Ophthalmol.* 101:1059–1068, 1983.

10. Nikoskelainen, E., Hoyt, W.F., Nummelin, K., et al. Fundus findings in Leber's hereditary optic neuroretinopathy. III. Fluorescein angiographic studies. *Arch. Ophthalmol.* 102:981–989, 1984.
This series of papers documents the presence and progression of the vascular changes before and during visual loss and in unaffected family members.

11. Novotny, E.J., Singh, G., Wallace, D.C., et al. Leber's disease and dystonia: A mitochondrial disease. *Neurology* 36:1053–1060, 1986.
Clinical study and biochemical analysis of mitochondrial DNA in a family with both neurologic disease (dystonia) and Leber's optic atrophy.

12. Pagès, M., Pagès, A.-M. Leber's disease with spastic paraplegia and peripheral neuropathy: Case report with nerve biopsy study. *Eur. Neurol.* 22:181–185, 1983.
Another neurologic association.

13. Stehouwer, A., Went, L.N. Leber's optic neuropathy. I. Clinical studies. *Doc. Ophthalmol.* 53:97–111, 1982.
Subtle clinical abnormalities were present in many members of 16 families known to be at risk.

14. Stehouwer, A., Oosterhuis, J.A., Renger-Van Dijk, A.H., et al. Leber's optic neuropathy. II. Fluorescein angiographic studies. *Doc. Ophthalmol.* 53:113–122, 1982.
Angiographic studies of patients at risk and those in the acute phase regularly demonstrated microangiopathy.

15. Syme, I.G., Bronte-Stewart, J., Foulds, W.S., et al. Clinical and biochemical findings in Leber's hereditary optic atrophy. *Trans. Ophthalmol. Soc. U.K.* 103:556–559, 1983.
The major advocates of cystine-hydroxocobalamin treatment draw only tentative conclusions based on a series of 49 patients. Their biochemical studies are also described.

54. TRAUMATIC OPTIC NEUROPATHY

Visual loss following head trauma may result from injury almost anywhere in the visual system, from the eye to the occipital lobes. Unilateral visual loss in the absence of significant ocular injury points to *traumatic optic neuropathy*. Bitemporal hemianopsia results from disruption of decussating axons in the chiasmal bar. The combination of a blind eye and an eye with temporal hemianopsia indicates simultaneous chiasmal and optic nerve involvement.

Pathogenesis

The severity of the injury varies widely. Most but not all of these patients have suffered concussions, but traumatic optic neuropathy is reported after even minor head trauma. With major trauma, the presence of multiple injuries may delay recognition of optic nerve injury. The swinging flashlight test, to look for the presence of a relative afferent pupillary defect, allows screening for optic neuropathy even in unconscious patients.

The mechanism for optic nerve damage by blunt head trauma is uncertain. The nerve seems most vulnerable as it passes through the optic canal in the lesser wing of the sphenoid bone. This intracanalicular portion, about 10 mm long, may be compressed against bone by edema or hemorrhage. Since it is fixed by its dura to the surrounding bone, its vascular supply is subject to disruption by shearing force.

Fractures of the optic canal are often associated with optic neuropathy. These fractures may be part of a more extensive facial injury or may be an isolated finding. An analysis of the distribution of stress when pressure is applied to the frontal bones of the intact skull indicates a concentration of forces in the orbital apex, perhaps explaining the peculiar vulnerability of the optic canal. These fractures are most easily demonstrated radiographically by computed tomography [4, 10].

Rarely, a previously uninvolved optic nerve may be injured during attempts to reduce facial fractures. Surgical manipulation of facial fractures traversing the orbital apex (Le Fort III fractures) may lead to retrobulbar hemorrhage or increased intraorbital pressure, with visual loss. Many surgeons will not attempt acute repair of facial fractures involving the orbital apex in a one-eyed patient [14].

Treatment

A considerable literature debates the management of traumatic optic neuropathy. With the exception of some Japanese series [8], most surgeons have experienced little success when surgical decompression of the optic canal has been undertaken in patients in whom complete visual loss was present at the initial examination. The failure to improve with decompression implies that optic nerve infarction is the explanation for the visual loss.

On the other hand, when there is evidence of progressive visual loss, compression is the more likely mechanism. In these cases, surgical decompression has sometimes been followed by restoration of vision. As is so often the case, evaluation of the effects of treatment is made difficult by the possibility of spontaneous improvement.

Neurosurgical subfrontal decompression has been used and may still be indicated if there are other reasons for craniotomy, but a transantral-transethmoidal removal of the medial wall of the optic canal has the advantage of being extracranial and therefore less invasive [5, 7]. The surgical skills for this procedure lie within the repertoire of many otolaryngologists [12].

An alternative approach is medical management. Several recent reports have described visual improvement after administration of corticosteroids in both megadose and conventional regimens [1, 2, 11]. Japanese workers add mannitol, urokinase, and oral vitamin B_{12} supplements [8]. A controlled prospective study of the treatment of traumatic optic neuropathy has been proposed [6]. Until the results of such a study are available, there is no clear evidence to support any specific approach.

1. Anderson, R.L., Panje, W.R., Gross, C.E. Optic nerve blindness following blunt forehead trauma. *Ophthalmology* 89:445–455, 1982.
   In seven cases of unilateral blindness following head trauma, treatment with megadose steroids seemed as effective as decompression. The authors recommend decompression if there is delayed visual loss unresponsive to 12 hours of megadose steroids or if there is initial return of vision with subsequent deterioration while the patient is on steroids.
2. Fujitani, T., Inoue, K., Takahashi, T., et al. Indirect traumatic optic neuropathy—visual outcome of operative and nonoperative cases. *Jpn. J. Ophthalmol.* 30:125–134, 1986.
   These workers report excellent results with both surgical and medical management.
3. Gross, C.E., DeKock, J.R., Panje, W.R., et al. Evidence for orbital deformation that may contribute to monocular blindness following minor frontal head trauma. *J. Neurosurg.* 55:963–966, 1981.
   Holographic interferometry of dried human skulls demonstrates transmission of forces applied in the frontal supraorbital area to the orbital apex.
4. Guyon, J.J., Brant-Zawadzki, M., Seiff, S.R. CT demonstration of optic canal fractures. *Am. J. Roentgenol.* 143:1031–1034, 1984.
   Computed tomography demonstrated 14 separate fractures in 10 patients, all of whom had visual loss.
5. Kennerdell, J.S., Amsbaugh, G.A., Myers, E.N. Transantral-ethmoidal decompression of optic canal fracture. *Arch. Ophthalmol.* 94:1040–1043, 1976.
   Delayed visual loss after subconcussive head trauma responded to decompression.

6. Kline, L.B., Morawetz, R.B., Swaid, S.N. Indirect injury of the optic nerve. *Neurosurgery* 14:756–764, 1984.
   The most comprehensive recent review of the problem, with 55 references.

7. Krausen, A.S., Ogura, J.H., Burde, R.M., et al. Emergency orbital decompression: A reprieve from blindness. *Otolaryngol. Head Neck Surg.* 89:252–256, 1981.
   In two cases of delayed visual loss following trauma, orbital decompression with a transantral approach resulted in restoration of vision. Mention is made of two other patients in whom a penetrating orbital injury produced blindness not relieved by orbital decompression.

8. Matsuzaki, H., Kunita, M., Kawai, K. Optic nerve damage in head trauma: Clinical and experimental studies. *Jpn. J. Ophthalmol.* 26:447–461, 1982.
   These authors favor a conservative medical approach. The considerable Japanese literature on this subject is referenced.

9. Ramsay, J.H. Optic nerve injury in fracture of the canal. *Br. J. Ophthalmol.* 63:607–610, 1979.
   A woman died 4 days after losing vision in one eye from trauma. Pathologic examination revealed infarction of the intracanalicular nerve underlying a fracture and epidural hemorrhage.

10. Seiff, S.R., Berger, M.S., Guyon, J., et al. Computed tomographic evaluation of the optic canal in sudden traumatic blindness. *Am. J. Ophthalmol.* 98:751–755, 1984.
    Five of nine patients had optic canal fractures. Three experienced some improvement in vision with or without steroid treatment or decompression.

11. Shakad, A., Hadani, M., Feinsod, M. CT and VER follow-up of reversible visual loss with fracture of the optic canal. *Acta Neurochirurg.* 62:91–94, 1982.
    Vision improved, as documented by visual evoked responses, in a 4-year-old girl treated with systemic corticosteroids after a head injury.

12. Sofferman, R.A. Sphenoethmoid approach to the optic nerve. *Laryngoscope* 91:184–196, 1981.
    A detailed description of the surgical technique from the otolaryngology literature.

13. Spoor, T.C., Mathog, R.H. Restoration of vision after optic canal decompression. *Arch. Ophthalmol.* 104:804–806, 1986.
    An unusual case in which visual loss caused by an orbital stab wound was partially restored by transethmoid-sphenoidotomy after 5 days of steroid treatment.

14. Weymuller, E.A. Jr. Blindness and Le Fort III fractures. *Ann. Otol. Rhinol. Laryngol.* 93:2–5, 1984.
    Results of a questionnaire indicate that most experienced surgeons are conservative in their approach to facial fractures when vision has been lost in one eye.

55. OPTIC GLIOMAS

Histologically, gliomas of the anterior visual pathways are low-grade (pilocytic) astrocytomas. Since they are generally tumors of childhood, probably diagnosis in adults represents the discovery of a long-standing tumor. Such *optic gliomas*, also called *anterior visual pathway gliomas*, should be distinguished from the much rarer *malignant optic glioma of adulthood*, a high-grade astrocytoma of poor prognosis that presents with rapid visual loss from a progressive optic neuropathy.

Optic gliomas can be subdivided according to their location. Tumors whose major bulk is located in the orbital optic nerve are called *optic nerve gliomas*, whereas more posterior tumors are designated as *chiasmal gliomas*. This distinction is of more than academic interest, since presentation, prognosis, and perhaps appropriate therapy depend on primary site.

Pathogenesis

Optic gliomas may be associated with neurofibromatosis; bilateral optic nerve gliomas are virtually diagnostic of this entity. Conversely, a significant number of patients with neurofibromatosis are found to have asymptomatic optic gliomas when appropriately evaluated [11].

Diagnosis

Optic nerve gliomas usually present as unilateral visual loss or proptosis. In young children, the visual loss may cause strabismus or nystagmus. Optic nerve gliomas also produce disk swelling and, less often, optic atrophy; optic atrophy is characteristic of chiasmal gliomas. Chiasmal gliomas present as visual loss or with signs of involvement of adjacent neural structures: hypopituitarism, diencephalic wasting, precocious puberty, or hydrocephalus.

The detection of optic gliomas has been greatly advanced by modern imaging techniques such as computed tomography and magnetic resonance [6]. In some patients, the picture is so characteristic that further evaluation is unnecessary (e.g., a fusiform enlargement of the optic nerve in a patient with known neurofibromatosis). When other diagnostic possibilities exist, biopsy may be required to establish the diagnosis. As in other areas of management of optic gliomas, thoughtful physicians disagree as to the precise indications for biopsy. The visual evoked potential, which is affected early in optic gliomas, may also prove useful in distinguishing this tumor from others of similar radiologic appearance.

Treatment

The controversy over the treatment of optic gliomas is a classic instance of the uncertainty inherent in clinical medicine. The interpretation of retrospective experience is difficult. For instance, two groups of physicians from the same institution have independently studied an overlapping series and drawn quite different conclusions. One group thought that their case material supported specific treatments [3]; the other group decided that no measures had been shown to be effective [1].

The two relevant variables in deciding whether or not to treat are the location of the neoplasm and its natural history. All reported series contain either a diagnostic or a treatment bias, and often both. Physicians who consider optic gliomas to be hamartomatous lesions, and therefore unlikely to progress, may neither biopsy nor treat. Physicians who believe that gliomas of the anterior visual pathways should be managed in much the same way as gliomas elsewhere both biopsy and treat. The former point to the fact that vision is stable or even improved with long-term follow-up in a majority of cases [9]. The latter report good results from their treatment, and cite instances of tumor progression when treatment has been withheld [7]. At present, the question whether an individual case should or should not be treated is unanswerable, as there are no prospective controlled series in the literature.

When there is radiologic evidence that the tumor is confined to the optic nerve, consideration must be given to removing the glioma in toto. Obviously, this leaves a blind eye, but if the cut margins of the nerve are clear of tumor involvement, the patient is presumed cured. Against this approach stand the observation that many patients with optic nerve gliomas have been followed for years without progression and the fact that many of these eyes have useful vision at the time the tumor is discovered.

In the case of chiasmal gliomas or predominately optic nerve gliomas that also involve the intracranial optic nerve and chiasm, there seems to be little justification for surgery beyond biopsy, with the exception of the rare patient who has hydrocephalus and requires shunting. In most of these patients, once the diagnosis is established, the alternatives are radiotherapy or observation. Cases in which radiotherapy has resulted in improvement of vision or radiologic regression of the tumor balance off against those with prolonged preservation of vision or even spontaneous regression [4, 12]. Also, radiotherapy is not without risk. Especially in very young children, radiation may produce hypopituitarism, growth retardation, and a generally adverse effect on the developing brain. Because of these side effects, some advocates of radiotherapy prefer to delay treatment until the child is at least 2 years old, if possible. Also, in some centers, chemotherapy is considered an alternative therapy.

The prognosis for life with optic nerve gliomas is good, with or without treatment. Chiasmal gliomas that invade adjacent neural structures decrease life expectancy, with or without treatment. The visual prognosis in an affected eye is uncertain. The biologic behavior of these tumors varies widely: some are indolent, some progressive. Those tumors associated with neurofibromatosis appear in general to have better prognoses than sporadic cases. Optimal management depends on determining which path an individual tumor is likely to follow, an assessment that is difficult prospectively, given current knowledge.

1. Borit, A., Richardson, E.P. Jr. The biological and clinical behaviour of pilocytic astrocytomas of the optic pathways. *Brain* 105:161–187, 1982.
   Analysis of 30 pathologically confirmed optic gliomas encountered at the Massachusetts General Hospital between 1931 and 1971 led these authors to conclude "the mortality and morbidity are much the same regardless of whether the patients have been treated surgically or by irradiation, or have received no treatment directed against the tumours."
2. Charles, N.C., Nelson, L., Brookner, A.R., et al. Pilocytic astrocytoma of the optic nerve with hemorrhage and extreme cystic degeneration. *Am. J. Ophthalmol.* 92:691–695, 1981.
   A case report demonstrating that enlargement of the tumor may not represent tumor growth per se.
3. Dosoretz, D.E., Blitzer, P.H., Wang, C.C., et al. Management of glioma of the optic nerve and/or chiasm. *Cancer* 45:1467–1471, 1980.
   Review of 20 of the same patients as Borit and Richardson (above) leads these authors to recommend resection if the disease is limited to the optic nerve, and biopsy and irradiation with more extensive lesions.
4. Frohman, L.P., Epstein, F., Kupersmith, M.J. Atypical visual prognosis with an optic nerve glioma. *J. Clin. Neuro-ophthalmol.* 5:90–94, 1985.
   Spontaneous improvement of vision occurred in a 13-year-old girl with the presumptive diagnosis of optic nerve glioma while she was awaiting surgery.
5. Grimson, B.S., Perry, D.D. Enlargement of the optic disk in childhood optic nerve tumors. *Am. J. Ophthalmol.* 97:627–631, 1984.
   In two cases, the optic disk was enlarged on the side of an optic nerve glioma.
6. Holman, R.E., Grimson, B.S., Drayer, B.P., et al. Magnetic resonance imaging of optic gliomas. *Am. J. Ophthalmol.* 100:596–601, 1985.
   These initial attempts to apply this imaging technique to the evaluation of optic gliomas show promise.
7. Horwich, A., Bloom, H.J.G. Optic gliomas: Radiation therapy and prognosis. *J. Radiat. Oncol. Biol. Phys.* 11:1067–1079, 1985.
   Twenty-nine of 30 patients with optic gliomas were treated by radiotherapy with a 93 percent 10-year survival.
8. Fletcher, W.A., Imes, R.K., Hoyt, W.F. Chiasmal gliomas: Appearance and long-term changes demonstrated by computerized tomography. *J. Neurosurg.* 65:154–159, 1986.
   The computed tomograms from 22 patients with chiasmal gliomas demonstrated a spectrum of findings. Tumors with a globular appearance must be part of a clinical picture that supports the diagnosis of glioma (i.e., be associated with diencephalic syndrome or neurofibromatosis) or undergo biopsy for definitive diagnosis.
9. Imes, R.K., Hoyt, W.F. Childhood chiasmal gliomas: Update on the fate of patients in the 1969 San Francisco study. *Br. J. Ophthalmol.* 70:179–182, 1986.
   Long-term follow-up of patients from Hoyt and Bahdassarian's seminal paper (Br. J. Ophthalmol. 53:793–798, 1969) supports the original proposition that an optic glioma is "congenital, non-neoplastic, and self-limiting, and has a good prognosis for life."

10. Klug, G.L. Gliomas of the optic nerve and chiasm in children. *Neuro-ophthalmology* 2:217–223, 1982.
    In some of the patients in this series from Australia, decompression of the optic nerve was performed, with no apparent benefit.
11. Lewis, R.A., Gerson, L.P., Axelson, K.A., et al. von Recklinghausen neurofibromatosis. II. Incidence of optic gliomata. *Ophthalmology* 91:929–935, 1984.
    Fifteen percent of patients with neurofibromatosis had optic gliomas; two-thirds of these gliomas were asymptomatic.
12. McDonnell, P., Miller, N.R. Chiasmatic and hypothalamic extension of optic nerve glioma. *Arch. Ophthalmol.* 101:1412–1415, 1983.
    An important case documenting the extension of an optic nerve glioma into the chiasm and hypothalamus, with resulting hydrocephalus. The tumor then responded to radiotherapy.
13. McFadzean, R.M., Brewing, T.B., Doyle, D., et al. Glioma of the optic chiasm and its management. *Trans. Ophthalmol. Soc. U.K.* 103:199–207, 1983.
    This series of nine cases led the authors to conclude that biopsy was not necessary and that radiotherapy was effective.
14. Rush, J.A., Younge, B.R., Campbell, R.J., et al. Optic glioma: Long-term follow-up of 85 histopathologically verified cases. *Ophthalmology* 89:1213–1219, 1982.
    This analysis of the Mayo Clinic experience carefully avoids unsupportable conclusions about treatment. All 10 patients with extended chiasmal involvement died, regardless of therapy.
15. Tenny, R.T., Laws, E.R., Younge, B.R., et al. The neurosurgical management of optic glioma: Results in 104 patients. *J. Neurosurg.* 57:452–458, 1982.
    Another perspective on the Mayo Clinic series. The discussion contains brief summaries of many previously published papers.
16. Wright, J.E., McDonald, W.I., Call, N.B. Management of optic nerve gliomas. *Br. J. Ophthalmol.* 64:545–552, 1980.
    The group from Moorfields Eye Hospital reports that biopsy is neither necessary nor particularly helpful in the management of optic nerve gliomas. About half of their patients had an indolent course; in half of the patients the tumor enlarged. Surgery is advocated only when growth is documented.

X. OCULAR MOTILITY AND PUPIL

John W. Gittinger, Jr.

Isolated paralysis of the superior oblique muscle, which is innervated by the fourth or trochlear nerve, is frequently encountered clinically and constitutes the most common cause of vertical strabismus. Fourth nerve palsies are often congenital and may run in families [1, 4]. Head trauma is the most commonly identified cause of acquired fourth nerve palsy. Another large group of transient fourth nerve palsies are attributed to vascular disease, particularly that associated with diabetes, and a significant number must be considered truly idiopathic.

Occasionally, fourth nerve palsies prove to be manifestations of other disease processes. Recent reports include cases caused by brain stem hemorrhage [19] and metastases [11], a cysticercal cyst [6], and posterior fossa tumors [7]. The publication of such papers attests to the rareness with which specific causes can be identified. Various other causes mentioned in large case series include aneurysms, *Herpes zoster ophthalmicus*, brain stem arteriovenous malformations, sinusitis, and neurosurgery. Multiple sclerosis is a rare cause of fourth nerve palsy, presumably because the nerve fasicles leave the brain stem dorsally, away from the major white matter tracts.

Unilateral Fourth Nerve Palsy

Unilateral fourth nerve palsy manifests as a hypertropia on the ipsilateral side that is greater when the hypertropic eye is adducted and that increases when the head is tilted toward the side of the palsy (Bielschowsky's test). For a right fourth nerve palsy, there is a right hypertropia that is greater on left gaze and greater on right head tilt; for a left fourth nerve palsy, there is a left hypertropia that is greater on right gaze and greater on left head tilt. This pattern is most consistent when the palsy is of recent onset; the well-known phenomenon of spread of comitance changes the examination with time. Bielschowsky's test depends on otolithic reflexes and will not be positive when the patient is in the supine position. Even with the head upright, an increase in the hypertropia on head tilt is not observed in some cases.

Another characteristic feature of fourth nerve palsies is excyclotropia. The involved eye is rotated around the visual axis away from the nose. This is usually measured by using a double Maddox rod in a trial frame. A potentially confusing adaptation occasionally occurs when the paretic eye is used for fixation: the noncyclotropic eye perceives images as torted [12]. In a few instances, torsion of the entire fundus is obvious ophthalmoscopically [16].

A person with unilateral fourth nerve palsies often carries his head in a position that relieves diplopia. For most, this means a head tilt away from the side of the palsy with the chin tucked down. Paradoxically, a few tilt their heads toward the palsy, increasing the vertical deviation. Presumably, this allows them to separate the diplopic images further and thus suppress one. This *ocular torticollis* is especially significant in young children, in whom a compensatory scoliosis may develop. Remarkably, for reasons that are not evident, many persons with unilateral fourth nerve palsies have no head tilt at all.

Bilateral Fourth Nerve Palsy

Bilateral fourth nerve palsies are more difficult to diagnose. In symmetric bilateral fourth nerve palsies there may be little or no vertical deviation in the primary position, only either a small horizontal deviation (esotropia or exotropia) or orthophoria. A diagnostic finding, when present, is a left hypertropia on right gaze and a right hypertropia on left gaze. There is no compensatory head tilt, and the head tilt test may be positive in both directions (right hypertropia on right head tilt and left hypertropia on left head tilt). Two other findings that suggest bilateral fourth nerve palsies are an esotropia that increases on down gaze (a V-pattern esotropia) and a large degree of excyclotropia. Unilateral fourth nerve palsy produces up to about 10 degrees of excyclotropia; bilateral fourth nerve palsy produces as much as 25 degrees, especially in down gaze.

Most bilateral fourth nerve palsies follow head trauma, probably either because the thin anterior medullary velum where the nerves decussate has been subject to shearing forces or because the delicate rootlets of the nerves have been torn away from the brain stem as they emerge. Even minor head trauma may cause unilateral palsy, but when there has been concussive head trauma, bilaterality should always be considered. In some cases, none of the typical findings is present, and surgery directed toward only the greater and therefore manifest palsy in bilateral cases serves to unmask the contralateral paresis.

Diagnosis

Vertical deviations occur in association with other types of strabismus and may be mistaken for fourth nerve palsies [8]. Graves' orbitopathy, inflammatory orbital pseudotumor, blow-out fractures, and skew deviations may mimic fourth nerve palsies. Occasionally, myasthenia gravis selectively involves the superior oblique muscle [15]. Other isolated vertical muscle palsies may represent partial nuclear third nerve palsies [13].

Often the differential problem is between congenital and acquired fourth nerve palsy. Many congenital fourth nerve palsies do not manifest until late childhood or even adulthood because fusional mechanisms have kept the deviation latent. For such patients, old photographs may show a compensatory head tilt, and the vertical fusional vergences measured with prisms will be unusually large. In addition, the patient with a congenital fourth nerve palsy is less likely to complain of torsional diplopia. The distinction is important both because an occasional acquired fourth nerve palsy is an indicator of more serious neurologic problems and because the surgeon operating on a congenital palsy should be aware that the superior oblique muscle may be absent [5].

Treatment

Because of the torsional component, prisms seldom adequately compensate for the deviation produced by fourth nerve palsies. Before surgery is undertaken, time, usually 4 to 6 months, should be allowed for the possibility of spontaneous recovery of an acquired palsy or recompensation of a congenital one. In a growing child with a significant head tilt, surgery is indicated even if the deviation is well compensated, because of the risk of scoliosis.

The existence of many surgical procedures suggests that none is totally satisfactory. The two most common operations used for treatment of fourth nerve palsies are a weakening of the ipsilateral inferior oblique muscle and a superior oblique tendon tuck to strengthen the palsied muscle. These may be combined on the same eye [14]. When cyclotropia is the major component, procedures have been developed to take advantages of the fact that the anterior parts of the oblique tendons are involved in cyclotorsion, while the posterior portions provide the vertical actions. Anterolateral displacement of the anterior portion of the superior oblique tendon (the Harada-Ito operation) serves to correct excyclotropia [10].

1. Astle, W.F., Rosenbaum, A.L. Familial congenital fourth cranial nerve palsy. *Arch. Ophthalmol.* 103:532–535, 1985.
   Three families, each with two members who had fourth nerve palsies, are reported.
2. Bixenman, W.W. Diagnosis of superior oblique palsy. *J. Clin. Neuro-ophthalmol.* 1:199–208, 1981.
   An excellent review of diagnostic features, including a discussion of the Knapp classification.
3. Coppeto, J.M., Lessell, S. Cryptogenic unilateral paralysis of the superior oblique muscle. *Arch. Ophthalmol.* 96:275–277, 1978.
   Fifteen of 43 cases of superior oblique palsy had no definable cause.
4. Harris, D.J. Jr., Memmen, J.E., Katz, N.N.K., et al. Familial congenital superior oblique palsy. *Ophthalmology* 93:88–90, 1986.
   Four more families with two or more cases.
5. Helveston, E.M., Giangiacomo, J.G., Ellis, F.D. Congenital absence of the superior oblique tendon. *Trans. Am. Ophthalmol. Soc.* 79:123–135, 1981.
   These surgeons found no superior oblique tendon in eight surgical cases, including one confirmed neuroradiologically. In the discussion, Parks notes that this had not

been his experience.

6. Keane, J.R. Trochlear nerve pareses with brainstem lesions. *J. Clin. Neuro-ophthalmol.* 6:242–246, 1986.
   Three cases in which brain stem lesions were identified radiologically, including a presumed cysticercal cyst of the fourth ventricle.

7. Krohel, G.B., Mansour, A.M., Petersen, W.L., et al. Isolated trochlear nerve palsy secondary to a juvenile pilocytic astrocytoma. *J. Clin. Neuro-ophthalmol.* 2:119–123, 1982.
   This 9-year-old child had a partial left fourth nerve palsy and papilledema.

8. Kushner, B.J. Simulated superior oblique palsy. *Ann. Ophthalmol.* 13:337–343, 1981.
   Kushner describes 44 cases in which a deviation fitting the pattern of a superior oblique palsy had another explanation, most often a hypertropia accompanying intermittent exotropia.

9. Lee, J., Flynn, J.T. Bilateral superior oblique palsies. *Br. J. Ophthalmol.* 69:508–513, 1985.
   A review of 18 consecutive cases from the Bascom Palmer Eye Institute.

10. Mitchell, P.R., Parks, M.M. Surgery for bilateral superior oblique palsy. *Ophthalmology* 89:484–488, 1982.
    A series of eight patients who had bilateral superior oblique tendon surgery, a modification of the Harada-Ito procedure.

11. Murray, R.S., Ajax, E.T. Bilateral trochlear nerve palsies: A clinicoanatomic correlate. *J. Clin. Neuro-ophthalmol.* 5:57–58, 1985.
    A 74-year-old man with bilateral fourth nerve palsies had a lesion in the anterior cerebellar vermis thought to represent metastatic lung carcinoma.

12. Olivier, P., von Noorden, G.K. Excyclotropia of the nonparetic eye in unilateral superior oblique muscle paralysis. *Am. J. Ophthalmol.* 93:30–33, 1982.
    An unusual sensory adaptation is described.

13. Pusateri, T.J., Sedwick, L.A., Margo, C.E. Isolated inferior rectus muscle palsy from a solitary metastasis to the oculomotor nucleus. *Arch. Ophthalmol.* 105:675–677, 1987.
    Autopsy confirmed a "subnuclear" third nerve location for the lesion in this vertical muscle palsy.

14. Reynolds, J.D., Biglan, A.W., Hiles, D.A. Congenital superior oblique palsy in infants. *Arch. Ophthalmol.* 102:1503–1505, 1984.
    In their 20 patients who were operated on before the age of 2 years, these surgeons obtained better results with a simultaneous weakening of the inferior oblique muscle and superior oblique tendon tuck.

15. Rush, J.A., Shafrin, F. Ocular myasthenia presenting as superior oblique weakness. *J. Clin. Neuro-ophthalmol.* 2:125–127, 1982.
    After presentation with a right hypertropia greater on left gaze, other ocular motor signs led to the diagnosis of myasthenia gravis.

16. Ruttum, M., von Noorden, G.K. Adaptation to tilting of the visual environment in cyclotropia. *Am. J. Ophthalmol.* 96:229–237, 1983.
    A discussion of the sensory adaptations in both congenital and acquired fourth nerve palsies.

17. Sydnor, C.F., Seaber, J.H., Buckley, E.G. Traumatic superior oblique palsies. *Ophthalmology* 89:134–138, 1982.
    Of 85 cases of superior oblique palsy treated at Duke, 33 were posttraumatic, 37 were congenital, and 15 had no known cause. Of the posttraumatic cases, 12 were bilateral and 21 were unilateral. Thirteen posttraumatic cases resolved spontaneously; the others required surgery.

18. von Noorden, G.K., Murray, E., Wong, S.Y. Superior oblique paralysis: A review of 270 cases. *Arch. Ophthalmol.* 104:1771–1776, 1986.
    This paper describes the largest and most extensively analyzed series to date.

19. Wise, J., Gomolin, J., Goldberg, L.L. Bilateral superior oblique palsy: Diagnosis and treatment. *Can. J. Ophthalmol.* 18:28–32, 1983.
    Three case reports (including one man with a hypertensive hemorrhage documented by computed tomography) of bilateral fourth nerve palsies.

57. OPSOCLONUS

The description of abnormal eye movements presents problems even for experienced observers. Although a consensus is emerging from data obtained by eye movement recordings, the nomenclature is not rigorously applied in much of the literature, especially that based on observation alone. The term *opsoclonus* denotes random, semiconjugate, chaotic movements of the eyes, often associated with fluttering movements of the lids. A more evocative word is *saccadomania,* since these movements are saccades or rapid eye movements. Other descriptions of the same or similar movements are dancing eyes, lightning eye movements, ataxic conjugate movements of the eyes, opsochoria, and opsoclonia. The characteristics of opsoclonus include variation in amplitude, initiation by blinking or closing the eyes, and persistence in sleep and coma.

Opsoclonus may be seen in association with other abnormalities of eye movements, especially *ocular dysmetria* (saccades that are too long and overshoot the visual target, the ocular equivalent of limb dysmetria) and *ocular flutter* (to-and-fro back-to-back horizontal saccades interrupting fixation). Since opsoclonus is a saccadic movement and therefore has no slow phase, it is not a true nystagmus. Also, unlike nystagmus, opsoclonus is arrhythmic. One form of nystagmus that is sometimes considered with opsoclonus is *ocular myoclonus.* Two types of ocular myoclonus have been described, both sometimes accompanied by movements of the palate and other facial and respiratory muscles (palatoocular myoclonus): bouncing ball eye movements, which are rapid (1–3 Hz), vertical, pendular oscillations, and jerky, nystagmoid movements with simultaneous oblique and rotatory components [10].

Pathogenesis

The pathophysiology of opsoclonus is poorly understood. Because ocular flutter and ocular dysmetria are cerebellar eye movement disorders, cerebellar dysfunction has been postulated. Autopsy studies, however, have failed to reveal specific cerebellar pathology [8]. This, of course, does not rule out a biochemical lesion, which would not be demonstrated by conventional neuropathologic methods [16]. One ingenious suggestion is that opsoclonus represents an inhibition of the pause neurons, cells that lie in the pontine reticular formation and fire continuously, except immediately before and during a saccade. Pause neurons are thought to inhibit burst neurons, which produce the immediate premotor command for saccades [17]. Damage to pause neurons might therefore result in excessive, random saccades from disinhibition of burst neurons.

Although no specific pathology is recognized for opsoclonus, ocular myoclonus is regularly associated with lesions in the connections of the inferior olivary nucleus, in particular the central tegmental (dentatoolivary) tract, connecting the inferior olive with the contralateral dentate nucleus of the cerebellum. The oblique and rotatory movements are associated with unilateral lesions; the bouncing ball eye movements appear with bilateral disease. The cause is usually a brain stem or cerebellar infarct, and there is characteristically a delay of 6 to 8 months before the abnormal movements appear. They then persist for life. On pathologic examination of the brain stem at postmortem, the olive is grossly hypertrophic, a finding picturesquely called the "stuffed olive."

Diagnosis

Since many abnormal eye movements can be precisely defined only by electrooculography, the clinical problem is the differential diagnosis of chaotic eye movements. Probably the most important association of opsoclonus is with remote malignancies. In children, opsoclonus may be the presenting sign of neuroblastomas, one of the more common tumors of childhood. There is a coexisting ataxia and often a history of irritability. Neuroblastomas arise in the adrenals and the sympathetic chains of the abdomen, thorax, and neck. Diagnosis is made by determination of excess urinary catecholamines and by computed tomography.

Opsoclonus may also be a paraneoplastic manifestation in an adult. The primary tumors identified include carcinomas of the lung, breast, uterus, and thyroid. An autoimmune mechanism is postulated, but has not been well defined. Anti-Purkinje cell antibodies have been detected in both paraneoplastic cerebellar degeneration and opsoclonus.

Most children with opsoclonus do not harbor neuroblastomas. In the neonatal period, constant or intermittent opsoclonus may be observed in otherwise normal babies. Also, opsoclonus, myoclonus, and truncal ataxia are manifestations of a viral or postinfectious encephalitis in both children and adults. Lumbar puncture usually reveals a slight, predominately mononuclear, cerebrospinal fluid pleocytosis. The largest series were collected before 1970 from Boston hospitals. Virologic studies on two children, also from Massachusetts, encountered in the 1980s suggested Coxsackie B3 virus infection [9]. Epidemics of St. Louis encephalitis in Iowa and Texas each had one instance of opsoclonus [4]. Most patients with opsoclonus and encephalitis have recovered without sequelae, although there is a small risk of permanent neurologic damage and even death.

Opsoclonus is also a feature of some toxic encephalopathies: amitriptyline, thallium, chlordecone (Kepone), the combination of haloperidol and lithium, and toluene abuse [10]. Finally, instances of brain stem structural lesions—tumor or hemorrhage—are occasionally encountered [7].

In blind infants, chaotic eye movements resembling opsoclonus develop, usually at about 3 months of age. These are sometimes inappropriately called "searching eye movements of the blind." The differential diagnosis of severe visual loss in young children with ophthalmoscopically normal eyes includes Leber's congenital amaurosis and optic glioma (see Chap. 55). Some children with opsoclonus and blindness never have a specific etiology defined. A point to consider in the differentiation of poor vision as a result of other causes from that caused by opsoclonus is the presence or absence of other neurologic findings such as ataxia.

Treatment

Treatment of opsoclonus depends on its cause. In many cases of opsoclonus, the disorder is self-limited and no intervention is required. Obviously, any underlying malignancy should be identified. Neuroblastomas are managed with radiotherapy and chemotherapy. The prognosis in patients with opsoclonus seems to be better than average for patients with neuroblastomas as a group. Remarkably, the opsoclonus may improve with or without treatment of the tumor. Corticosteroids sometimes improve opsoclonus, and thiamine administration was followed by remission in one patient with paraneoplastic opsoclonus [12].

1. Cogan, D.G. Opsoclonus. In P.J. Vinken and G.W. Bruyn (eds.), *Handbook of Clinical Neurology*, Vol 39. New York: Elsevier Science Publishing, 1978. Pp. 611–617.
   Cogan considers the opsoclonus-palatal myoclonus syndrome a clinical subtype of opsoclonus.
2. Digre, K.B. Opsoclonus in adults: Report of three cases and review of the literature. *Arch. Neurol.* 43:1165–1175, 1986.
   One of these patients had a high titer of anti-Purkinje cell antibodies. Digre also provides an extensive tabular review and 105 references.
3. Dropscho, E., Payne, R. Paraneoplastic opsoclonus-myoclonus: Association with medullary thyroid carcinoma and review of the literature. *Arch. Neurol.* 43:410–415, 1986.
   Dropscho and Payne add another type of primary tumor to the list of associated tumors and speculate on the etiology of the syndrome.
4. Evans, R.W., Welch, K.W.A. Opsoclonus in a confirmed case of St. Louis encephalitis. *J. Neurol. Neurosurg. Psychiatry* 45:660–661, 1982.
   One of the specific viral associations of opsoclonus.
5. Hoyt, C.S., Mousel, D.K., Weber, A.A. Transient supranuclear disturbances of gaze in healthy neonates. *Am. J. Ophthalmol.* 89:708–713, 1980.
   Opsoclonus, skew deviation, and transient downward deviation of the eyes in otherwise healthy neonates may resolve spontaneously.
6. Hunter, S., Kooistra, C. Neuropathologic findings in idiopathic opsoclonus and my-

oclonus: Their similarity to those in paraneoplastic cerebellar cortical degeneration. *J. Clin. Neuro-ophthalmol.* 6:236–241, 1986.
Structural lesions were found only in the cerebellum and inferior olives. Etiologies and previous autopsy cases are tabulated.

7. Keane, J.R. Transient opsoclonus with thalamic hemorrhage. *Arch. Neurol.* 37:423–424, 1980.
Keane, who previously described opsoclonus in glioma, reports three patients with thalamic hemorrhage and transient opsoclonus.

8. Kilgo, G.R., Schwartze, G.M. Opsoclonus: Update on clinical and pathologic associations. *J. Clin. Neuro-ophthalmol.* 4:109–113, 1984.
Another autopsied case reveals no specific lesion.

9. Kuban, K.C., Ephros, M.A. Syndrome of opsoclonus-myoclonus caused by coxsackie B3 infection. *Ann. Neurol.* 13:69–71, 1983.
Two children from Cape Cod evaluated at Children's Hospital in Boston within 2 weeks of each other had evidence of encephalitis caused by Coxsackie virus.

10. Lazar, R.B., Ho., S.U., Melen, O., et al. Multifocal central nervous system damage caused by toluene abuse. *Neurology* 33:1337–1340, 1983.
Three young toluene abusers had opsoclonus, ocular flutter, and ocular dysmetria.

11. Nakada, T., Kwee, I.L. Oculopalatal myoclonus. *Brain* 109:431–441, 1986.
Analysis of the eye movements in five cases of palatooocular myoclonus leads to a separation into two types. The oscillations may be the result of malfunctioning vestibuloocular reflex adaptation by the flocculus of the cerebellum.

12. Nausieda, P.A., Tanner, C.M., Weiner, W.J. Opsoclonic cerebellopathy: A paraneoplastic syndrome responsive to thiamine. *Arch. Neurol.* 38:780–781, 1981.
Truncal ataxia and opsoclonus improved within 24 hours of thiamine administration.

13. Rivner, M.H., Jay, W.M., Green, J.B., et al. Opsoclonus in *Hemophilus influenzae* meningitis. *Neurology* 32:661–663, 1982.
Opsoclonus in an infant with hemophilus meningitis was associated with evidence of an abnormal immune response.

14. Rosenberg, N.L. Hearing loss an initial symptom of the opsoclonus-myoclonus syndrome. *Arch. Neurol.* 41:998–999, 1984.
Bilateral hearing loss thought to be the result of diffuse involvement of brain stem auditory pathways preceded the development of opsoclonus and myoclonus.

15. Warrier, R.P., Kini, R., Besser, A., et al. Opsomyoclonus and neuroblastoma. *Clin. Pediatr. (Phila.)* 24:32–34, 1985.
Recent case reports of this association.

16. Wertenbaker, C., Behrens, M.M., Hunter, S.B., et al. Opsoclonus—a cerebellar disorder? *Neuro-opthalmology* 2:73–83, 1981.
Another autopsy and review suggest that "the responsible lesion is biochemically specific but anatomically diffuse."

17. Zee, D.S., Robinson, D.A. A hypothetical explanation of saccadic oscillations. *Ann. Neurol.* 5:405–421, 1979.
Zee and Robinson suggest that instability in both the horizontal and vertical saccadic pulse generators is the basis for opsoclonus.

58. DOWNBEAT NYSTAGMUS

Nystagmus refers to rhythmic oscillations of the eyes. To be a true nystagmus, each oscillation must contain a slow phase. By convention, however, nystagmus is named according to the direction of the fast phase, when it is present. (Nystagmus with two slow phases is termed pendular or elliptical.) Thus, jerk nystagmus may be described as left-beating, right-beating, up-beating, or down-beating. Some years ago Cogan [3] observed that *downbeat nystagmus* had unique characteristics and associations. These observations have been confirmed and refined by additional clinical experience and modern electrooculography.

Pathogenesis

The precise physiologic basis for downbeat nystagmus is not agreed upon, but dysfunction in the vestibulocerebellum (the flocculus and nodulus) is postulated. This region, which includes the so-called cerebellar tonsils, is selectively affected in the congenital anomaly called cerebellar ectopia, one part of the Arnold-Chiari malformation.

Arnold-Chiari malformation type II is an extensive hindbrain maldevelopment regularly associated with lumbar meningomyelocele and spina bifida that presents in childhood as hydrocephalus. By contrast, Arnold-Chiari malformation type I is a caudal displacement of the cerebellar tonsils, variably associated with bony abnormalities at the craniocervical junction (basilar impression, Klippel-Feil deformity). This is often asymptomatic until adulthood, when it presents as foramen magnum compression (cerebellar signs and lower cranial nerve palsies), central cord syndromes (syringohydromyelia), or a pure cerebellar syndrome in which downbeat nystagmus is a prominent finding. Adults with Arnold-Chiari malformation type I may complain of incoordination, especially after neck extension; symptoms are also increased by straining, coughing, or sneezing [9].

A primary, paraneoplastic, or toxic cerebellar degeneration may also feature downbeat nystagmus [2]. In many series, familial cerebellar degeneration is the most common cause of downbeat nystagmus [3, 6]. Other etiologies reported include anticonvulsant and lithium intoxication [1], magnesium depletion [12], encephalitis [7], and vitamin B_{12} deficiency [9]. Only a relatively small proportion of patients with downbeat nystagmus have multiple sclerosis, posterior fossa tumor, or stroke. In a number of cases, no etiology is ever defined.

Diagnosis

The most striking feature of downbeat nystagmus is that it violates Alexander's law, which states that nystagmus is enhanced with gaze deviation in the direction of the fast phase. Downbeat nystagmus increases in amplitude with gaze down and laterally, rather than just down. When downbeat nystagmus is present, smooth pursuit downward is impaired more than smooth pursuit upward. This has been considered by some to be a clue to the pathogenesis of downbeat nystagmus (as the major representative of the class of pursuit-defect nystagmus). Recently, it has also been demonstrated that downbeat nystagmus is in some cases posturally dependent [5].

Persons with downbeat nystagmus may complain of vertical oscillopsia (illusory movement of the environment), blur, or even vertical diplopia. The latter is probably the result of an accompanying skew deviation. These complaints are exaggerated by looking down, as in reading, and may lead to abnormal head posturing—holding the chin down so that the eyes are elevated.

The evaluation of a patient with downbeat nystagmus must include a complete neurologic examination. In the past the neuroradiologic demonstration of cerebellar ectopy was difficult. Vertebral angiography and pneumoencephalography are uncomfortable procedures with significant morbidities. Conventional computed tomography does not delineate the foramen magnum well, and until recently, metrizamide myelography was the procedure of choice. The advent of magnetic resonance imaging permits Arnold-Chiari type I abnormalities to be detected with relative ease by multiplanar visualization of this region [14].

Treatment

Once the diagnosis of Arnold-Chiari malformation is made, consideration must be given to surgical decompression. Suboccipital craniectomy has been successful in a number of cases in relieving symptoms and producing objective remission of downbeat nystagmus [15, 16]. Complications of such surgery include respiratory depression and lower cranial nerve damage. Another surgical procedure reported to relieve downbeat nystagmus is transoral removal of the odontoid process [13].

Medical treatment is also an alternative. Obviously, when the downbeat nystagmus is a toxic manifestation, the toxin should be withdrawn. Magnesium supplementation should be provided when this mechanism is suspected, and alcoholic cerebellar degeneration may respond to thiamine. Oscillopsia or visual blurring produced by downbeat nystagmus improves in some cases after the administration of clonazepam [4] or with the use of base-out prisms in glasses [8].

1. Berger, J.R., Kovacs, A.G. Downbeat nystagmus with phenytoin. *J. Clin. Neuro-ophthalmol.* 2:209–211, 1982.
   Two cases and a tabular differential diagnosis are presented.
2. Bogousslavsky, J., Regli, F. Monocular downbeat nystagmus. *J. Neurol.* 232:99–101, 1985.
   A monocular case in a woman with sporadic pontocerebellar degeneration.
3. Cogan, D.G. Down-beat nystagmus. *Arch. Ophthalmol.* 80:757–768, 1968.
   About one-third of Cogan's cases were due to Arnold-Chiari malformation, one-third were due to cerebellar degeneration, and one-third were due to other causes or were idiopathic.
4. Currie, J.N., Matsuo, V. The use of clonazepam in the treatment of nystagmus-induced oscillopsia. *Ophthalmology* 93:924–932, 1986.
   Clonazepam improved symptoms in all seven patients with downbeat nystagmus receiving long-term therapy.
5. Gresty, M., Barratt, H., Rudge, P., et al. Analysis of downbeat nystagmus: Otolithic vs semicircular canal influences. *Arch. Neurol.* 43:52–55, 1986.
   The effect of head position on the vestibuloocular reflex was assessed electrooculographically.
6. Halmagyi, G.M., Rudge, P., Gresty, M.A., et al. Downbeating nystagmus: A review of 62 cases. *Arch. Neurol.* 40:777–784, 1983.
   A large series is carefully analyzed.
7. Hirst, L.W., Clark, A.W., Wolinsky, J.S., et al. Downbeat nystagmus: A case report of herpetic brain stem encephalitis. *J. Clin. Neuro-ophthalmol.* 3:245–249, 1983.
   Downbeat nystagmus developed preterminally. No specific lesions were found at autopsy.
8. Lavin, P.J.M., Traccis, S., Dell'Osso, L.F., et al. Downbeat nystagmus with a pseudocycloid waveform: Improvement with base-out prisms. *Ann. Neurol.* 13:621–624, 1983.
   Hyperemesis gravidarum resulted in Wernicke's encephalopathy and an unusual variant of downbeat nystagmus that increased on up gaze and was damped by convergence.
9. Mayfrank, L., Thoden, U. Downbeat nystagmus indicates cerebellar or brain-stem lesions in vitamin B_{12} deficiency. *J. Neurol.* 233:145–148, 1986.
   Two patients with pernicious anemia had downbeat nystagmus.
10. Paul, K.S., Lye, R.H., Strange, F.A., et al. Arnold-Chiari malformation: Review of 71 cases. *J. Neurosurg.* 58:183–187, 1983.
    An overview of the manifestation of Arnold-Chiari malformation type I in adults.
11. Rosenberg, M.L. Reversible downbeat nystagmus secondary to excessive alcohol intake. *J. Clin. Neuro-ophthalmol.* 7:23–25, 1987.
    Primary position downbeat nystagmus in three alcoholics without structural lesions improved or resolved with abstinence.
12. Saul, R.F., Selhorst, J.B. Downbeat nystagmus with magnesium depletion. *Arch. Neurol.* 38:650–652, 1981.
    Downbeat nystagmus was associated with hypomagnesemia in two patients.
13. Senelick, R.C. Total alleviation of downbeat nystagmus in basilar impression by transoral removal of the odontoid process. *J. Clin. Neuro-ophthalmol.* 1:265–267, 1981.
    Brief description of an unusual surgical approach.
14. Spinos, E., Laster, D.W., Moody, D.M. MR evaluation of Chiari I malformations at 0.15 T. *Am. J. Radiol.* 144:1143–1148, 1985.
    Describes the uses of magnetic resonance imaging in 12 patients with Arnold-Chiari malformation type I.

15. Spooner, J.W., Baloh, R.W. Arnold-Chiari malformation: Improvement in eye movements after surgical treatment. *Brain* 104:51–60, 1981.
    This and the next paper are the most quantitative of the papers describing improvement in the nystagmus after suboccipital decompression.
16. Yee, R.D., Baloh, R.W., Honrubia, V. Episodic vertical oscillopsia and downbeat nystagmus in a Chiari malformation. *Arch. Ophthalmol.* 102:723–725, 1984.
    In this case, the eye movements were almost normal between the episodes of oscillopsia.
17. Zasorin, N.L., Baloh, R.W. Downbeat nystagmus with alcoholic cerebellar degeneration. *Arch. Neurol.* 41:1301–1302, 1984.
    In this patient, the findings were not reversed by treatment with thiamine.

59. SPASMUS NUTANS

The description *spasmus nutans* (literally "nodding spasms") is applied to a disorder of early childhood with three components: nystagmus, head nodding, and head tilting. Spasmus nutans has been recognized for about a century and for most of this time was considered a benign, self-limited problem. Recently, the significance of this complex of signs has undergone a reevaluation.

Spasmus nutans usually presents in infants aged 3 to 8 months and lasts between 4 and 36 months. Nystagmus is the most consistent finding. The striking feature of the nystagmus is its asymmetry, being much more prominent in one eye, even at times monocular [17]. The most frequent description is of a rapid, small-amplitude, horizontal, pendular nystagmus. The nystagmus of spasmus nutans may be evoked by the near reflex [3].

The head nodding and tilting appear to be compensatory, as both damp the nystagmus. The head tilting is sometimes called torticollis but bears only a superficial resemblance to the "wry neck" of extrapyramidal movement disorders. Head tilt develops during attempts at fixation in only about one-third of cases. Both head nodding and head tilting disappear before the nystagmus as spasmus nutans resolves.

Pathogenesis

Spasmus nutans is thought to represent a disorder in the maturation of the ocular motor system. Historically, various etiologic factors including poor lighting, low birth weight, and stress have been invoked as causes for spasmus nutans. The only associations confirmed by statistical study are a family history of nystagmus and the presence of various nonspecific neurologic abnormalities (cerebral palsy, mental retardation) [9]. In addition, many children who have had spasmus nutans subsequently develop strabismus. Sets of identical twins with spasmus nutans have been reported [7, 8].

Diagnosis

The differential diagnosis of nystagmus in childhood includes congenital nystagmus, visual loss, and spasmus nutans. Congenital nystagmus, despite its appellation, is not often recognized at birth, but rather becomes apparent during the first few months of life. Like spasmus nutans, congenital nystagmus is sometimes accompanied by head nodding. Unlike spasmus nutans, its wave form is variable, even changing with time in the same person, and it is usually binocular, although occasionally it is asymmetric or even monocular. Congenital nystagmus often damps with convergence or has a null point or position of gaze where it is diminished.

The most important consideration in a child with nystagmus is whether the nystagmus is a manifestation of visual loss. Large-amplitude nystagmus, sometimes considered a variant of opsoclonus, may result from bilateral blindness in early life (see Chap. 57). Vertical, slow, pendular oscillations develop in some adults with monocular visual loss, often after a long latent period (the so-called Heimann-Bielschowsky phenomenon).

These oscillations are usually subclinical, but may be large enough to attract attention Monocular vertical or horizontal nystagmus may be a sign of unilateral visual loss in children. The diagnostic problem is compounded by the fact that the cause of the visual loss may not be apparent, since optic atrophy or retinal pigmentary changes may not have evolved at the time of initial examination.

When visual loss manifests as nystagmus in a child, the possiblity of an optic glioma should be considered. While other associated findings (optic atrophy, anomalies of the optic nerve, or a diencephalic syndrome) simplify the diagnosis, there are now several cases in which a clinical syndrome considered classic for spasmus nutans has proved to be the presentation of an optic glioma [2, 5, 13, 14]. Many physicians who have studied this problem recommend that all patients with the diagnosis of spasmus nutans have computed tomography as part of their evaluation, even when other findings are not present [16]. Others believe that computed tomography may not be necessary when the nystagmus is typical, i.e., fine and horizontal, and there are no other abnormalities [11] The visual evoked potential may prove to be a useful diagnostic tool, since it is usually markedly abnormal in patients with optic gliomas [1]. Visual evoked potentials, however, have not been studied in patients with true spasmus nutans.

Treatment

Because isolated spasmus nutans is a self-limited process, no treatment is necessary The appropriate management of optic glioma is uncertain (see Chap. 55). The discovery through the use of computed tomography of a number of optic gliomas presenting as spasmus nutans within the last decade suggests that the older series may have contained such patients but that the diagnosis was never made because of the indolence of the tumor.

1. Albright, A.L., Sclabassi, R.J., Slamovits, T.L., et al. Spasmus nutans associated with optic gliomas in infants. *J. Pediatr.* 105:778–780, 1984.
   Abnormal visual evoked potentials were a prominent finding in the two cases described in this paper.

2. Antony, J.H., Ouvrier, R.A., Wise, G. Spasmus nutans: A mistaken identity. *Arch Neurol.* 37:373–375, 1980.
   Three cases of gliomas presenting as spasmus nutans. In one instance, there was even spontaneous improvement of the nystagmus.

3. Chrousos, G.A., Ballen, A.E., Matsuo, V., et al. Near-evoked nystagmus in spasmus nutans. *J. Pediatr. Ophthalmol. Strab.* 23:141–143, 1986.
   Further studies of the same two patients as in the following reference. There is no note of computed tomography for either one.

4. Chrousos, G.A., Reingold, D.R., Chu, F.C., et al. Habitual head turning in spasmus nutans: An oculographic study. *J. Pediatr. Ophthalmol. Strab.* 22:113–116, 1985.
   The head tilt damped the nystagmus.

5. Donin, J.F. Acquired monocular nystagmus in children. *Can. J. Ophthalmol.* 2:212–215, 1967.
   One of the first papers to recognize explicitly an association between findings resembling spasmus nutans and optic glioma.

6. Farmer, J., Hoyt, J. Monocular nystagmus in infancy and early childhood. *Am. J Ophthalmol.* 98:504–509, 1984.
   In this series of 11 children with monocular nystagmus, 6 had chiasmal tumors, 4 had spasms nutans, and 1 had an ocular anomaly.

7. Hoefnagel, D., Biery, B. Spasmus nutans. *Dev. Med. Child Neurol.* 10:32–35, 1968.
   One of the few modern series of true spasmus nutans. Neuroradiologic evaluation is not mentioned. Two sets of twins are included; in one set, both twins had similar findings.

8. Hoyt, C.S., Aicardi, E. Acquired monocular nystagmus in monozygous twins. *J. Pediatr. Ophthalmol. Strab.* 16:115–118, 1979.
   Spasmus nutans in identical twins.

9. Jayalakshmi, P., Scott, T.F.M., Tucker, S.H., et al. Infantile nystagmus: A prospec

tive study of spasmus nutans, congenital nystagmus, and unclassified nystagmus of infancy. *J. Pediatr.* 77:177–187, 1970.
These authors attempt to apply statistical methods to a population of children with nystagmus.

0. Katzman, B., Lu, L.W., Tiwari, R.P. Spasmus nutans in identical twins. *Ann. Ophthalmol.* 13:1193–1195, 1981.
Another set of identical twins had spasmus nutans.

1. King, R.A., Nelson, L. B., Wagner, R.S. Spasmus nutans: A benign clinical entity. *Arch. Ophthalmol.* 104:1501–1504, 1986.
In a series of 14 patients studied with computed tomography, none had chiasmal gliomas. Two did have other anomalies of the brain (empty sella with arachnoid cyst and porencephalic cyst). These authors question whether computed tomography is always necessary in typical cases.

2. Lavery, M.A., O'Neill, J.F., Chu, F.C., et al. Acquired nystagmus in early childhood: A presenting sign of intracranial tumor. *Ophthalmology* 91:425–435, 1984.
A series of 10 patients collected from various centers documenting the difficulty and delay in making the diagnosis.

3. Koenig, S.B., Naidich, T.P., Zaparackas, Z. Optic glioma masquerading as spasmus nutans. *J. Pediatr. Ophthalmol. Strab.* 19:20–24, 1982.
A "classic" case of spasmus nutans was the presentation of a chiasmal glioma.

4. Schulman, J.A., Shults, W.T., Jones, J.M. Jr. Monocular vertical nystagmus as an initial sign of chiasmal glioma. *Am. J. Ophthalmol.* 87:87–90, 1979.
Another instance of chiasmal glioma mistaken for spasmus nutans.

5. Sedwick, L.A., Burde, R.M., Hodges, F.J. III. Leigh's subacute necrotizing encephalomyelopathy manifesting as spasmus nutans. *Arch. Ophthalmol.* 102:1046–1048, 1984.
Computed tomography of a child with asymmetric, pendular, vertical nystagmus with a see-saw component. The child also had motor incoordination and demonstrated bilateral basal ganglia lucencies. The diagnosis of subacute necrotizing encephalomyelopathy was made at autopsy.

6. Smith, J.L., Flynn, J.T., Spiro, H.J. Monocular vertical oscillations of amblyopia: The Heimann-Bielschowsky phenomenon. *J. Clin. Neuro-ophthalmol.* 2:85–91, 1982.
Three adults with reduced vision from trauma, hypothalamic-pituitary sarcoidosis, or amblyopia had monocular pendular vertical oscillations. The authors state that childhood brain tumors are more common in their practices than spasmus nutans.

7. Weissman, B.M., Dell'Osso, L.F., Abel, L.A., et al. Spasmus nutans: A quantitative prospective study. *Arch. Ophthalmol.* 105:525–528, 1987.
Characteristics of the nystagmus—a dissociated, pendular nystagmus with variable differences in the phases in each eye—may distinguish spasmus nutans from other ocular oscillations of early childhood.

0. TONIC PUPIL

he term *tonic pupil* is usually applied to any postganglionic parasympathetic dener-
ation of the intraocular muscles. *Adie's tonic pupil, Adie's syndrome,* the *Holmes-Adie*
yndrome, or *pupillotonic pseudotabes* are all designations for the combination of tonic
upil and loss of deep tendon reflexes. The combination of tonic pupil and segmental
nhidrosis or hypohidrosis has been called *Ross's syndrome* [14].

athogenesis
here are three processes that may produce tonic pupils. First, local orbital disorders
iay damage the parasympathetic ganglion of the eye, the ciliary ganglion, or its post-
anglionic parasympathetic efferents in the short ciliary nerves. Tonic pupils occasion-
lly appear after orbital surgery (including panretinal photocoagulation) or trauma,

with orbital cellulitis, or in orbital ischemia associated with giant-cell arteritis [3]. Sec ond, bilateral tonic pupils are a feature of many parasympathetic neuropathies, includ ing those associated with diabetes mellitus, syphilis, primary familial amyloidosis, an Fisher's syndrome.

The third and most common type of tonic pupil is that of Adie's syndrome. Partiall because tonic pupils may occasionally be seen with varicella-zoster virus and measle a viral etiology for Adie's syndrome is suspected, but has never been proven. Adie's syr drome usually presents in young females, and a relationship to migraine has been pos tulated [10]. The loss of deep tendon reflexes that forms the other half of Adie's syr drome most often involves the ankles and knees, and occasionally the biceps or triceps Loss of neurons in the dorsal root ganglia of the spinal cord has been demonstrate neuropathologically in the few available autopsies, suggesting a "ganglionitis" as th underlying process [18].

Diagnosis

The typical patient with Adie's syndrome is a young woman presenting for the evalua tion of anisocoria. The involved pupil is generally larger than the uninvolved pupil i room light, but may be smaller in dim illumination. The reaction to light is diminishe or absent in the tonic pupil. With bright light and magnification, such as provided by slit lamp, part of the pupil may be seen to react to light, indicating a segmental paralysi of the iris sphincter. Irregular contractions of the sphincter were sometimes describe as vermiform movements. Such segmental sphincter palsy is characteristic but no pathognomonic of Adie's syndrome, since it may occur in other situations, includin trauma, partial third nerve palsy, and aberrant regeneration of the third nerve, and wit midbrain and supranuclear involvement [15].

In most Adie's tonic pupils that are not acute, there is also light-near dissociation that is, the pupillary constriction to light is poor or absent, and the near response, al though slow ("tonic"), is present. The other major cause of light-near dissociation is up per brain stem disease, i.e., the dorsal midbrain syndrome. The light-near dissociatio of the Argyll Robertson pupil of tertiary syphilis is also attributed to midbrain disease Of course, a blind eye's pupil will not react to light, but it may react to a near stimulus The basis for the light-near dissociation observed with Adie's tonic pupil is probabl aberrant regeneration of fibers that previously innervated the ciliary muscle or the con strictor pupillae [8].

Another feature of diagnostic importance is denervation hypersensitivity. Most, bu not all, tonic pupils constrict in reaction to topically applied dilute solutions of parasym pathomimetics. Methacholine was the first drug of this type to be used diagnostically When methacholine became difficult to obtain, dilute pilocarpine (0.125%) was found t be superior in demonstrating supersensitivity, probably because it is a slightly stronge miotic than 2.5% methacholine [2]. Care must be taken in performing these pupillo pharmacologic tests that the patient is not accommodating or has not become drows while waiting for the drug to work, since accommodation and drowsiness cause refle miosis.

With the exceptions of deep tendon reflexes and those cases in which the pupillar findings are a manifestation of a more generalized autonomic dysfunction, most toni pupils are not associated with neurologic disease. Any patient with bilateral tonic pupil or decreased pupillary reactions to light should, however, have a syphilis serology [5] Tonic pupils tend to become smaller with time. In unilateral cases, 4 percent of fellow pupils become involved each following year [16].

Treatment

In Adie's syndrome, accommodation may be reduced initially, but often recovers witl time. In a young person, the temporary use of reading glasses or monocular occlusio may be helpful. A few patients experience cramps in the eye when attempting accom modation. These cramps may be relieved by cycloplegic agents. Occasionally, other com plaints have been relieved by the chronic administration of dilute parasympathomimeti [4] or anticholinesterase [19] solutions. Often the only therapy necessary is to reassure the patient that the anisocoria, which may have resulted in an unnecessary neurologic evaluation before the correct diagnosis was made, is benign.

1. Bell, T.A.G. Adie's tonic pupil in a patient with carcinomatous neuromyopathy. *Arch. Neurol.* 104:331–332, 1986.
   A unilateral tonic pupil not really Adie's syndrome, was one manifestation of a polyneuropathy in a 51-year-old man with anaplastic metastatic carcinoma.
2. Bourgon, P., Pilley, S.F.J., Thompson, H.S. Cholinergic hypersensitivity of the iris sphincter in Adie's tonic pupil. *Am. J. Ophthalmol.* 85:373–377, 1978.
   A 2.5% methacholine test was positive in 64 percent of tonic pupils; 0.125% pilocarpine was positive in 80 percent.
3. Currie, J., Lessell, S. Tonic pupil with giant cell arteritis. *Br. J. Ophthalmol.* 68:135–138, 1984.
   A case report with speculations on why the ciliary ganglion is usually spared in an ischemic orbitopathy (anastomotic blood supply) and why tonic pupil is not recognized more often in temporal arteritis (it is not looked for).
4. Flach, A.J., Dolan, B.J. Adie's syndrome: A medical treatment for symptomatic patients. *Ann. Ophthalmol.* 16:1151–1154, 1984.
   In their single case, the administration of 0.125% pilocarpine three times a day produced a grateful patient.
5. Fletcher, W.A., Sharpe, J.A. Tonic pupils in neurosyphilis. *Neurology* 36:188–192, 1986.
   There were positive serologic findings in five patients with bilateral tonic pupils.
6. Korczyn, A.D., Rubenstein, A.E., Yahr, M.D., et al. The pupil in familial dysautonomia. *Neurology* 31:628–629, 1981.
   In these patients with a familial dysautonomia, tonic pupils were not found.
7. Lepore, F.E. Diagnostic pharmacology of the pupil. *Clin. Neuropharmacol.* 8:27–37, 1985.
   A straightforward review of the use of clinical pupillopharmacologic testing.
8. Loewenfeld, I.E., Thompson, H.S. Mechanism of tonic pupil. *Ann. Neurol.* 10:276–277, 1981.
   A "lost" paper by H.K. Anderson is rediscovered and provides elegant experimental verification of the aberrant reinnervation mechanism for light-near dissociation.
9. Maitland, C.G., Scherokman, B.J., Schiffman, J., et al. Paraneoplastic tonic pupils. *J. Clin. Neuro-ophthalmol.* 5:99–104, 1985.
   Tonic pupils were a minor manifestation of a paraneoplastic dysautonomic process in two patients.
10. Massey, E.W. Pupillary dysautonomia and migraine: Is Adie's pupil caused by migraine? *Headache* 21:143–146, 1981.
    Both migraine and tonic pupil are relatively common in young women, but the significance of this association is uncertain.
11. Ponsford, J.R., Bannister, R., Paul, E.A. Methacholine pupillary responses in third nerve palsy and Adie's syndrome. *Brain* 105:583–597, 1982.
    In this study, pupillary sensitivity to methacholine did not distinguish between a preganglionic and a postganglionic lesion.
12. Ramsay, D.A. Dilute solutions of phenylephrine and pilocarpine in the diagnosis of disordered autonomic innervation of the iris: Observations in normal subjects, and in the syndromes of Horner and Holmes-Adie. *J. Neurol. Sci.* 73:125–134, 1986.
    Pupillary sensitivity to 1% phenylephrine and 0.05% pilocarpine was tested in normal, Horner's, and tonic pupils. As in other studies, the sensitivity of tonic pupils was quite variable.
13. Rubenstein, A.E., Yahr, M.D., Mytilineou, C., et al. Orthostatic hypotension in the Holmes-Adie syndrome. *Mt. Sinai J. Med.* 47:57–61, 1980.
    These authors believe that, on the basis of their single case, the Holmes-Adie syndrome should be expanded to include baroreceptor dysfunction.
14. Spector, R.H., Bachman, D.L. Bilateral Adie's tonic pupil with anhidrosis and hyperthermia. *Arch. Neurol.* 41:342–343, 1984.

The twelfth reported case of progressive anhidrosis and tonic pupil, also known as Ross's syndrome.

15. Thompson, H.S. Segmental palsy of the iris sphincter in Adie's syndrome. *Arch. Ophthalmol.* 96:1615–1620, 1978.
Thompson allows us to look at the tonic pupil through new eyes, so to speak.

16. Thompson, H.S. (ed.). *Topics in Neuro-ophthalmology.* Baltimore: Williams & Wilkins, 1979. Pp. 95–123.
A symposium on the tonic pupil.

17. Thompson, H.S. Light-near dissociation of the pupil. *Ophthalmologica (Basel)* 189:21–23, 1984.
A brief discussion of the clinical problem.

18. Ulrich, J. Morphological basis of Adie's syndrome. *Eur. Neurol.* 19:390–395, 1980.
A rare autopsy case confirms previous findings.

19. Wirthschafter, J.D., Herman, W.K. Low concentration eserine therapy for the tonic pupil (Adie) syndrome. *Ophthalmology* 87:1037–1043, 1980.
Very dilute solutions of a reversible anti-cholinesterase provided variable symptomatic relief in three of five patients.

61. HORNER'S SYNDROME

Oculosympathetic paresis is termed *Horner's syndrome* in Great Britain and the United States; in Europe it is often referred to as the *syndrome of Claude Bernard.* Clinically, Horner's syndrome manifests as ptosis, miosis, and decreased sweating ipsilaterally. The ptosis is incomplete—usually 1 to 2 mm—and the lower lid may be elevated, so-called upside-down ptosis. The resulting narrowing of the palpebral fissure results in the false appearance of enophthalmos, just as widening of the palpebral fissure is often incorrectly interpreted as exophthalmos. Additionally, in congenital Horner's syndrome or in an occasional acquired Horner's syndrome of long standing, the iris of the involved eye may be hypopigmented, producing heterochromia iridis.

Pathogenesis
The sympathetic pathways arise in the hypothalamus, and the central neuron passes through the brain stem to synapse in the spinal cord gray matter between C8 and T2. The second neuron, usually referred to as the *preganglionic neuron,* passes out the ventral root and joins the cervical sympathetic chain after passing through part of the brachial plexus. Some of the axons follow the subclavian ansa, whose course takes them near the apex of the lung. The next synapse is in the superior cervical ganglion, which is the sympathetic ganglion of the eye and is located over the transverse processes of the C1 and C2 vertebrae. The third or *postganglionic neuron* then sends its axons into the sympathetic plexus surrounding the carotid artery, where it eventually reaches the eye via the long posterior ciliary nerves. Interruption of this pathway at any point produces a Horner's syndrome, although some consider oculosympathetic paresis from postganglionic lesions a partial Horner's syndrome, since sweating is minimally involved.

Diagnosis
The miosis and resulting anisocoria are best seen in dim light. The pupils are still reactive, and bright light makes them more equal in size. The anisocoria is exaggerated after 5 seconds of darkness compared with that after 15 seconds of darkness (dilation lag). This must be demonstrated either photographically or by infrared pupillometry [7].

Although ptosis and miosis are obvious clinically, decreased sweating must be specifically elicited. Various techniques are used (dermal galvanic resistance, wetting of powders spread on the skin [8]), but none are part of most physicians' diagnostic armamentarium. The distribution of decreased sweating, provides information as to the localization of the lesion producing the Horner's syndrome.

The initial step in the evaluation of a patient with anisocoria and ptosis is to establish whether sympathetic denervation is present. Although not infallible, pupillopharmacologic testing is the easiest technique available [12]. A solution of 4 to 10% cocaine is instilled in both eyes, two drops about 5 minutes apart. Cocaine dilates normally innervated pupils by blocking the reuptake of norepinephrine in the synaptic cleft on the pupillary dilator muscle. If Horner's syndrome is present, the pupil fails to dilate. False-positives are encountered with darkly pigmented irides.

Central Neuron

Once the diagnosis is made, the next step is to determine where the lesion is located in the sympathetic pathways. Central Horner's syndromes are usually accompanied by other neurologic signs, as when Horner's syndrome is part of the lateral medullary syndrome. Both preganglionic and postganglionic Horner's syndromes may be isolated findings. After the effects of a cocaine test have worn off (at least 24 hours), instillation of 1% hydroxyamphetamine into both eyes should dilate the normal pupil or that of an eye with a central or preganglionic Horner's syndrome. If the lesion is in the postganglionic neuron, hydroxyamphetamine—which acts by releasing norepinephrine into the synapse—does not dilate the pupil. The combination of a positive cocaine test and a positive hydroxyamphetamine test (involved pupil fails to dilate while uninvolved pupil does) points to a lesion in the postganglionic neuron. Pupillopharmacologic localization has not proved to be reliable with congenital Horner's syndrome [14].

Preganglionic Neuron

Traditionally, it has been thought that an isolated preganglionic Horner's syndrome is likely to be the result of a malignant disease, whereas postganglionic Horner's syndromes are benign. This view has been challenged recently by the observation that, although tumors are still the most common cause of oculosympathetic paresis, only a small minority of Horner's syndromes are the initial manifestation of tumors [7]. Also, an increasing number of instances of postganglionic Horner's syndrome with underlying disease are being reported. These are rarely tumors but include carotid aneurysms, dissections [12], and fibromuscular dysplasia.

The evaluation of a patient with a Horner's syndrome localized to the preganglionic neuron should include chest radiography and perhaps computed tomography of the upper thorax and neck. When an undetected malignant disease is the cause, the most likely site is the pulmonary apex. Pain in the ipsilateral arm is usually associated (so-called Pancoast's syndrome).

Postganglionic Neuron

The most commonly recognized cause of a postganglionic Horner's syndrome is vascular headache, an entity for which there is a strong male predominance. The description *Raeder's paratrigeminal syndrome* [3] is applied to painful Horner's syndrome. As with many other eponyms, Raeder's syndrome has been attached to more than one set of findings, and care must be taken in interpreting the literature. When more than a postganglionic Horner's syndrome and trigeminal involvement confined to the ophthalmic division are present, parasellar mass lesions such as tumors or aneurysms must be considered as likely causes.

The description *cluster headache* refers to a unilateral, severe headache that recurs up to several times daily for periods of weeks to months and then remits (the "cluster"). Ipsilateral conjunctival injection with ptosis and miosis may be present during the headache, and a permanent postganglionic Horner's syndrome evolves in a minority of patients. These headaches, although representing a significant disability by themselves, are not ordinarily associated with other systemic diseases. Various pharmacologic manipulations, including treatment with systemic steroids, methysergide, and lithium, may abort the cluster.

The appropriate evaluation of patients with a postganglionic Horner's syndrome is under discussion. Except for a careful physical examination and history, workup is probably not required in the typical case of cluster headache in a middle-aged man. When there are atypical features, consideration should be given to angiography, especially intravenous digital subtraction studies, which have a low risk and can be performed on outpatients. When there is doubt as to the localization of the lesion producing the Horner's syndrome, other evaluation may be indicated.

Treatment

Horner's syndrome itself requires no treatment. Once specific causes have been excluded, the patient should be reassured that the ptosis is unlikely to progress.

1. Fisher, C.M. The headache and pain of spontaneous carotid dissection. *Headache* 22:60–65, 1982.
   Fisher briefly describes the clinical picture in 21 cases of spontaneous carotid dissection. Headache and neck pain accompanied by oculosympathetic paresis, a subjective bruit, pain on swallowing, or visual scintillations suggested the diagnosis.
2. Frieman, J.R., Whiting, D.W., Kosmorsky, G.S., et al. The cocaine test in normal patients. *Am. J. Ophthalmol.* 98:808–810, 1984.
   Testing of normal eyes with topical 10% cocaine revealed asymmetry of up to 0.5 mm between normal fellow eyes in pupillary dilation. The pupils of black persons did not dilate reliably with cocaine.
3. Grimson, B.S., Thompson, H.S. Raeder's syndrome. A clinical review. *Surv. Ophthalmol.* 24:199–210, 1980.
   The syndrome is discussed from both the historical and practical points of view.
4. Heitman, K., Bode, D.D. The Paredrine test in normal eyes: A controlled study. *J. Clin. Neuro-ophthalmol.* 6:228–231, 1986.
   Hydroxyamphetamine (1%) dilates light irides more than dark irides in normal eyes, and the fellow pupil becomes miotic.
5. Keane, J.R. Oculosympathetic paresis: Analysis of 100 hospitalized patients. *Arch. Neurol.* 36:13–16, 1979.
   This series, largely neurology inpatients, is dominated by strokes, especially brain stem infarcts.
6. Kline, L.B., Vitek, J.J., Raymon, B.C. Painful Horner's syndrome due to spontaneous carotid artery dissection. *Ophthalmology* 94:226–230, 1987.
   In the three cases reported here and on review of the literature, spontaneous carotid dissection has a good prognosis, with or without treatment.
7. Maloney, W.F., Younge, B.R., Moyer, N.J. Evaluation of the causes and accuracy of pharmacologic localization in Horner's syndrome. *Am. J. Ophthalmol.* 90:394–402, 1980.
   Four hundred and fifty cases from the Mayo Clinic were identified because infrared pupillography was performed. No cause for the Horner's syndrome was found in 40 percent of the cases. The leading identifiable causes were tumor, cluster headache, and iatrogenic (primarily neck surgery and carotid angiography). Only 3 percent were the initial sign of a tumor.
8. Morris, J.G.L., Lee, J., Lim, C.L. Facial sweating in Horner's syndrome. *Brain* 107:751–758, 1984.
   This Australian group used alizarin powder to map anhidrosis in Horner's syndrome. Loss of sweating on the medial aspect of the forehead and the side of the nose was found in patients with postganglionic Horner's syndrome. Preganglionic Horner's syndrome caused by brachial plexus avulsions often had no associated anhidrosis, possibly because the sympathetic nerves to sweat glands leave via different roots from those to the pupil.
9. Stone, W.M., de Toledo, J., Romanul, F.C.A. Horner's syndrome due to hypothalamic infarction: Clinical, radiologic, and pathologic correlations. *Arch. Neurol.* 43:199–200, 1986.
   Clinicopathologic correlation of a central Horner's syndrome.
10. Thompson, B.M., Corbett, J.J., Kline, L.B., et al. Pseudo-Horner's syndrome. *Arch. Neurol.* 39:108–111, 1982.
    Eighteen patients with ptosis and miosis not representing oculosympathetic paresis are reported, with a tabulation of the differential diagnosis.

11. Van der Wiel, H.L., Van Gijn, J. Localization of Horner's syndrome. *J. Neurol. Sci.* 59:229–235, 1983.
    Forty control pupils had a mean dilation of 1.5 mm with hydroxyamphetamine, with anisocoria up to 1.0 mm. In a series of 20 patients with Horner's syndrome only 4 of 10 patients with postganglionic Horner's syndrome had positive hydroxyamphetamine tests (that is, 1.0 mm or more of relative miosis). Thus, there were six false-negatives, but no false-positives, among the other 14 patients.

12. Van der Wiel, H.L., Van Gijn, J. The diagnosis of Horner's syndrome: Use and limitations of the cocaine test. *J. Neurol. Sci.* 73:311–316, 1986.
    Using a similar methodology as in their hydroxyamphetamine study, these authors found that a relative miosis of more than 1.0 mm in the affected eye was reliably associated with Horner's syndrome. On the other hand, only a little more than half of the patients thought actually to have Horner's syndrome achieved this amount of anisocoria.

13. Vijayan, N., Watson, C. Evaluation of oculocephalic sympathetic function in vascular headache syndromes. Part II: Oculocephalic sympathetic function in cluster headache. *Headache* 22:200–202, 1982.
    Six of seven patients with cluster headache had evidence of sympathetic denervation during a cluster period. This is a subject of considerable interest to physicians concerned with headaches (see also O. Sjaastad's editorial in Cephalalgia *5:59–61, 1985, and P. Herman's article in* Headache *23:102–105, 1983).*

14. Weinstein, J.M., Zweifel, T.J., Thompson, H.S. Congenital Horner's syndrome. *Arch. Ophthalmol.* 98:1074–1078, 1980.
    All patients with congenital Horner's syndrome had positive hydroxyamphetamine tests, suggesting the possibility of transsynaptic degeneration in those with preganglionic lesions.

XI. VISUAL PATHWAYS

John W. Gittinger, Jr.

In evaluating transient visual loss, the physician must rely on the patient's description of a brief, alarming, and unexpected event. Probably the most difficult subjective distinction is whether the loss was monocular or binocular: a transient homonymous hemianopsia is often misinterpreted as visual loss in the eye to the side of the hemianopsia. Only if the patient has thought to cover one eye during an episode can the localization be accepted with any confidence. With the scinitillating scotoma of migraine, even sophisticated observers may experience as a monocular event what is almost certainly an occipitally generated homonymous hallucination.

The duration of the visual loss is also relevant. Momentary loss of vision is referred to as a *transient obscuration,* whereas visual loss confined to one eye and lasting more than a few seconds but less than 30 minutes is called *amaurosis fugax,* literally "fleeting blindness" [6]. The visual loss varies from blur to complete blindness and may be described in various terms: a fog, a curtain falling or a shadow rising, loss of quadrants or hemifields, loss of peripheral vision sparing central acuity, or a constriction of the field until vision is absent.

Pathogenesis

Amaurosis fugax is recognized as one type of transient ischemic attack and, therefore, as an indicator of ipsilateral carotid disease and a predictor of impending stroke. There are, however, many other causes of transient monocular blindness. The heart is also a source of emboli that transiently interrupt the retinal circulation. Underlying cardiac pathologies include atrial myxoma, subacute bacterial endocarditis, rheumatic valvular disease, and mitral valve prolapse. Both abnormalities of the blood itself (polycythemia, thrombocytosis, anemia, macroglobulinemia, and sickle cell trait) and local ocular disease and anomalies (peripapillary staphylomas, optic disk drusen), hypopyon and hyphema from intraocular lens implants [8], and angle-closure glaucoma [12] sometimes cause transient visual loss. Almost any cause of disk swelling, including papilledema, ischemic optic neuropathy, and inflammation, may produce transient obscurations of vision, either monocularly or binocularly. Transient monocular blindness that occurs only when the eye is in a particular position of gaze (gaze-evoked amaurosis) is a symptom of optic nerve meningiomas and orbital cavernous hemangiomas [9].

Recurrent amaurosis fugax in otherwise healthy young people has often been attributed to migraine. An alternative explanation is embolization from prolapsing mitral valves [7]. Mitral valve prolapse is present in about 6 percent of normal young women and up to 40 percent of young patients with cerebral and retinal strokes. The diagnosis is ordinarily made by echocardiography, but there is no unanimity as to the applicable echocardiographic criteria. The importance of mitral valve prolapse remains uncertain.

Diagnosis

The evaluation of a patient with transient monocular visual loss depends on the age at presentation. In a person under the age of 40 years, carotid disease is unlikely unless there are additional risk factors such as hypertension, hyperlipoproteinemia, and perhaps acquired immune deficiency syndrome (AIDS) [16]. If an ophthalmic examination and appropriate blood work exclude other vascular and local causes, then echocardiography may be indicated. Empirical treatment with platelet antiaggregants should be considered.

When the patient is over the age of 50 years, carotid disease is the most important consideration. The likelihood of carotid disease increases considerably when there are other signs (carotid bruit or visible retinal emboli) or symptoms (hemispheric transient ischemic attacks). The recent onset of a combination of amaurosis fugax and hemispheric transient ischemic attacks such as extremity or facial weakness, tingling or numbness of the fingers, or speech difficulties lends an urgency to the evaluation, as the risk of stroke is greatest in the first 2 months after transient ischemic attacks begin.

Treatment

Management depends on assessment by the clinician of the effectiveness of surgical treatment in carotid disease. Despite the fact that over 100,000 carotid endarterectomies are performed each year in the United States, there is no convincing evidence that this surgery prevents stroke or decreases morbidity and mortality [18]. In the absence of a proven effective therapy, no firm recommendations for evaluation are possible. Noninvasive techniques may help to demonstrate carotid stenosis and occlusion, but normal studies do not exclude the possibility of a symptomatic carotid plaque. If a surgeon who has a low operative mortality is available and the clinician favors endarterectomy, then consideration must be given to carotid arteriography, which is still the definitive study. Occasionally, a vascular disease other than atherosclerosis (fibromuscular dysplasia) is demonstrated. Even when there are retinal emboli, the carotid angiogram may be normal, suggesting that the source of the emboli is other vessels or the heart.

Although bilateral visual loss may occasionally represent disease of both carotid arteries, the association of bilateral blurred vision or transient homonymous hemianopsia and diplopia points to ischemia in the basilar artery distribution. The situation in regard to basilar artery ischemia is relatively simple, for there is no widely accepted surgical treatment for vertebrobasilar insufficiency, and angiography is not usually done.

Bilateral visual loss in young persons may represent *basilar artery migraine.* In an episode of basilar artery migraine, the visual disturbance is followed by vertigo and unsteadiness of gait, speech difficulty, and bilateral tingling and numbness in the hands and around the mouth. The patient may fall to the ground (so-called drop attacks) or lose consciousness. Bickerstaff, who described this syndrome, thinks that it is a variant of classic migraine [2] (see Chap. 64).

1. Adams, H.P. Jr., Putman, S.F., Corbett, J.J., et al. Amaurosis fugax: The results of arteriography in 59 patients. *Stroke* 14:742–744, 1983.
   In this series, about one-third of the patients had normal carotid arteriograms on the affected side, about one-third had atherosclerotic lesions potentially treatable by endarterectomy, and one-third had untreatable lesions. Two had fibromuscular dysplasia.
2. Bickerstaff, E.R. Basilar artery migraine. In F.C. Rose (ed.), *Handbook of Clinical Neurology,* Vol 4(48):*Headache.* Amsterdam: Elsevier Science Publishers, 1986. Pp. 135–140.
   Bickerstaff discusses "Bickerstaff's migraine."
3. Fawcett, I.M., Barrie, T., Sheldon, C., et al. The prevalence of carotid artery disease in patients presenting with amaurosis fugax. *Trans. Ophthalmol. Soc. U.K.* 104:787–791, 1985.
   These investigators found stenosis of greater than 25 percent or occlusion of the ipsilateral extracranial carotid artery in over half of their patients with amaurosis fugax by using Doppler ultrasonography. The question not addressed is how many of the patients with normal noninvasive studies would have carotid disease if arteriography were performed.
4. Fisher, M., Yellin, A. Bilateral visual loss in carotid artery disease. *J. Clin. Neuroophthalmol.* 5:109–111, 1985.
   Asymmetric bilateral transient visual loss in a patient with bilateral carotid disease. (See also L. Caplan's letter to the editor, Arch. Neurol. 42:839–840, 1985.)
5. Gaul, J.J., Marks, S.J., Weinberger, J. Visual disturbance and carotid artery disease. 500 symptomatic patients studied by non-invasive carotid artery testing including B-mode ultrasonography. *Stroke* 17:393–398, 1986.
   Transient visual disturbances of various types are correlated with the results of noninvasive testing.
6. Hedges, T.R. The terminology of transient visual loss due to vascular insufficiency. *Stroke* 15:907–908, 1984.
   Hedges attempts to sort out the nomenclature.
7. Jackson, A.C. Neurologic disorders associated with mitral valve prolapse. *Can. J. Neurol. Sci.* 13:15–20, 1986.

This review discusses diagnosis and cerebral and retinal ischemia, but also mentions a number of other postulated associations.

8. Kosmorski, G.S., Rosenfeld, S.I., Burde, R.M. Transient monocular obscuration—? Amaurosis fugax: A case report. *Br. J. Ophthalmol.* 69:688–690, 1985.
   Examination of a patient during an episode of transient blurred vision and erythropsia revealed microhyphema following cataract extraction and lens implantation.

9. Orcutt, J.C., Tucker, W.H., Mills, R.P., et al. Gaze-evoked amaurosis. *Ophthalmology* 94:213–218, 1987.
   Three patients with optic nerve meningiomas and three with cavernous hemangiomas presented with gaze-evoked amaurosis, probably caused by pressure-induced optic nerve ischemia.

10. Parkin, P.J., Kendall, B.E., Marshall, J., et al. Amaurosis fugax: Some aspects of management. *J. Neurol. Neurosurg. Psychiatry* 45:1–6, 1982.
    This series of 51 patients provides a perspective on one approach to amaurosis fugax in the late 1970s.

11. Poole, C.J.M., Ross Russell, R.W. Mortality and stroke after amaurosis fugax. *J. Neurol. Neurosurg. Psychiatry* 48:902–905, 1985.
    A series of 110 patients was managed medically. The greatest risk of death was from myocardial infarction.

12. Poole, C.J.M., Ross Russell, R.W., Harrison, P., et al. Amaurosis fugax under the age of 40 years. *J. Neurol. Neurosurg. Psychiatry* 50:81–84, 1987.
    All 16 patients in this series had normal angiograms, and aspirin did not affect the frequency of their amaurosis fugax, even when there was evidence of abnormal platelet function.

13. Ravits, J., Seybold, M.E. Transient monocular visual loss from narrow-angle glaucoma. *Arch. Neurol.* 41:991–993, 1984.
    Three patients with angle closure had their visual loss initially attributed to other causes.

14. Ropper, A.H. Transient ipsilateral paresthesias (TIPs) with transient monocular blindness. *Arch. Neurol.* 42:295–296, 1985.
    Ropper documents the unusual occurrence of simultaneous hemispheric transient ischemic attacks and transient monocular blindness.

15. Sadun, A.A., Currie, J.N., Lessell, S. Transient visual obscurations with elevated optic discs. *Ann. Neurol.* 16:489–494, 1984.
    Brief visual loss was encountered in patients with disk edema and vitritis, optic nerve sheath meningioma, Fuchs's coloboma, and optic disk drusen.

16. Schwartz, N.D., So, Y.T., Hollander, H., et al. Eosinophilic vasculitis leading to amaurosis fugax in a patient with acquired immunodeficiency syndrome. *Arch. Intern. Med.* 146:2059–2060, 1986.
    Transient monocular visual loss was the presenting manifestation of an eosinophilic vasculitis in a 49-year-old man with AIDS.

17. Tomsak, R.L., Jergens, P.B. Benign recurrent transient monocular blindness: A possible variant of acephalgic migraine. *Headache* 27:66–69, 1987.
    Twenty-four more people, ranging in age from 19 to 61 years, who had recurrent transient monocular blindness and negative work-ups.

18. Warlow, C. Carotid endarterectomy: Does it work? *Stroke* 15:1068–1076, 1984.
    Warlow concludes that further studies are necessary to establish the effectiveness of carotid endarterectomy. See also editorials by Dyken (Stroke 17:355–358, 1986) and Barnett, Plum, and Walton (Stroke 15:941–943, 1984).

63. HOMONYMOUS HEMIANOPSIA

Loss of visual field to the same side in both eyes is known as a *homonymous hemianopsia,* as distinct from binasal or bitemporal hemianopsia. If an entire hemifield is lost in both eyes, this is a *complete* homonymous hemianopsia. Incomplete homonymous hemianopsias are described as either *congruous,* if the field loss is the same in both eyes, or *incongruous,* if it is not. The combination of a left and right homonymous hemianopsia is called a *bilateral homonymous hemianopsia.* A unilateral homonymous hemianopsia alone does not reduce visual acuity; a bilateral homonymous hemianopsia may decrease acuity to the same degree in both eyes or even produce complete blindness.

Pathogenesis

Homonymous hemianopsia results from a lesion in the visual pathways on the opposite side anywhere behind the chiasmal semidecussation: the optic tract, lateral geniculate, optic radiations, or occipital lobe. Most homonymous hemianopsias in older patients are the consequence of arteriosclerotic vascular disease in the posterior cerebral artery distribution or arise from a cardiac source, especially atrial fibrillation [7]. Of course, tumor and trauma may also cause hemianopsias, and degenerative or demyelinating disease is occasionally implicated. In younger persons, myxomatous or mitral valve emboli from the heart, vasculitis, migraine, and other nonarteriosclerotic vascular disorders are more often recognized. Occipital infarction may follow cervical manipulation [3] or be a remote effect of electrical shock [2]. Congenital hemianopsias may be the sequelae of early life trauma and vascular events or have an undefined developmental etiology [12].

Diagnosis

Tract hemianopsias are relatively uncommon and tend to be incongruous. Because the axons in the optic tract originate in the ganglion cell layer of the retina, optic atrophy is often associated. Visual acuity is sometimes reduced because of involvement of the adjacent chiasm. Most optic nerve hemianopsias are associated with tumors or aneurysms acting as mass lesions [8]; a posttraumatic parasellar hematoma has also been described [4].

If tract hemianopsias are uncommon, geniculate hemianopsias must be considered rare. In some reported cases, there is either a selective involvement or a sparing of the wedge of field just above and below the horizontal meridian, thought to reflect the distribution of the lateral choroidal artery [9].

Hemianopsias from lesions in the optic radiations may be congruous or perhaps slightly incongruous. Superior wedge-shaped quadrantanopsias, sometimes described as "pie-in-the-sky" defects, point to temporal lobe involvement; inferior quadrantanopsias point to parietal lobe lesions. When the parietal lobe is involved, asymmetric optokinetic responses are the rule; the optokinetic response is diminished to targets going toward the side of the lesion.

Most homonymous hemianopsias encountered clinically are the result of occipital infarctions [11]. The posterior cerebral arteries supply the occipital cortex, and the primary manifestation of thromboembolic vascular disease in their distribution is a complete or very congruous hemianopsic field defect. In addition, the occipital cortices are metabolically active tissues and are susceptible to sudden changes in oxygenation, as occurs with hypotension or metabolic poisons.

Congruous paracentral scotomata (visual field defects that do not extend into the periphery) pointing at fixation are characteristic of occipital infarction or injury. Similarly, since the most peripheral parts of the temporal visual field are represented by cortex along the opposite calcarine fissure that receives information from only one eye, selective sparing or involvement of the monocular temporal crescent points to an occipital process.

A finding that is suggestive of, but not specific to, occipital hemianopsias is *macular sparing,* the preservation of a few degrees of field around fixation in an otherwise complete homonymous hemianopsia. This is in contrast to *macular splitting,* in which the field loss respects the vertical meridian through fixation. Visual acuity is normal in both macular sparing and macular splitting hemianopsias. The basis for macular sparing is not well understood. Several degrees of macular sparing may be the result of a blood supply to the occipital pole of the brain, where the calcarine cortex representing the macula is located, by branches of the middle cerebral artery. On the other hand, a degree or two of macular sparing is sometimes found in hemianopsias that are the result of occipital lobectomy.

The correspondence of the vertical meridian through fixation with the separation of the visual pathways into the right and left hemispheres is not absolute, since there is up to 15 degrees of tilt across the vertical meridian even in unilateral lesions [13]. Involvement of both hemifields in both eyes, however, suggests bilateral homonymous hemianopsia. If the blind spots and the temporal crescents are ignored, the perimetric defects in the two eyes should be superimposable. Rarely, bilateral homonymous hemianopsia presents as central scotomata, reducing acuity but preserving peripheral field.

Bilateral occipital infarction and other processes may also produce *cortical blindness*. Clinically, the patient cannot see, but the pupillary reactions are normal. This is also the picture of functional blindness; the differential diagnosis must be made by the clinical context (see Chap. 65). Numerous causes of cortical blindness have been reported: occipital infarction, vasospasm in migraine or after angiography, postictal, posttraumatic, and meningitis and degenerative diseases. As a rule, patients with cortical blindness experience visual improvement spontaneously or die as the result of their extensive neurologic injury. Permanent, complete cortical blindness is uncommon [1].

Most homonymous hemianopsias can be accurately localized on the basis of their perimetric characteristics and associated neurologic signs. The discovery of a hemianopsia should, however, prompt neuroradiologic imaging with either computed tomography or magnetic resonance. Positron emission tomography is currently under investigation as an imaging technique [5].

Treatment

Treatment of homonymous hemianopsia is largely limited to the management of the underlying cause, if it can be defined. A few patients have benefited from prism glasses, which optically expand the peripheral field [10]. Because of the importance of peripheral vision in detecting moving objects, the patient with a complete homonymous hemianopsia should be advised that driving is dangerous. Persons who are otherwise neurologically intact often function surprisingly well with hemianopsias. There is some evidence that training increases the ability to detect objects in the "blind" field, perhaps through facilitation of subcortical visual systems. This technique has seen only limited clinical application [14].

1. Aldrich, M.S., Alessi, A.G., Beck, R.W., et al. Cortical blindness: Etiology, diagnosis, and prognosis. *Ann. Neurol.* 21:149–158, 1987.
   In this series of 25 patients, complete visual loss and bioccipital abnormalities on computed tomography were poor prognostic signs.
2. Gans, M., Glaser, J.S. Homonymous hemianopia following electrical injury. *J. Clin. Neuro-ophthalmol.* 6:218–221, 1986.
   Four days after an electrical injury, a 53-year-old man evolved a right homonymous hemianopsia from an occipital infarct.
3. Gittinger, J.W. Jr. Occipital infarction following chiropractic cervical manipulation. *J. Clin. Neuro-ophthalmol.* 6:11–13, 1986.
   A case report with references to the various causes of homonymous hemianopsias in young people.
4. Katayama, Y., Yoshida, K., Ogawa, H. et al. Traumatic homonymous hemianopsia associated with a juxtasellar hematoma after acute closed head injury. *Surg. Neurol.* 24:289–292, 1985.
   A hemianopsia thought to be caused by compression of the optic tract by a hematoma cleared spontaneously.
5. Kiyosawa, M., Mizuno, K., Hatazawa, J., et al. Metabolic imaging in hemianopsia using positron emission tomography with ^{18}F-deoxyfluoroglucose. *Am. J. Ophthalmol.* 101:310–319, 1986.
   Metabolic mapping with positron emission tomography was more sensitive than computed tomography or magnetic resonance imaging in detecting occipital dysfunction

in eight patients with hemianopsias. This technique has poorer resolution and is both more expensive and more time consuming than the other imaging methods.

6. Miller, N.R. *Walsh and Hoyt's Clinical Neuro-Ophthalmology* (4th ed.). Baltimore: Williams & Wilkins, 1982. Pp. 127–152.
   The pages cited contain a review of hemianopsias with illustrative fields and extensive references.

7. Pessin, M.S., Lathi, E.S., Cohen, M.B., et al. Clinical features and mechanism of occipital infarction. *Ann. Neurol.* 21:290–299, 1987.
   Thirty-five consecutive patients identified as having unilateral occipital infarction on computed tomography were retrospectively reviewed. A cardiac source was found in 10 patients, vertebrobasilar atheroma in 6, migraine in 5, and systemic illness associated with hypercoagulability in 3. The largest group (11 patients) had no identifiable source of emboli.

8. Savino, P.J., Paris, M., Schatz, N.J., et al. Optic tract syndrome: A review of 21 patients. *Arch. Ophthalmol.* 96:656–663, 1979.
   Craniopharyngioma, aneurysm, and pituitary adenoma lead the list of etiologies.

9. Shacklett, D.E., O'Connor, P.S., Dorwart, R.H., et al. Congruous and incongruous sectoral visual field defects with lesions of the lateral geniculate nucleus. *Am. J. Ophthalmol.* 98:283–290, 1984.
   Two cases that suggest that vascular lesions of the geniculate cause congruous wedge-shaped defects, whereas infiltration may produce incongruous defects.

10. Smith, J.L., Weiner, I.G., Lucero, A.J. Hemianopic Fresnel prisms. *J. Clin. Neuro-ophthalmol.* 2:19–22, 1982.
    A description of a technique to expand the visual field of patients with hemianopsias.

11. Trobe, J.D., Lorber, M.L., Schlezinger, N.S. Isolated homonymous hemianopia: A review of 104 cases. *Arch. Ophthalmol.* 89:377–381, 1973.
    Vascular lesions predominate in white males between the ages of 50 and 70 years.

12. Tychsen, L., Hoyt, W.F. Occipital lobe dysplasia: Magnetic resonance findings in two cases of isolated congenital hemianopia. *Arch. Ophthalmol.* 103:680–682, 1985.
    Magnetic resonance imaging demonstrated occipital dysplasia in two patients with congenital hemianopsias and normal computed tomography.

13. Younge, B.R. Midline tilting between seeing and nonseeing areas in hemianopia. *Mayo Clin. Proc.* 51:563–568, 1976.
    Younge found that in 24 of 200 patients with hemianopsias the visual field defect by kinetic perimetry did not respect the vertical meridian through fixation.

14. Zihl, J., Werth, R. Contributions to the study of "blindsight." II. The role of specific practice for saccadic localization in patients with postgeniculate visual field defects. *Neuropsychologica* 22:13–22, 1984.
    In these three patients with hemianopsia, the accuracy of saccades into their blind field improved with practice.

64. MIGRAINE

The term *migraine* is applied to various headache syndromes and to the neurologic phenomena that accompany them. Ophthalmologic symptoms and findings may be important components of *classic migraine, migraine equivalents,* and *complicated migraine* (including *ophthalmoplegic migraine*). Basilar artery migraine is a type of complicated migraine in which visual symptoms may be prominent [18]. Some authorities also consider *cluster headache* (see Chap. 61) a variant of migraine.

Classic migraine is recurrent headache preceded by a visual aura. This aura characteristically lasts 15 to 30 minutes and usually consists of an expanding hemianopsic scotoma with scintillating borders. The pattern of lines at the edge of the scotoma (cheveux de frise) is said to resemble medieval fortification plans—thus, the description *fortification spectra.* Other visual aurae include transient homonymous hemianopsia and various positive and negative scotomata, even including transient monocular and binocular blindness (see Chap. 62).

Pathogenesis

The pathogenesis of classic migraine is uncertain. One useful model has been that the aura represents vasoconstriction and that the headache represents vasodilation. There is now, however, some evidence that the circulatory changes are secondary to primary metabolic alterations in the brain, perhaps mediated through platelet serotonin. The classic migranous aura may represent a propagating occipital cortical dysfunction. Attempts have been made to correlate the structural features of the primary visual cortex with the subjective sensations described.

In rare instances, the usually temporary cortical dysfunction becomes permanent, producing a hemianopsia. This is one type of complicated migraine—what Fisher prefers to call a permanent migraine accompaniment [8]. Computed tomography demonstrates cerebral infarction not necessarily confined to the occipital cortex.

Diagnosis

Another type of complicated migraine with ophthalmologic significance is ophthalmoplegic migraine [1], which Fisher [8] would call a prolonged migraine accompaniment because the deficit lasts days to weeks. Ophthalmoplegic migraine consists of transient, recurrent third nerve palsies usually beginning in childhood. The diagnosis is one of exclusion, although there are few other causes of recurrent third nerve palsy in children. The mechanism of ophthalmoplegic migraine is uncertain.

When the aura of migraine occurs without the headache, this is considered a migraine equivalent (also called *acephalgic migraine* or *migraine dissociée*). Some patients have classic migraine as young adults, a period of years free of symptoms, and then acephalgic migraine in middle life. Acephalgic migraine may also present independently of classic migraine in patients in any age group [11].

Most migraines are not associated with structural lesions in the central nervous system or with any underlying systemic disease. There is frequently a family history of migraine, and many adult migraneurs experienced episodes of car sickness in childhood. Migraine may be precipitated by exogenous estrogens, such as birth control pills. Migraine in women is characteristically associated with menstruation and ameliorated by pregnancy. Migranous scotomata are encountered in patients with systemic lupus erythematosus [9], and occasional cases of classic migraine seem to be related to intracranial arteriovenous malformations [3]. Atypical features or other findings such as a bruit, seizure, or field defect should suggest the latter diagnosis. Computed tomography is probably not warranted in the evaluation of typical cases of classic migraine.

Especially when they present in older persons, migranous scotomata may be confused with transient ischemic attacks. There is little evidence at present that embolism or transient alterations in blood flow from cerebrovascular disease are the cause of acephalgic migraine in a large proportion of older persons [4]. Unless there are other signs or symptoms prompting evaluation for carotid or cerebrovascular disease, these patients should probably be considered as having migraine equivalents.

Treatment

The treatment of migraine raises complex issues. A variety of medications are available: ergots and clonidine probably act to constrict extracranial arteries; cyproheptadine and methysergide affect serotonin pathways. Propranolol, the paradigmatic beta-adrenergic blocker, acts both as a direct vasoconstrictor and to alter serotonin metabolism, either of which could account for its antimigraine activity. Not all beta blockers are effective in migraine prophylaxis, and beta-adrenergic agonists may abort the visual aura of migraine [12]. There is also considerable current interest in the calcium channel blockers (e.g., nifedipine, verapamil, and diltiazem), vasodilators that are used primarily to treat angina. Amitriptyline and monoamine oxidase inhibitors have antimigraine effects that are independent of their antidepressant actions.

Vasoconstrictors are probably contraindicated in patients with acephalgic migraine, since the aura may represent ischemia. How much vasoconstrictors actually increase the risk of permanent stroke is uncertain, since most are not thought to act on intra-cranial vessels. Often, these patients respond well to reassurance. Some physicians recommend simple, conservative measures such as aspirin or caffeine (in the form of coffee or tea) [15]. Stress is an important precipitant of migraine, and it is clearly desirable to reduce stress if possible.

1. Bailey, T.D., O'Connor, P.S., Tredici, T.J., et al. Ophthalmoplegic migraine. *J. Clin. Neuro-ophthalmol.* 4:225–228, 1984.
   These authors argue that, with a classic history and normal high-resolution computed tomography, arteriography is not necessary to make the diagnosis of ophthalmoplegic migraine.
2. Bartleson, J.D. Transient and persistent neurological manifestations of migraine. *Stroke* 15:383–386, 1984.
   This brief review classifies and comments on the various neurologic manifestations of migraine.
3. Bruyn, G.W. Intracranial arteriovenous malformation and migraine. *Cephalalgia* 4:191–207, 1984.
   Bruyn reviews 57 reported instances and 7 personal cases of migraine associated with arteriovenous malformations and attempts to identify features that suggest the diagnosis.
4. Cohen, G.R., Harbison, J.W., Blair, C.J., et al. Clinical significance of transient visual phenomena in the elderly. *Ophthalmology* 91:436–442, 1984.
   Strokes were not encountered in a cohort of 43 patients with transient visual disturbances beginning after the age of 40 years (thus, the word "elderly" in the title is somewhat misleading). Most of these visual phenomena were attributed to migraine.
5. Corbett, J.J. Neuro-ophthalmic complications of migraine and cluster headaches. *Neurol. Clin.* 1:973–995, 1983.
   A review with 101 references.
6. Dalessio, D.J. Is there a difference between classic and common migraine? What is migraine, after all? *Arch. Neurol.* 42:275–276, 1985.
   This editorial addresses the concerns of neurologists about the definition and pathogenesis of migraine.
7. Featherstone, H.J. Clinical features of stroke in migraine: A review. *Headache* 26:128–133, 1986.
   In the 64 reported cases reviewed here, the typical patient was a young adult with a history of migraine who experienced increased headache and then developed a hemianopsia or hemiplegia or both.
8. Fisher, C.M. Late-life migraine accompaniments as a cause of unexplained transient ischemic attacks. *Can. J. Neurol. Sci.* 7:9–17, 1980.
   Fisher reports a series of 120 patients with transient neurologic and visual phenomena other than isolated scintillating scotoma who had normal arteriograms. These are explained as transient migraine accompaniments.
9. Honda, Y. Scintillating scotoma as the first symptom of systemic lupus erythematosus. *Am. J. Ophthalmol.* 99:607, 1985.
   A brief case report emphasizes the importance of recognizing this association. (Essentially the same article is published in Metabolic, Pediatric and Systemic Ophthalmology *10:22–23, 1987, along with a reviewer's comments.)*
10. Katz, B. Migrainous central retinal artery occlusion. *J. Clin. Neuro-ophthalmol.* 6:69–71, 1986.
    The case of a 29-year-old migraneur who developed a central retinal artery occlusion one day after starting on low-dose propranolol excites no fewer than two accompanying editorials.
11. Kunkel, R.S. Acephalgic migraine. *Headache* 26:198–201, 1986.
    A brief review that includes discussions of visual, neurologic, abdominal, and cardiac symptoms.
12. Kupersmith, M.J., Hass, W.K., Chase, N.E. Isoproterenol treatment of visual symptoms in migraine. *Stroke* 10:299–305, 1979.

Treatment with a beta-adrenergic agonist is recommended when visual symptoms are prominent in migraine.

13. O'Connor, P.S., Tredici, T.J. Acephalgic migraine: Fifteen years experience. *Ophthalmology* 88:999–1003, 1981.
    Sixty-one Air Force men with acephalgic migraine were evaluated, some quite extensively, without significant underlying disease being discovered.

14. Olsen, T.S., Firberg, L., Lassen, N.A. Ischemia may be the primary cause of the neurologic deficits in classic migraine. *Arch. Neurol.* 44:156–161, 1987.
    Regional cerebral blood flow studies both precipitated auras in migraineurs and demonstrated significant reduction in local perfusion. None of these auras were visual, and 6 of 11 patients had apparently preexisting neurologic deficits, making interpretation of this study difficult. (See also the editorials in Arch. Neurol. *44:321–327, 1987.)*

15. Sacks, O. *Migraine: Understanding a Common Disorder.* Berkeley: University of California Press, 1985.
    This monograph, written in an anecdotal style with the lay reader in mind, offers the insights of one neurologist into the nature and management of migraine.

16. Selby, G. *Migraine and Its Variants.* Sydney: ADIS Health Science Press, 1983.
    In contrast to Sacks' book above, this traditional medical treatise emphasizes pharmacotherapy.

17. Spector, R.H. Migraine. *Surv. Ophthalmol.* 29:193–207, 1984.
    A succinct review with 121 references.

18. Sturzenegger, M.H., Meienberg, O. Basilar artery migraine: A follow-up study of 82 cases. *Headache* 25:408–415, 1985.
    The clinical features of 82 cases that met these authors' criteria for basilar artery migraine; visual symptoms were prominent.

65. FUNCTIONAL VISUAL LOSS

Visual loss without identifiable organic cause has been variously described as *hysterical, factitious, malingering,* or *functional.* The last of these adjectives is preferable, since functional implies neither motive nor psychiatric diagnosis.

Pathogenesis
Except in unusual circumstances, there are no objective criteria to distinguish nonorganic visual loss consciously feigned ("malingering") from that in which the patient is unaware of the nature of the deficit ("hysteria"). Psychiatric evaluation of patients with functional visual loss often fails to uncover specific psychopathology [4]. Clinicians have long been aware that functional visual loss is more common in military conscripts during time of war, suggesting somatization, the conversion of anxiety into physical symptoms.

Diagnosis
The diagnosis and management of functional visual loss is every bit as challenging as that of organic visual loss. Like any other patient, the patient with functional visual loss must be approached with an open but questioning mind. The coexistence of organic and functional disease must always be considered. To make the diagnosis of functional visual loss, the examiner must demonstrate that the results of the examination are incompatable with visual physiology or that they can be improved by suggestion or persistence. Correct diagnosis is made more difficult because functional visual loss may be superimposed on organic visual loss and because some organic causes of visual loss may not be readily apparent.

Monocular Visual Loss
Complete loss of vision in one eye with normal visual acuity in the fellow eye is encountered most often in persons seeking compensation for an injury. The preservation of normal, symmetric pupillary reactions is strong evidence that the blindness is not organic. This may be confirmed by various maneuvers to confuse the patient as to which eye is being tested, resulting in correct identification of material visible only to the "blind" eye. Examples of such procedures are the measurement of stereopsis with polarizing glasses, the use of a red filter over the good eye to obscure material printed on a green background, and cycloplegia with placement of a plus lens in front of the "blind" eye with testing of distance and near vision binocularly (only the uncyclopleged "blind" eye would be able to read at near). When the test used is not part of the routine eye examination, it is imperative that the examiner have the mechanics and expected results clearly in mind. Testing for functional visual loss should confuse the patient, not the examiner.

Binocular Visual Loss
Binocular reduction in acuity in the presence of a normal anatomic examination is more difficult to prove as functional than is unilateral visual loss. One clue to the nature of the visual loss is the behavior of the patient. A distinction has often been made between hysterics, who may seem unconcerned with severe visual loss and ambulate normally, avoiding objects placed in their paths, and malingerers, who resent the examination and exaggerate the effects of poor vision. An example of such exaggeration is patients who, when asked to look at their own hand held in front of them, are unable to locate it, unaware that limb position is available from both proprioception and vision.

Bilateral visual loss with normal pupillary reactions and ophthalmoscopic examination may represent central (cortical) blindness or certain retinal degenerations in which ophthalmoscopy is normal in the early stages, such as progressive cone dystrophy or Stargardt's disease. Visual field testing helps in making the differential diagnosis. Central scotomata are rarely functional, and full peripheral isopters should direct attention to the macula. Constriction of the peripheral visual field is encountered both in functional visual loss and after bilateral occipital infarction. The bilateral homonymous hemianopsia of occipital infarction is often discontinuous at the vertical meridian through fixation, since the infarctions are only rarely perfectly symmetric in the two hemispheres (see Chap. 63).

Visual Fields
With functional visual loss, the fields are constricted, usually to between 10 and 20 degrees from fixation. They also fail to expand physiologically at increased testing distances (so-called *tubular fields*). Tubular fields are best elicited with a tangent screen. Testing commences with the patient seated 1 m from the tangent screen. The limits of the field are measured along multiple meridians by using one of the larger test objects such as a 5-mm white sphere, and the responses are clearly marked on the screen with pins. The patient is then moved 2 m away from the screen, and the procedure is repeated with a stimulus twice as large (in this example, a 10-mm white sphere) to keep the visual angle of the target presented constant. Since the testing distance has been doubled and light travels in straight lines, the diameter of the field should double. Most people with functional visual loss respond by keeping the diameter of the field at the two testing distances equal.

Other patterns of functional field loss are observed. Some (spiraling of isopters in toward fixation or star-shaped fields from variable responses) are also encountered as testing artifacts. Constriction of the visual fields may also be a testing artifact, warranting retesting on another day and with two testing distances.

Certain types of hemianopsias are now recognized as characteristic functional deficits [2]. Complete binasal hemianopsias are so rarely the result of organic lesions that a functional disorder should be suspected. A complete monocular temporal hemianopsia that becomes an homonymous hemianopsia on binocular testing and is unassociated with a relative afferent pupillary defect is functional. Homonymous and bitemporal hemianopsias should be presumed to be organic unless proven otherwise.

Treatment

Bilateral reduction in acuity is often encountered in older children [1, 8]. Some of these children simply want glasses, and vision improves dramatically when lenses of equal but opposite power are placed before their eyes. Others respond to encouragement and patience. Insisting that the child "guess" at lines he initially cannot read may dramatically improve poor acuity. Shuffling of small lenses in and out of the trial frame or Phoropter encourages this process.

In the military, marathon refractions by persistent ophthalmologists often result in marked visual improvement. An extreme approach, not applicable in civilian life, consists of bilateral patching in a quiet room. This "retinal rest" is in fact a form of sensory deprivation and usually produces remission within a day or two [7].

Treatment of functional visual loss is often difficult. Psychotherapy has no proven value, and referral to a psychiatrist may be resisted by the patient. Excessive neuroradiologic evaluations or placebo treatments seem to magnify the patient's anxiety. A good approach is to provide reassurance that the eye does not appear permanently damaged and that vision will probably improve [10]. Confrontations or accusations usually accomplish little except to alienate the patient from the physician. Third parties, such as insurers or targets of damage suits, should be protected by specifying the functional nature of the complaints in medical reports. Be aware that the psychiatric diagnosis *hysteria* is potentially compensable.

1. Catalano, R.A., Simon, J.W., Krohel, G.B., et al. Functional visual loss in children. *Ophthalmology* 93:385–390, 1986.
   Twenty-three children aged 6 to 15 years presented with blurred vision without organic cause. When the child and parents were reassured, visual complaints resolved in all but one patient, who had intercurrent psychiatric disease.
2. Gittinger, J.W. Jr. Functional monocular temporal hemianopsia. *Am. J. Ophthalmol.* 101:226–231, 1986.
   I report four cases and review hemianopsias as functional deficits.
3. Hesterberg, R.C., Jr., Tredici, T.J. A review of ocular malingering and hysteria for the flight surgeon. *Aviat. Space Environ. Med.* 54:934–936, 1983.
   More a position paper than a review, this work still has a few clinical pearls.
4. Kathol, R.G., Cox, T.A., Corbett, J.J., et al. Functional visual loss: Follow-up of 42 cases. *Arch. Ophthalmol.* 101:729–735, 1983.
   This analysis of a group of patients evaluated in a neuroophthalmology clinic concludes that few patients had social or economic impairment despite persistence of their defect unless there was an associated psychiatric disorder.
5. Keane, J.R. Neuro-ophthalmic signs and symptoms of hysteria. *Neurology* 32:757–762, 1982.
   Brief case reports illustrate the protean manifestations of functional disease, including eye movement and pupillary abnormalities.
6. Keltner, J.L., May, W.N., Johnson, C.A., et al. The California syndrome: Functional visual complaints with potential economic impact. *Ophthalmology* 92:427–435, 1985.
   This series of 84 patients emphasizes the medicolegal problem.
7. Kramer, K.K., La Piana, F.C., Appleton, B. Ocular malingering and hysteria. *Surv. Ophthalmol.* 24:89–96, 1979.
   An outline of the approach in a military referral center, including the various testing techniques that distinguish organic from functional visual loss.
8. Mantyjarvi, M.I. The amblyopic schoolgirl syndrome. *J. Pediatr. Ophthalmol. Strab.* 18:30–33, 1981.
   About 2 percent of the school children in a Finnish town had functional amblyopia, with a peak incidence in girls around the age of 10 years.
9. Slavin, M.L. The use of the red Amsler grid and red-green lenses in detecting spurious paracentral visual field defects. *Am. J. Ophthalmol.* 103:338–339, 1987.
   Another maneuver to elicit functional field loss.

10. Thompson, H.S. Functional visual loss. *Am. J. Ophthalmol.* 100:209–213, 1985.
    In this excellent summary, Thompson offers the philosophy of an experienced clinician toward dealing with functional disease, including a classification of clinical types.

66. VISUAL HALLUCINATIONS

In a *visual hallucination,* something is seen that is not there. This is in contrast to an *illusion,* when something actually seen is misinterpreted. *Formed* visual hallucinations are of identifiable objects; *unformed* visual hallucinations are of lights or amorphous images. This distinction is not absolute; both formed and unformed hallucinations may coexist. A common and interesting type of formed hallucination is that of a younger self *(autoscopia).* The content of visual hallucinations does not in general have localizing value.

Pathogenesis
Many persons who experience visual hallucinations avoid discussing them openly, fearing psychiatric attribution. When visual hallucinations are unassociated with auditory hallucinations, psychiatric disease is unlikely. Among the many nonpsychiatric causes of visual hallucinations are alcohol and other drugs, sensory deprivation, visual loss, and seizures. Probably the most frequently encountered visual hallucination is the migranous aura (see Chap. 64).

Healthy people may have visual hallucinations under conditions of fatigue or sensory deprivation (e.g., mountain climbers, long-distance drivers, or house officers experiencing sleep deprivation). Some normal persons also have hallucinations while going to sleep *(hypnagogic hallucinations)* or upon awakening *(hypnopompic hallucinations)* [10]. Unlike hallucinations from organic disease, hypnagogic and hypnopompic hallucinations may be pleasant experiences.

Visual hallucinations of light flashes are termed *phosphenes* or *photisms.* Digital pressure on the globe will produce a phosphene, as does vitreous traction on the retina. (Note that floaters are not, strictly speaking, hallucinations, as they represent images of actual vitreous discontinuities on the retina.) Phosphenes may be induced by sound in normal persons as part of a startle reaction; for example, a drowsy person in a dim room who experiences a flash of light with a sudden, sharp sound [7, 11]. The phosphene is localized in the direction of the origin of the sound and may represent intersensory spread of the auditory stimulus. This phenomenon is exaggerated in persons with anterior visual pathway disease, in which the phosphene appears in the area of defective vision. Similar phosphenes occur with optic neuritis upon eye movement, in this situation presumably representing a mechanical supersensitivity of the inflamed nerve.

Visual hallucinations from organic disease are classified as either *irritative* (ictal, stimulation) or *release* phenomena. Hallucinations that are the result of seizure activity tend to be intermittent, sterotyped, and associated with other seizure activity. In contrast, release hallucinations are continuous, variable, and not accompanied by other motor or sensory changes. Patients with release hallucinations have some disorder of the visual sensory system, such as decreased visual acuity or field. The loss of normal sensory input appears to release spontaneous central nervous system activity, actuating the hallucinations.

Release hallucinations develop in a minority of patients with blindness or visual field defects. The speculation that the patients who tend to develop visual hallucinations have more diffuse cerebral disease is contravened by cases in young, otherwise healthy persons. Release hallucinations may have their onset during visual loss and disappear with complete blindness or may develop after blindness. These hallucinations are both formed and unformed. The vivid descriptions found in the literature make fascinating reading, but the subjective experience is almost always unpleasant and disturbing. Even if the content of the hallucinations is not intrinsically alarming (e.g., spiders, prehistoric monsters), affected individuals find it difficult to concentrate or sleep and may consider suicide to escape from the display.

Diagnosis

Hallucinations in a visual field defect, when both ictal and release mechanisms may obtain, have been well studied. The most common context for such hallucinations is homonymous hemianopsia from occipital infarction. In large series of hemianopsias, the incidence of hallucinations was on the order of 10 to 15 percent [8, 9]. The hallucinations may be formed or unformed. Colored images of pyramids or tetrahedrons often develop just before or at the onset of the hemianopsia. When they are a release phenomenon, the hallucinations tend to fade with time.

Formed visual hallucinations may be of remembered scenes (déjà vu) or of novel situations (jamais vu). The persistence of a recently seen image is known as *palinopsia* or *paliopsia*. A related phenomenon is *visual allesthesia,* the transfer and persistence of an image from a normal to a defective portion of the visual field [5]. Such visual preservation is often associated with other visual sensory disturbances, including illusory visual spread, polyopia, and central metamorphopsia. The majority of patients reported have had right hemispheric pathology. Visual allesthesia is clearly an ictal event in some cases and may disappear with anticonvulsant therapy.

Treatment

With ictal hallucinations, treatment of the underlying seizure disorder is indicated. Management of release hallucinations is very difficult; a trial of anticonvulsants may be warranted. Fortunately, many release hallucinations are transient.

1. Bachman, D.M. Formed visual hallucinations after metrizamide myelography. *Am. J. Ophthalmol.* 97:78–81, 1984.
   Visual hallucinations thought to be a toxic effect of metrizamide administration as part of an evaluation of an Arnold-Chiari malformation in an elderly patient.
2. Cogan, D.G. Visual hallucinations as release phenomena. *Albrecht v. Graefes Arch. Klin. Exp. Ophthalmol.* 188:139–150, 1973.
   Cogan clearly delimits the concept of release hallucinations.
3. Duke-Elder, S., Scott, G.I. *System of Ophthalmology.* Vol. 9. *Neuro-ophthalmology.* St. Louis: Mosby, 1971. Pp. 562–573.
   This is the System *at its best: a brief, critical review of visual hallucinations and synesthesias.*
4. Dunn, D.W., Weisberg, L.A., Nadell, J. Peduncular hallucinations caused by brain-stem compression. *Neurology* 33:1360–1361, 1983.
   A brief case report that raises the difficult question of peduncular hallucinosis. Removal of a craniopharyngioma in an already blind child with a sleep disturbance resulted in cessation of microzoologic hallucinosis (snakes).
5. Eretto, P.A., Schoen, F.S., Krohel, G.B., et al. Palinoptic visual allesthesia. *Am. J. Ophthalmol.* 93:801–803, 1982.
   This brief case report of ictal allesthesia leads back into the surprisingly large literature on this subject.
6. Gittinger, J.W. Jr., Miller, N.R., Keltner, J.L., et al. Sugarplum fairies. Visual hallucinations. *Surv. Ophthalmol.* 27:42–48, 1982.
   A case of ictal autoscopia with a middle fossa meningioma occasions discussion of hallucinations. The first author hereby disavows the reference to dreams in the title.
7. Jacobs, L., Karpik, A., Bozian, D., et al. Auditory-visual synesthesia: Sound induced photisms. *Arch. Neurol.* 38:211–216, 1981.
   This series of nine cases confirms the observations of Lessell and Cohen (below) and suggests the relationship of photisms to the startle response.
8. Kolmel, H.W. Coloured patterns in hemianopic fields. *Brain* 107:155–167, 1984.
9. Kolmel, H.W. Complex visual hallucinations in the hemianopic field. *J. Neurol. Neurosurg. Psychiatry* 48:29–38, 1985.

Dr. Kolmel's two papers are based on observations on his personal series of hemianopsias.

10. Lessell, S. Higher disorders of visual function: Positive phenomena. In J.S. Glaser and J.L. Smith (eds.), *Neuro-ophthalmology*, Vol 8. St. Louis: Mosby, 1975. Pp. 27–44.

    An excellent review of the subject of hallucinations.

11. Lessell, S., Cohen, M.M. Phosphenes induced by sound. *Neurology* 29:1524–1527, 1979.

    Sound-induced phosphenes are described as a transient symptom of decreased vision from unilateral ocular disease.

Index